Metabolic Disorders of Bone

Metabolic Disorders of Bone

C. R. PATERSON

MA, BSc, DM, MRCPath

Senior Lecturer in Clinical Chemistry
University of Dundee

BLACKWELL SCIENTIFIC PUBLICATIONS

OXFORD LONDON EDINBURGH MELBOURNE

© 1974 Blackwell Scientific Publications
Osney Mead, Oxford,
3 Nottingham Street, London W1
9 Forrest Road, Edinburgh,
P.O. Box 9, North Balwyn, Victoria, Australia.

ISBN 0 632 00281 6

First published 1974

Distributed in the United States of America by
J. B. Lippincott Company, Philadelphia
and in Canada by
J. B. Lippincott Company of Canada Ltd., Toronto

Printed in Great Britain by
Billing & Sons Ltd, Guildford
and bound by
Kemp Hall Bindery, Oxford

Contents

Preface

Just over a year ago I felt that there was a need for a new account of metabolic bone disease. Existing texts had become seriously dated and there had been major advances in our understanding of the physiology of calcium metabolism, and of the pathophysiology, investigation and management of this group of disorders. I hope that this book will be useful to anyone who has to deal with patients with metabolic bone disease.

Previous books on this subject have included a substantial and critical account of the physiology of calcium metabolism. I felt that it was no longer possible for a single author to provide a critical account both of the physiology and of the clinical disorders. However some understanding of the new physiology is an essential background to the discussion of the changes found in disease. Accordingly I have given in chapter 1 a brief outline of those aspects of physiology which are most relevant to the clinical problems.

I am indebted to Professor P.D.Griffiths and my colleagues in the Department of Clinical Chemistry for their remarkable tolerance of my preoccupation with bone and to my clinical colleagues in and around Dundee for their kindness in letting me investigate their patients. For helpful criticism of some chapters in draft I am grateful to Dr A.J.Hedley, Mr A.Gunn, Dr J.R.Evans, Dr P.Zarembski, Professor D.Kashiwagi and Miss Margaret Browning and especially to my wife who looked at the whole text. They saved me from many errors of content or style; those which remain are all my own work.

I owe a great debt to Miss Mary Benstead for many fine figures and also to Miss M.McCathie, Mrs E.Rough and Mr T.King for help with the illustrations. The staff of the University Library in Dundee were most helpful; in addition I had the assistance of Mrs E.Hutchison, Mrs E.Adamson and Mr A.Ashcroft in assembling and checking the references. Mrs Eleanor Mudie typed the whole book in draft and prepared the index; I am greatly in her debt for her speed and accuracy. I thank Mrs M.Bonar, Mrs M.Simpson and Miss E.Flett for their help. The editor of the *Postgraduate Medical Journal* kindly allowed me to re-use a review article as part of chapter 4.

Finally I need to thank my wife, who not only criticised the whole text and checked the proofs, but also gave constant encouragement.

March 1974   Colin Ralston Paterson

Chapter 1: Physiological Aspects of Calcium Metabolism

Bone is a living tissue with two main functions. It provides a supporting structure which is both strong and light but also remarkable in that it grows and remodels itself to withstand normal or new stresses. Secondly bone serves as a depository of calcium and phosphorus which are themselves important for the function of all tissues. The physiology of bone and calcium metabolism has been fully covered in recent books (Rasmussen 1970, Vaughan 1970, Bourne 1972, Hancox 1972b) and this discussion will be limited to a few aspects which are relevant to metabolic bone disease and its investigation. I shall outline the composition of bone, the normal metabolism of calcium and phosphorus and cover in greater detail the physiological control of the plasma calcium.

THE CELLS OF BONE

Four main types of cell are associated with bone: osteoblasts, osteocytes, osteoclasts and fibroblasts (fig. 1.1). All are derived embryologically from primitive mesenchymal reticulum cells. Good electron-microscope pictures of bone cells are to be found in Cooper et al (1966) and Bourne (1972).

Osteoblasts
Osteoblasts line all bone surfaces except those with active osteoclastic resorption and a few bone surfaces in the skull sinuses which are lined with epithelium. There are two forms of osteoblasts: 'resting' osteoblasts and 'active' osteoblasts. Resting osteoblasts are flattened spindle-shaped cells which are nevertheless metabolically active and respond rapidly to changes in circulating parathyroid hormone or calcitonin. Active osteoblasts are larger cells and have a variety of shapes. They are active in the synthesis of both collagen and mucopolysaccharides. They are rich in alkaline phosphatase

1

which, as a pyrophosphatase, probably has an important role in calcification. Active and resting osteoblasts together form a membrane which appears to have the properties of an epithelial membrane. This

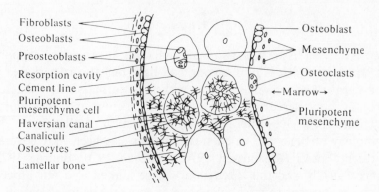

Fibroblasts
Osteoblasts
Preosteoblasts
Resorption cavity
Cement line
Pluripotent mesenchyme cell
Haversian canal
Canaliculi
Osteocytes
Lamellar bone

Osteoblast
Mesenchyme
Osteoclasts
←Marrow→
Pluripotent mesenchyme

FIGURE 1.1. Diagram of cross-section of adult cortical bone to indicate the arrangement of Haversian canals, the resorption cavities, the osteocytes with their canaliculi, and the different cells lining the bone surfaces. The periosteal surface is on the left, the endosteal surface on the right. From Vaughan (1970) by permission.

is indicated by the differences in the composition of the extracellular fluid on either side, by the secretion of collagen on one side only and by the remarkable differences between the ion-exchange activity of living and dead bone (Neuman 1969, Pritchard 1972b).

Osteoclasts

Osteoclasts have a remarkable appearance (Hancox 1972a, Cameron 1972). They are large or very large multinucleate cells. Most have ten to twenty nuclei but osteoclasts with several hundred have been described. Osteoclasts are mobile and their histological appearances are therefore variable. Next to the bone, the cell membrane forms a 'brush' border or 'ruffled' border of finger-like processes which reach down to the bone surface. Between the processes are cytoplasmic channels adjacent to which are vacuoles within the cell. In the channels and vacuoles electron-microscopy has demonstrated both bone salts and collagen. The bone adjacent to the osteoclasts shows recognisable resorption-pits visible under quite low magnification and known as Howship's lacunae.

Osteocytes

Osteocytes (Kleeman et al 1971, Pritchard 1972a, Hancox 1972b) are derived from osteoblasts during bone formation but mature by losing some of their cytoplasm. Each osteocyte occupies a lacuna in the bone and gives out cytoplasmic processes which reach out to a bone territory of the order of 100 μm in diameter and also communicate with similar processes derived from osteoblasts (fig. 1.2). The role of the osteocyte is not yet entirely clear but it is probably responsible for rapid exchanges of calcium between bone and extracellular fluid. It is likely that the osteocyte, rather than the osteoclast, has the major role in the response to parathyroid hormone and thus in blood calcium homeostasis. Enlargement of osteocyte lacunae is said to be a feature of hyperparathyroidism.

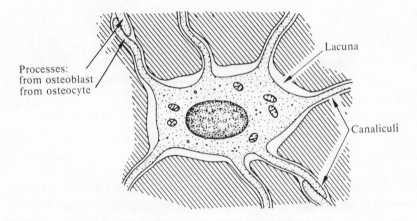

FIGURE 1.2. Osteocyte to illustrate manner in which cytoplasmic processes communicate with similar processes from other osteocytes and from osteoblasts on the bone surface.

Fibroblasts

Fibroblasts are found on the surface of bone outside the layer of osteoblasts and pre-osteoblasts. They seem to be relatively inactive except perhaps after fractures, but there is no evidence that they turn into osteoblasts or vice-versa.

CHEMICAL COMPOSITION OF BONE

Bone matrix

About 90% of the matrix from mature bone is collagen. The remaining matrix consists of mucopolysaccharides, other proteins, peptides and lipids (table 1.1). The organic matrix is known histologically as osteoid.

TABLE 1.1. Composition of adult bovine cortical bone, derived from data collected by Herring (1972). Comparable data for human bone is not available.

	Percent of weight of whole dry bone
Inorganic matter	76·0
Organic matter	24·0
	Percent by weight of organic matter
Collagen	88·5
Bone sialoprotein	1·0
Chondroitin sulphate	0·8
Peptides	0·5
Lipids	0·4
Other proteins, glycoproteins and matter not accounted for	8·8

Collagen This is a structural protein of great tensile strength which is found in skin, tendons, cartilage and bone. About 50% of the collagen in man is in the bone. It is a protein of unusual structure and composition (Herring 1972, Grant & Prockop 1972). The amino-acid composition is remarkable in that one third of the residues are glycine while nearly another quarter consists of the imino-acids, proline and hydroxyproline. Apart from a small proportion of hydroxyproline in elastin, hydroxyproline and hydroxylysine are unique to collagen. The basic 'tropocollagen' molecule is a rod 1·5 nm in diameter and 300 nm long and consists of three peptide chains wound helically round each other.

The synthesis of collagen is also unusual. The hydroxyproline and hydroxylysine are not incorporated directly into the peptide chain in the usual manner with specific codons and transfer RNA's. Proline and lysine molecules are incorporated and hydroxylated subsequently in the microsomes; vitamin C is required for this hydroxylation. Tropocollagen molecules are extruded from the cell and further maturation takes place extracellularly (fig. 1.3). With increasing perfection of packing the microfibrils visible by electron microscopy show a characteristic periodic banding.

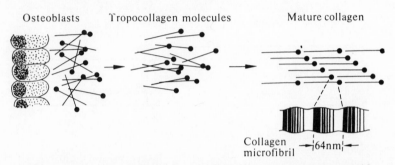

Osteoblasts   Tropocollagen molecules   Mature collagen

Collagen microfibril   64nm

FIGURE 1.3. Tropocollagen molecules (each with three peptide chains) are extruded from the osteoblast or fibroblast and further maturation takes place outside the cell. Mature collagen fibrils have a characteristic banded appearance by electron microscopy and this corresponds to the regular (fifth-stagger) arrangement of the tropocollagen molecules.

Carbohydrate-protein complexes (Herring 1972) These substances are a major constituent of the ground substance of bone. They are of clinical importance because bone abnormalities are found in rare inherited disorders of, for example, mucopolysaccharide metabolism. In the future defects in the ground substance may be demonstrated in other bone disorders.

Two main groups of carbohydrate-protein complexes are described. These are firstly protein-polysaccharides consisting of a protein attached to acid mucopolysaccharide chains, and secondly glycoproteins, in which protein is linked to an oligosaccharide. The most thoroughly investigated of these is bone sialoprotein whose main constituents are protein, sialic acid, galactose, galactosamine and glucosamine. It has a strong affinity for heavy metals but its physiological function is not known.

Bone mineral

The mineral phase of bone consists of crystalline hydroxyapatite and amorphous calcium phosphates. The proportion of amorphous material varies; it is greatest in new bone and in bone from young animals.

TABLE 1.2. Mineral constituents of bone from the data of Pellegrino and Biltz (1965). The totals are calculated on the basis of a total bone mass of 4,460 grams.

	As percent of bone mass	Total Grams	Total Gram-equivalents
Calcium	25·7	1146	57·3
Phosphate (PO₄)	34·5	1539	48·6
Carbonate (CO₃)	5·8	258	8·6
Sodium	0·65	29·0	1·26
Magnesium	0·32	14·4	1·20
Chloride	0·12	5·3	0·15
Fluoride	0·03	1·6	0·08
Potassium	0·02	0·8	0·02

The composition of hydroxyapatite crystals corresponds to the formula: $Ca_{10}(PO_4)_6(OH)_2$. In bone there are several other ions which become substituted within the crystal or adsorbed on the surface. These include sodium, magnesium, strontium, fluoride, carbonate and citrate in addition to trace elements such as copper and zinc and, on occasion, toxic metals such as lead and radium. The fluoride occupies the same position in the crystal as the hydroxy-group and a small proportion of fluoride improves the stability of the crystal, reducing its loss from dentine in caries and from bone with aging. The sodium content of bone is quite large and much of it is rapidly exchangeable. The main constituents of bone mineral are shown in table 1.2. The bones contain 99% of the body's calcium, 88% of the phosphorus, 50% of the magnesium, 35% of the sodium and 9% of the water.

Calcification

The history of this subject is littered with discarded theories which it would be unprofitable to discuss. The mechanism of calcification is still not understood but some factors are known (Walker 1973). The collagen fibres of the matrix play an important role; crystallisation can be induced on the native collagen of decalcified bone but not on reconstituted collagen. There are probably similar differences between newly synthesised collagen at bone-forming surfaces and the more mature collagen which four or five days later suddenly begins to calcify. Cameron (1972) has published elegant electron-microscope pictures of early calcification of bone matrix.

The role of the osteoblasts in forming a biological membrane on the bone surfaces has already been mentioned. This membrane must be important for calcification for it maintains an extracellular fluid of specialised composition adjacent to the bone surfaces. However blood plasma and extracellular fluid are supersaturated with respect to bone crystal and the problem, therefore, is not why osteoid calcifies but why other tissues do not. Recent evidence suggests that pyrophosphate $(PO_3-O-PO_3)^{4-}$ is an important naturally occurring inhibitor of calcification (Russell & Fleisch 1970). Human bone contains pyrophosphate and bone alkaline phosphatase has pyrophosphatase activity. It is suggested that inactive bone surfaces are covered with a layer of pyrophosphate which is hydrolysed by pyrophosphatase from osteoblasts when bone formation is taking place.

Pyrophosphate probably has an important physiological role in preventing inappropriate calcification in bone and other tissues and perhaps also contributes normally to the prevention of urinary calculi. Pyrophosphate cannot be administered therapeutically but analogous compounds, the diphosphonates (with a $-P-C-P-$ core), have shown promise in the management of certain bone disorders, notably Paget's disease (Fleisch et al 1972).

CALCIUM METABOLISM IN MAN

Calcium requirements

In most Western communities the daily calcium intake in the diet is 500–1,000 mg principally from milk and milk products, flour with added calcium, and vegetables. In many developing countries the dietary intake of calcium is much lower; among South African negroes the general range of calcium intake is between 175 mg and 475 mg daily. There have been many attempts by official bodies to define a minimum requirement for calcium; typical recommendations have been 400 mg/day for adults with substantially higher figures, such as 1,500 mg/day, in pregnancy and lactation.

There is very little evidence that a low calcium intake causes any harm in otherwise healthy people or that calcium supplements have any value in people with low intakes (Walker 1972a). In particular there is no evidence of poor growth, poor teeth or thin bones in communities with a low intake, but whose diet is otherwise adequate. There is no evidence that supplementing the diet with calcium confers any benefit either while growing or during pregnancy or lactation. There is little evidence of the 'ravages of calcium depletion' from child-bearing or rearing in underprivileged societies claimed in some official reports. The possibility that calcium deficiency contributes to the bone loss of aging in man has been widely discussed but here again the evidence is inadequate (chapter 14).

In health calcium absorption in the intestine adapts in a remarkably efficient way to wide changes in dietary calcium or calcium requirement (see below). In Western communities, of a calcium intake of say 1,000 mg, the net absorption is only 100–200 mg. The calcium intake therefore must be extremely low before a negative calcium balance is likely. Even in pregnancy in underprivileged societies calcium absorption rises so that there is little calcium depletion (Shenolikar 1970). Calcium depletion only contributes to the clinical problem in patients with vitamin D deficiency, intestinal disease, gross malnutrition with marasmus, or starvation. In these cases there is evidence of disordered calcium absorption in the intestine and so of failure of the adaptation mechanism.

Calcium absorption

In man calcium is absorbed throughout the small intestine (Avioli 1972, Wills 1973b). The greatest calcium absorbing capacity is in the duodenum where there is active transport. However the greater part of the calcium is absorbed in more distal parts of the small intestine where the evidence for active transport is less good. In these segments passive diffusion or facilitated diffusion are the mechanisms employed. In the duodenum the active transport depends on the availability of vitamin D and is controlled by its metabolite 1 : 25-dihydroxycholecalciferol. This hormone probably operates by controlling the synthesis of intestinal calcium-binding proteins and so contributes to the adaptation to a low or a high calcium intake (p. 26).

Net absorption is the result of two unidirectional fluxes of calcium and the size of these is not always appreciated. In man, in balance on a diet containing 1,000 mg of calcium daily, the net absorption is about 150 mg; this is the result of a total inflow from lumen to blood of 350 mg with an excretion from blood into lumen of 200 mg (fig. 1.4). During starvation calcium continues to be secreted into the gut and so lost from the body.

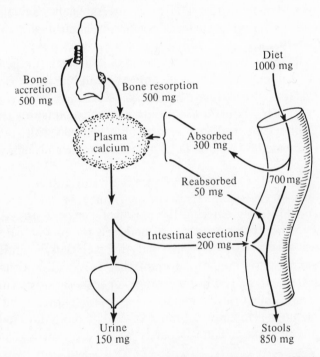

FIGURE 1.4. Calcium turnover in man. The figures (mg/day) have been rounded off in the intests of clarity and show that in health the urinary and faecal calcium excretion together equal the dietary calcium while bone resorption and bone accretion are equal. (*After* Jackson (1967)). Teachers of this subject will find the series of diagrams in that book helpful.

It has been known for more than thirty years that, with a low intake of calcium, the proportion of calcium absorbed from the diet increases. For example Hegsted et al (1952), using volunteers from among the inmates of a Peruvian prison, demonstrated that intestinal absorption of calcium was adequate to maintain calcium balance even on diets with as little as 100–200 mg calcium. Rats on a low calcium diet respond within a week with increased efficiency of calcium absorption but vitamin D deficient rats fail to do so (Nicolaysen et al 1953). Adaptation is also responsible for the enhanced calcium absorption at times when a positive calcium balance is needed as in growing children, pregnancy and after fractures. Nicolaysen suggested that this adaptation was mediated by an endocrine factor which he called the endogenous factor. It now seems likely that 1 : 25-di-hydroxycholecalciferol contributes to the mechanism of adaptation (Boyle et al 1972).

Many factors affect calcium absorption in man. It is greatly reduced in vitamin D deficiency, uraemia and in malabsorption syndromes. It is also reduced by the administration of phytic acid, phosphate or steroids or in the presence of excess unabsorbed fatty acids in the intestine. Calcium absorption diminishes with advancing age. It is increased by vitamin D, antibiotics, lactose and some amino-acids.

Plasma calcium

Calcium is constantly entering the plasma from bone and gut and leaving it for bone, gut or urine. Nonetheless the plasma calcium is maintained within narrow limits and the mechanisms underlying calcium homeostasis are so important that they will be considered in a separate section. The normal range for total serum calcium depends to some extent on the method employed (chapter 3) but most modern methods give a normal range of 2·2–2·6 mmol/litre (8·8–10·4 mg/100 ml). Plasma calcium is partly bound to protein, especially

TABLE 1.3. State of calcium in normal human plasma (data of Walser (1961)).

	mmol/l	mg/100 ml	% of total
Free calcium ions	1·18	4·72	47·5
Protein-bound	1·14	4·56	46·0
CaHPO$_4$	0·04	0·16	1·6
Calcium citrate	0·04	0·17	1·7
Unidentified	0·08	0·32	3·2
Total	2·48	9·93	100

albumin. The extent of this binding is affected by pH; it is reduced in acidosis and increased in alkalosis. Table 1.3 shows the main forms of calcium in normal human plasma.

Calcium in bone

The total body calcium is in the range 1,000–1,500 grams and more than 98% of it is in the bone. Even in adults skeletal remodelling continues and, in balance, bone accretion and bone resorption are each of the order of 500 mg/day. Kinetic studies (Nagant de Deuxchaines & Krane 1967, Harris & Heaney 1969 or 1970) have shown an exchangeable calcium pool of about four grams which, in various models, has been divided into two or more compartments according to the speed of equilibration. The anatomical basis of this pool is not clear, but it has been estimated that bone crystal surfaces exposed to extracellular fluid on the walls of the lacunae, canaliculi and Haversian canals amount to 1,500 to 5,000 square metres in the average man (Robinson 1964).

Urinary excretion of calcium

The glomerulus filters the plasma diffusible calcium (ionised and complexed calcium) so that about 9 grams of calcium are filtered daily. The renal tubule reabsorbs almost all of the ionised calcium but a smaller proportion of the complexed calcium. As a result, of a total urine calcium of 100–400 mg/day, only 20–30% is ionised, while the rest is bound to sulphate, phosphate and organic anions such as glucuronate and citrate. A normal range for daily calcium excretion is difficult to define and depends on age, sex and, to a small extent, dietary calcium intake (chapter 3).

The tubular reabsorption of calcium is increased by parathyroid hormone and by thiazide diuretics. It is reduced by frusemide, acetazolamide, phosphorus depletion and during a diuresis, especially when sodium excretion is increased. Various tests have been devised for the assessment of tubular calcium reabsorption particularly in relation to hypo- and hyperparathyroidism (chapter 3).

Calcium in sweat

The loss of calcium through the skin varies with many factors. It ranges between 20 mg and 365 mg per day and so could be a serious source of error in balance studies (Isaksson et al 1967).

THE HOMEOSTASIS OF CALCIUM

A constant concentration of ionic calcium in the extracellular fluid is important for the normal function of all tissues especially the heart, other muscles, and nerves. At least four distinct mechanisms contribute to the maintenance of a normal plasma calcium concentration: chemical equilibrium, parathyroid hormone, calcitonin and $1:25$-dihydroxycholecalciferol, a metabolite of vitamin D_3.

CHEMICAL EQUILIBRIUM

The role of chemical equilibrium in the maintenance of the extracellular fluid calcium concentration is controversial, particularly now that it is appreciated that bone crystal is in contact with a special extracellular compartment bounded by the bone cells. Despite this

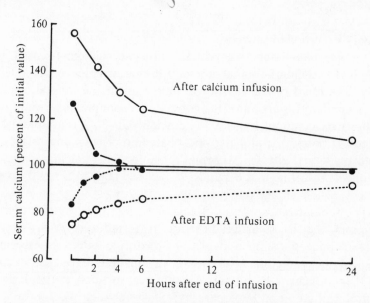

FIGURE 1.5. The change in plasma calcium concentration induced by infusions of calcium or EDTA into normal dogs (●) and dogs whose thyroid and parathyroid glands had been removed (○). The intact animal restores its plasma calcium to normal very quickly but the plasma calcium in the operated animal also slowly returns to the base line figures (data of Sanderson et al 1960).

fact, dynamic chemical equilibrium probably does play a part in calcium homeostasis. Figure 1.5 shows the effect of a calcium load or an infusion of EDTA (a calcium chelating agent) on the plasma calcium in normal dogs or dogs whose thyroid and parathyroid glands had been removed. The intact animal restores its plasma calcium to normal very rapidly. The plasma calcium in the operated animal also returns to the base-line value but takes much longer. This slow homeostasis is probably the result of chemical equilibrium which, in man, maintains the plasma calcium after parathyroidectomy in the range 1·5–1·8 mmol/1 (6–7 mg/100 ml).

Parathyroid Hormone

The parathyroid glands were first described in an Indian rhinoceros by Owen in 1850 and in man by Virchow in 1863. In 1880 Sandström clearly demonstrated the four glands. The association between parathyroidectomy, tetany and hypocalcaemia in experimental animals was worked out between 1900 and 1910. The first effective extracts of parathyroid glands were prepared by Hanson and by Collip in 1923–1925. The history of this subject was well reviewed by Fourman and Royer (1968) and by Potts and Deftos (1969).

Anatomy of the parathyroid glands

The parathyroid glands are derived from the endoderm of the third and fourth branchial pouches. There are ordinarily four glands, two upper and two lower, although patients with five or even more glands have been described. The upper pair of glands have a relatively constant position behind the middle third of the thyroid. The glands of the lower pair are more variable in position; they are related embryologically to the thymus and are sometimes at the lower pole of the thyroid or even in the mediastinum. Both pairs of glands are commonly supplied by the inferior thyroid artery (Alveryd 1968, Heimann et al 1971).

The normal parthyroid gland is round or oval, about 6 mm in length and about 30 mg in weight. It is yellowish-brown because of its fat-content and thus not always easy to distinguish from surrounding adipose tissue. Microscopically the glands contain chief cells, which are responsible for the secretion of parathyroid hormone, oxyphil cells whose function is not known, fat cells and fibrous tissue (p. 80).

Chemistry of parathyroid hormone

Parathyroid hormone (PTH) is a peptide and the amino-acid sequence of bovine and porcine PTH is known (fig. 1.6). In bovine PTH the fragment with the 29 amino-acid residues from the amino-terminal part of the molecule has biological activity (Keutman et al 1972). The sequence of human PTH has not yet been fully worked out but figure 1.7 shows the amino-terminal sequence.

NH_2-**Ala-Val-Ser-Glu-Ile-Gln-Phe-Met-His-Asn-Leu-Gly-Lys-His-Leu** (15)-
-**Ser-Ser-Met-Glu-Arg-Val-Glu-Trp-Leu-Arg-Lys-Leu-Gln**-Asp (30)-
-Val-His-Asn-Phe-Val-Ala-Leu-Gly-Ala-Ser-Ile-Ala-Tyr-Arg-Asp (45)-
-Gly-Ser-Ser-Gln-Arg-Pro-Arg-Lys-Lys-Glu-Asp-Asn-Val-Leu-Val (60)-
-Glu-Ser-His-Gln-Lys-Ser-Leu-Gly-Glu-Ala-Asp-Lys-Ala-Asp-Val (75)-
-Asp-Val-Leu-Ile-Lys-Ala-Lys-Por-Gln-COOH

FIGURE 1.6. Amino-acid sequence of bovine parathyroid hormone. The bold lettering indicates the biologically active portion of the molecule. (Potts et al 1971b).

NH_2-Ser-Val-Ser-Glu-Ile-Gln-Leu-Met-His-Asn-Leu-Gly-Lys-His-Leu (15)
-Asn-Ser-Met-Glu-Arg-Val-Glu-Trp-Leu-Arg-Lys-Lys-Leu-Gln-Asp (30)
-Val-His-Asn-Phe-Val-Ala-Leu ...

FIGURE 1.7. Amino-terminal sequence of human parathyroid hormone (Niall et al 1973). At the time of going to press, there was some uncertainty about positions 22, 28 and 30 (Brewer et al 1972).

There appear to be differences both in molecular weight and in immunological reactivity between the circulating hormone and that which is extracted from the parathyroid glands. It seems likely that the gland hormone is cleaved within the peripheral blood between C33 and C34. It is controversial whether any of the amino-terminal fragment can be detected in the plasma but the carboxy-terminal fragment ('PTH-7') is a major part of the immunoreactive PTH in the plasma (Oldham et al 1972, Canterbury et al 1973, Potts 1974).

Secretion of parathyroid hormone

The secretion of parathyroid hormone into the blood is principally controlled by the plasma ionic calcium. A fall or rise in plasma calcium results in detectable changes in plasma parathyroid hormone levels within 10 minutes. Oldham et al (1972) found evidence that this rapid response to changes in the plasma calcium was due to changes in the enzymatic conversion of the glandular to the secreted form of PTH. The glandular form of PTH may itself be derived from a precursor with a molecular weight of about 12,000 (Habener & Kemper 1972).

The secretion of PTH is also affected by the plasma magnesium content: it is increased by hypomagnesaemia and reduced by hypermagnesaemia (Sherwood et al 1970, Massry et al 1970, Altenähr & Leonhardt 1972). There is some evidence from studies *in vitro* that calcitonin has a direct effect on parathyroid tissue to promote PTH secretion (Oldham et al 1971). The phosphate concentration in the plasma does not influence PTH secretion by itself but phosphate administration in man causes a small fall in plasma calcium, which in turn stimulates PTH secretion (Reiss et al 1970). PTH secretion is promoted by alkalosis but only as a result of the fall in ionised calcium (Kaplan et al 1972).

Parathyroid hormone metabolism
The half-life of plasma PTH is between 30 and 60 minutes. Studies with isotopically labelled PTH show that it is localised in the bone cells and in the kidney; the kidney appears to be the main organ responsible for PTH hydrolysis (Fujita et al 1970, Zull & Repke 1972).

Actions of parathyroid hormone
The traditional view is that the principal role of PTH is the homeostasis of calcium. This view has been challenged by Wills (1970a) and Bernstein et al (1970) who suggested the possibility that PTH was mainly concerned with acid-base homeostasis and that its action on calcium metabolism was incidental. PTH has direct and independent actions on the bone and the kidney (Arnaud & Tenenhouse 1970). It is controversial whether it also has a direct action on the intestine. At least in the bone and the kidney the action of PTH is mediated by an increase in the concentration of cyclic adenosine 3', 5' monophosphate (cyclic AMP) (Aurbach et al 1971). One result of this is that the urinary excretion of cyclic AMP is increased in hyperparathyroidism and decreased in hypoparathyroidism (Taylor et al 1970).

In the bone, PTH causes increased resorption both by osteoclasts and by osteocytes. That this is a direct action of PTH is clear from the work of Barnicot (1948) and Gaillard (1965). Barnicot transplanted parathyroid glands into the brains of mice and found that bone near the implants developed typical evidence of PTH-induced resorption with proliferation of osteoclasts. Gaillard grew embryonic mouse bones in tissue culture and demonstrated a direct action of parathyroid extract. The early response to PTH is seen in bone culture with, within 30 seconds, activation of the enzyme adenyl cyclase which converts adenosine triphosphate (ATP) to cyclic AMP. This in turn leads to the release of the enzymes responsible for bone resorption. More steps may be involved as the action of PTH, and of dibutyryl cyclic 3', 5' AMP which mimics cyclic AMP, is blocked by the carbonic anhydrase inhibitor, acetazolamide (Waite et al 1970). Another early effect of PTH is the uptake of calcium by bone cells (Parsons & Robinson 1971), so that a transient fall precedes the rise in serum calcium after injection of PTH. The action of PTH on bone is inhibited by oestrogens and enhanced by oophorectomy (Orimo et al 1972, Atkins et al 1972).

The administration of PTH causes rapid changes in the kidney. There is an increase in the excretion of phosphate, sodium, potassium and bicarbonate and a decrease in the excretion of hydrogen ion, calcium, magnesium and ammonia (Arnaud & Tenenhouse 1970, Vainsel 1973). These changes are also mediated by cyclic AMP and urinary cyclic AMP is derived from the kidney. The action of PTH on the excretion of phosphate has been studied most extensively and probably results from an inhibition of phosphate reabsorption in the proximal tubule (Agus et al 1971). The effect of PTH on calcium reabsorption has sometimes been regarded as unimportant. Nordin and Peacock (1969) however have emphasised that this action may be as important or more important than the action on the bone in calcium homeostasis.

Intestinal calcium absorption is increased in hyperparathyroidism (Avioli et al 1965) but experimental studies designed to examine the effect of PTH on calcium absorption have given conflicting results. It is likely that PTH has an action on the active transport of calcium but not on passive diffusion of calcium which may be more important with diets of normal calcium content (Shah & Draper 1966, Clark & Rivera-Cordero 1971).

In addition to its action on bone, kidney and gut, PTH may have actions on the transport of calcium and phosphorus across cell-membranes in other tissues (Arnaud & Tenenhouse 1970, Chausmer et al 1972). PTH in quite small doses increases blood flow in hepatic and renal arteries but the significance of this is not clear (Charbon & Pieper 1972).

Inter-relationship with vitamin D It has long been recognised that some of the actions of PTH, notably those on bone and gut are not found in vitamin D deficiency (Arnaud & Tenenhouse 1970). Recent evidence suggests that PTH controls the conversion of 25-hydroxy-cholecalciferol to 1 : 25-dihydroxycholecalciferol by the kidney (p. 25).

CALCITONIN

The story of calcitonin began in the years 1958–1960 when it was shown both in Copp's laboratory and by Sanderson et al (1960) (fig. 1.5) that total thyro-parathyroidectomy in the dog impaired the response to a calcium load. In 1961 Copp and his colleagues showed that when the thyroid and parathyroid were perfused with blood of a high calcium content a hypocalcaemic factor was released. This they named calcitonin (Copp et al 1962). In 1963 Hirsch et al showed that cautery of the thyroid gland caused hypocalcaemia in parathyroid-ectomised rats. They extracted a hypocalcaemic factor from the thyroid and called it thyrocalcitonin because they could not then be certain of its identity with Copp's calcitonin. Since then progress has been rapid; the new hormone has been isolated, its amino-acid sequence has been determined, it has been synthesised and its place in therapeutics is beginning to be defined. The history of calcitonin has been reviewed by Copp (1969) and Savage (1969); recent general reviews have been provided by Anast & Conaway (1972) and Foster (1973). The name thyrocalcitonin is falling into disuse; it is recognised that the hormone is produced by cells which are not limited to the thyroid even in mammals so that the original and shorter name is preferred. Entries on calcitonin however are still indexed under thyrocalcitonin in *Index Medicus*.

Source

In man calcitonin is produced by C-cells which are principally found in the thyroid but also in the parathyroid and thymus (Galante et al 1968). The C-cells, or para-follicular cells, of the thyroid were first noted in 1876 and were later described by J. F. Nonidez in 1932. He observed that these cells were larger than the follicular cells, had clear vesicular nuclei and a cytoplasm containing argentaffin granules (fig. 1.8). He even suggested that the granules indicated an endocrine function for the cells (Pearse 1968).

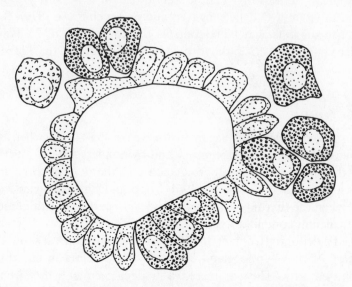

FIGURE 1.8. Parafollicular cells (C-cells) in the thyroid gland of a 35 day old puppy. The parafollicular cells are larger than the follicular cells and, with a silver nitrate stain, are seen to have many argentaffin granules. Some parafollicular cells lie in the follicular walls but most form clusters in the interfollicular spaces. *After* Nonidez (1932).

Recent work has made it clear that the C-cells are derived embryologically from the ultimobranchial body which remains a separate gland in fish, amphibians, reptiles and birds. There is now evidence from very elegant studies that ultimobranchial cells, and some other cells producing polypeptide hormones, are in turn derived from the neural crest (Le Douarin & Le Lievre 1972, Pearse & Polak 1972).

Chemistry

Calcitonin is a peptide with 32 amino-acids and a molecular weight of about 3,400 (Potts et al 1971a). There are extensive differences in the amino-acid sequence between calcitonins from different species, and that of human calcitonin is shown in figure 1.9. Calcitonin extracted from medullary-cell carcinoma of the thyroid includes a Calcitonin M with 32 amino-acids and a dimer, Calcitonin D.

Calcitonin concentrations in serum have been measured both by bioassay and by radio-immunoassay (p. 47).

```
 S————————————————S
 |                 |
NH₂-Cys-Gly-Asn-Leu-Ser-Thr-Cys-Met-Leu-Gly-Thr-Tyr-Thr-Gln-Asp
    Phe-Asn-Lys-Phe-His-Thr-Phe-Pro-Gln-Thr-Ala-Ile-Gly-Val-Gly
    Ala-Pro-CONH₂
```

FIGURE 1.9. Amino-acid sequence of human calcitonin (Potts et al 1971a).

Secretion

The principal stimulus for calcitonin release is hypercalcaemia, just as hypocalcaemia promotes PTH production from the parathyroid glands (fig. 1.10). However when the thyroid is removed from an

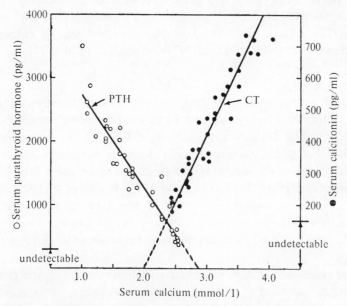

FIGURE 1.10. Serum levels of immunoreactive calcitonin and parathyroid hormone as a function of serum calcium in the pig. From Arnaud et al (1970a) with permission.

experimental animal little change is noted in serum calcium in contrast to the major changes which are the consequence of parathyroidectomy. For this reason the physiological importance of calcitonin has been questioned. It is clear however that the thyroidectomised animal restores its serum calcium to normal more slowly after a calcium load than does an intact animal (Munson & Gray 1970). Furthermore it is now clear that calcitonin release is not only provoked by hypercalcaemia but also by pancreozymin-cholecystokinin and by gastrin (Care et al 1971). Thus calcitonin release anticipates and prevents the rise in serum calcium which might follow a meal.

Other hormones also stimulate calcitonin relase, notably glucagon and adrenaline. It is likely that the adenyl cyclase system is involved in the response by the C-cells to these hormones (Care et al 1970). Intravenous infusions of magnesium cause hypocalcaemia and, at least in the pig, calcitonin release by the hypermagnesaemia is likely to be the mechanism (Littledike & Arnaud 1971).

Metabolism

When porcine calcitonin is infused into humans it disappears from the plasma with an initial half time of $2\frac{1}{2}$ minutes but later more slowly. The kidney appears to be the principal site of calcitonin breakdown in man (Riggs et al 1971a, Ardaillou et al 1971).

Actions

Calcitonin acts at least on the bone and the kidney. Its action on bone is to inhibit bone resorption and in this way it is an antagonist to PTH (fig. 1.11). It does not block the PTH induced activation of adenyl cyclase or the early uptake of calcium by bone cells but it does block calcium mobilisation and osteoclast proliferation which are later effects of PTH (Robinson et al 1972, Kallio et al 1972). Calcitonin *in vivo* has only a small effect on normal human subjects but in patients with Paget's disease of bone it causes a marked reduction in bone turnover and so in the urinary excretion of hydroxyproline (p. 250).

In man administration of human calcitonin causes an increase in the urinary excretion of calcium, sodium, phosphate, potassium and magnesium. These changes are direct effects of calcitonin, and not secondary actions mediated by PTH, because there is no change in the excretion of cyclic AMP in the urine and because the same changes can be demonstrated in patients with hypoparathyroidism (Bijvoet et al 1971, Haas et al 1971).

The mechanism of the action of calcitonin on any cell is not clear; it apparently does not activate adenyl cyclase (Aurbach et al 1971). Its action on osteoclasts includes the reversal of the effects of PTH on RNA synthesis and calcium transport across cellular and subcellular membranes (Mears 1972).

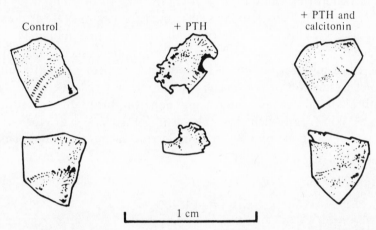

Control   + PTH   + PTH and calcitonin

1 cm

FIGURE 1.11. Mouse calvaria in tissue culture to show effect of calcitonin on the bone resorption induced by parathyroid hormone. (*Courtesy of Dr. Jennifer Nisbet*).

VITAMIN D AND 1,25-DIHYDROXYCHOLECALCIFEROL

It is not clear when rickets was first recognised but it was certainly known in the middle ages and by the seventeenth century it was so common in London that the Europeans called it the English disease. It was at that time a disease of urban communities with their atmospheric pollution and lack of sunlight. In the nineteenth century rickets was even found among the animals in London zoo. The antirachitic value of cod-liver oil and of sunlight was clearly demonstrated in human and experimental rickets between 1915 and 1925 by Hess and Ungar, by Sir Edward Mellanby and by Dame Harriet Chick among others. The anti-rachitic substance was soon distinguished from vitamin A and named vitamin D. The role of sunlight became clear when it was found that ultraviolet irradiation of the food

rendered it anti-rachitic. It became clear that ultraviolet light converted a precursor in the skin or in the food into vitamin D. The
history of this subject has been reviewed by McCollum (1967) and
by Fourman and Royer (1968).

Sources of vitamin D

Two forms of vitamin D are of importance in human nutriton:
ergocalciferol or vitamin D_2 and cholecalciferol or vitamin D_3 (fig.
1.12). The word calciferol was once used for vitamin D_2; at present
it is used by chemists to describe all sterols of the vitamin D type.
Ergocalciferol is present in artificially fortified foods such as margarine
and dried milk for infants; it is produced commerically by the ultraviolet irradiation of ergosterol, a plant sterol. Cholecalciferol is the
natural vitamin D found in fish and dairy products; it is also formed
in the skin from 7-dehydrocholesterol (7-DHC). Weight for weight
vitamin D_2 and vitamin D_3 have similar anti-rachitic activities in man.

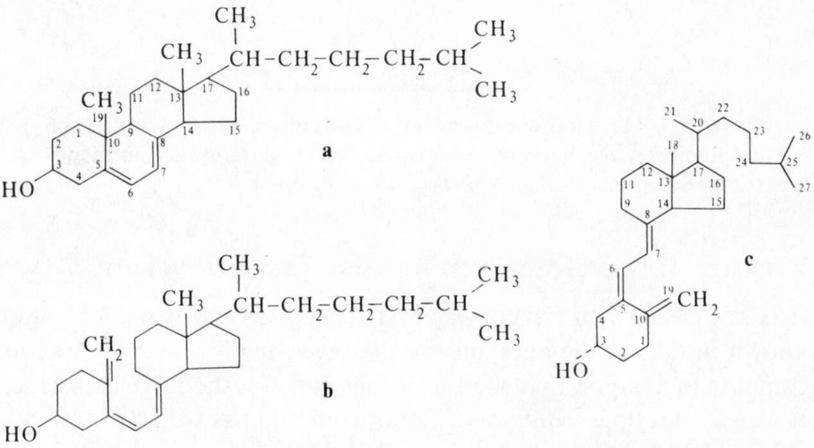

FIGURE 1.12. Structures of 7-dehydrocholesterol (a) and of vitamin
D_3 (b & c). The single bond between C6 and C7 in vitamin D allows
free rotation and it is likely that in solution and in crystals, vitamin D
takes up the elongated form (c). The system of numbering is based on
that used for steroids and is included to provide a framework for
subsequent discussion of metabolites and analogues. Vitamin D_2 differs
from vitamin D_3 only in that there is a double bond at C22–23 and an
additional methyl group (C28) at C24.

The average British diet contains 3·7 μg (144 iu) of vitamin D, with margarine as an important source (table 1.4). Many people take much less than 2·5 μg (100 iu) daily without getting clinical vitamin D deficiency (National Food Survey Committee 1964). Most depend, therefore, on exposure to ultraviolet light, rather than on diet for their vitamin D. The effective range of ultraviolet light is 250 to 305 nm (Knudson & Benford 1938) and the penetration of these short waves is limited by the obliquity of the rays (and thus the latitude, season and time of day) and also by atmospheric pollution. Even in the

TABLE 1.4. Proportion of the daily intake of vitamin D contributed by different foods in the British diet in 1962 (Greaves & Hollingsworth 1966). Total daily intake: 3·1 μg (126 iu).

Margarine	32%
Fish	26%
Eggs	16%
Butter	12%
Milk, cream and cheese	9%
Cereals	3%

north of England, (latitude 53°N) sunlight is sufficient to prevent rickets in 'white' children if there is no atmospheric pollution (Chisholm 1933, Loomis 1970). In the United States vitamin D consumption is generally higher than in Britain not least because of the addition of vitamin D to cow's milk in most states (Seelig 1970). In many other parts of the world dietary vitamin D is low; rickets develops readily when children are deprived of their exposure to sunlight (p. 168).

The causes of vitamin D deficiency are discussed in Chapter 10. The problems of the definition of the international unit of the various forms of vitamin D are discussed by Norman (1972).

Vitamin D requirements
In children the daily requirement for vitamin D appears to be between 2·5 μg and 5 μg so that the allowance of 10 μg (400 iu) daily recommended by official bodies in Britain, Canada and the United States is likely to be adequate even for children who have no exposure to

sunlight (Yendt 1970a). In adults there is much less information on vitamin D requirements. Smith and Dent (1969) suggested that adults require less than 2·5 μg (100 iu) per day and they may well be correct because osteomalacia after gastrectomy responds to parenteral doses of vitamin D as small as 2·5 μg daily (Morgan et al 1965b).

Public health authorities have found it very difficult to devise a system of vitamin D fortification of foods which will eliminate both rickets and infantile hypercalcaemia from the population (p. 125).

Vitamin D: absorption, distribution and storage

Vitamin D is absorbed at least in the duodenum and jejunum in man and, like other fat soluble vitamins, bile salts are required (Hollander et al 1971, Heaton et al 1972).

In the plasma antirachitic activity is associated with an α_1 globulin which is also found in urine and cerebrospinal fluid (Peterson 1971). The antirachitic activity of plasma has been measured by bioassays but the normal levels are difficult to define. Some populations have an adequate vitamin D intake and mean plasma antirachitic activities equivalent to 25 μg vitamin D/litre (1 iu/ml). Much lower results are compatible with health: some healthy Swiss babies had plasma antirachitic activities equivalent to 5·5 μg vitamin D/litre and low figures have also been noted among student nurses in Michigan and in hospital staff in Manchester (Lumb et al 1971).

Vitamin D or its metabolites are stored in the plasma and in many tissues but it is likely that adipose tissue and muscle are the most important (Lumb et al 1971, Rosenstreich et al 1971). The stores of vitamin D may be sufficient to postpone the onset of clinical vitamin D deficiency for several years: after partial gastrectomy osteomalacia seldom appears before a lapse of five years (p. 172).

Vitamin D metabolism

It has long been recognised that a direct effect of vitamin D on gut or bone from deficient animals could not be demonstrated *in vitro*. Furthermore calcium absorption *in vitro* in gut from deficient animals could not be altered by vitamin D unless the vitamin was given to the animals more than ten hours prior to sacrifice. It is now clear that this lag period is occupied partly by the further metabolism of vitamin D into more active polar derivatives (Norman 1971, Kodicek 1972, De Luca & Steenbock 1972).

Vitamin D_3 (cholecalciferol) is converted in the liver to 25-hydroxy-cholecalciferol (25-HCC) which is nearly twice as effective as cholecalciferol weight for weight in promoting calcium absorption in the intestine. It is likely to be the main form of vitamin D circulating in the plasma (Stamp 1973). 25-HCC is in turn converted in the kidney either to 1,25-dihydroxycholecalciferol (1,25-DHCC) or to 24,25-dihydroxycholecalciferol (24,25-DHCC). 1,25-DHCC is nearly five times as active in promoting calcium absorption as vitamin D_3; it is also the most rapidly acting of the vitamin D metabolites. Other polar vitamin D metabolites, such as 25,26-DHCC have been identified but these have little biological activity; their function is not yet clear but they may be forms in which vitamin D is excreted in the bile. The metabolism of vitamin D_2 (ergocalciferol) has not been so extensively studied but appears to be similar to that of vitamin D_3.

The production of 25-HCC by the liver is regulated to some extent; a thousand-fold increase in cholecalciferol dosage leads only to a ten-fold increase in 25-HCC production. The production of 1,25-DHCC by the kidney is closely regulated by the serum calcium and thus the dietary calcium (Omdahl et al 1972). When the serum calcium is low the increased production of parathyroid hormone promotes the secretion of 1,25-DHCC. When the serum calcium is high, the kidney changes within six hours to the production of 24,25-DHCC which has little biological activity on calcium absorption (fig. 1.13) (Cuisinier-Gleizes et al 1972, De Luca 1972, Fraser & Kodicek 1973, Omdahl & De Luca 1973).

Dihydrotachysterol$_3$ (DHT$_3$) is also hydroxylated in the liver; the product, 25-hydroxy-DHT$_3$ is itself metabolically active and requires no further hydroxylation in the kidney (Hallick & De Luca 1972). Recent research has also indicated that analogues of 1,25-DHCC, may be found which are more active on one target tissue than another. Such substances could be very valuable in clinical medicine.

Actions of 1,25 dihydroxycholecalciferol

There is no evidence that vitamin D has a direct action on any tissue; the changes seen when rickets or osteomalacia are treated with vitamin D are outlined in chapter 10. 25-HCC has a direct action on bone and on gut *in vitro* but only at concentrations some 100 times greater than those at which 1,25-DHCC is effective. Thus it is clear that the physiological actions of vitamin D_3 result from its conversion

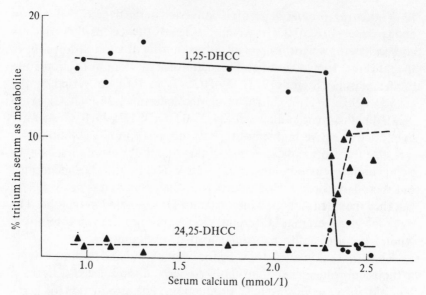

FIGURE 1.13. Relationship between the serum calcium at the time of injection of tritiated 25-HCC into rats and the relative amounts of the more polar metabolites in the serum twelve hours later. *After* Boyle et al (1972) with permission. The metabolites were separated by chromatography on Sephadex LH20 (Holick & De Luca 1971) and the 1,25-DHCC fraction may include 25,26-DHCC.

to 1,25-DHCC and perhaps other metabolites. When isotopically labelled vitamin D_3 is given to rats, the isotope is detectable in the liver within 15 minutes and soon afterwards in the intestinal mucosa, the bone cells, the cells of the proximal convoluted tubules and in the muscle cell-membranes (Callow et al 1966, Neville & De Luca 1966). It seems likely that these are the sites of action of 1,25-DHCC.

In the intestine 1,25-DHCC promotes the active transport of calcium in the duodenum and upper jejunum. The mechanism of this action is not clear but 1,25-DHCC is preferentially taken up by the cell nucleus and probably promotes the synthesis of a calcium-binding protein (Tanaka et al 1971, Omdahl & Thornton 1972, Avioli 1972, Alpers et al 1972, Tsai et al 1972). In quite small doses calcitonin *in vitro* inhibits the vitamin D-dependent element of intestinal calcium absorption (Olson et al 1972).

1,25-DHCC is preferentially localised in the nuclear fraction of bone cells and has a direct action on bone in tissue culture to promote bone resorption (Weber et al 1971, Holick et al 1972, Raisz et al 1972a, Wong et al 1972). The mechanism of the physiological action of vitamin D to permit normal bone mineralisation is not yet clear; it is possible that a metabolite other than 1,25-DHCC is responsible (Bordier et al 1973a).

The evidence for a direct action of 1,25-DHCC on the renal tubule is indirect. Patients with vitamin D deficiency often have impaired tubular phosphate reabsorption and this improves with the administration of vitamin D. While the tubular defect could be the result of secondary hyperparathyroidism this seems unlikely because in several clinical studies, the improvement in tubular phosphate handling took place rapidly and without any change in the serum calcium. Studies on experimental animals have also shown that an effect of vitamin D or of 25-HCC on tubular phosphate reabsorption could be demonstrated in parathyroidectomised animals. These studies used vitamin D in pharmacological doses on animals which were not vitamin D deficient. For this reason we cannot yet claim that there is conclusive evidence of a physiological action of 1,25-DHCC on the renal reabsorption of phosphate (Morgan et al 1965b, Gekle et al 1969, Puschett et al 1972).

CALCIUM METABOLISM IN NORMAL PREGNANCY AND IN THE NEWBORN

The skeleton of a newborn infant contains about 25 g of calcium and most of this is acquired during the third trimester of pregnancy. Balance studies and kinetic studies with a stable isotope of calcium (^{48}Ca) have indicated that in normal pregnancy there is an increase in intestinal calcium absorption and a decrease in calcium excretion in the urine. Thus pregnant women have no more net calcium loss than would have occurred during the same period in the non-pregnant state (Heaney & Skillman 1971). This conclusion is consistent with the evidence that in elderly women the amount of bone in the skeleton bears no relationship to parity, and that dietary calcium supplements in pregnancy confer no advantage (Walker 1972a).

The physiological basis of the changes in pregnancy is not fully understood. A modest fall in the total serum calcium has often been noted in the late months of pregnancy, and this fall is accompanied by a fall in the serum ionised calcium (Tan et al 1972). These changes are not the consequence of a suppression of parathyroid function; quite the opposite: in late pregnancy there is maternal parathyroid hyperplasia and an increase in circulating immunoreactive parathyroid hormone (Albright & Reifenstein 1948, Cushard et al 1972b). The rise in serum PTH, which may be the cause of the increased intestinal calcium absorption and decreased urine calcium excretion is presumably in response to the fall in serum calcium. The cause of this fall is not clear but it could result from the very large increase in the oestrogen content of the blood.

By term the maternal blood calcium returns to normal or nearly normal values while the infant's cord blood has a significantly higher total calcium and ionic calcium concentration, some values being greater than 2·6 mmol/l. These differences between mother and fetus reflect real differences in the ionic calcium concentration and could be the result of small transplacental differences of electrical potential (Tan & Raman 1972). The parathyroid glands appear to be active and responsive to changes in plasma calcium from an early stage of fetal life (Smith et al 1972a).

After birth, the infant's total and diffusible serum calcium concentrations fall and reach values below 2·2 mmol/l in as many as half of the infants (Bergman 1972). The reason for the physiological fall is not yet known: factors suggested include the sudden loss of placental calcium supply and delay in obtaining calcium from the feeds. In a few infants, severe hypocalcaemia occurs with fits or tetany. The factors contributing to this disorder are discussed on page 147.

Calcium metabolism in women on oral contraceptives

Women on oral progestational contraceptives have small but significant reductions in the serum levels of calcium and phosphorus (Simpson & Dale 1972).

PHOSPHORUS METABOLISM

Phosphorus is an essential constituent of all living organisms. An adult man has about 800 grams of phosphorus; four-fifths of this is in bone and most of the rest is in cells as organic phosphates, phospholipids or nucleic acids. The state of phosphorus in plasma is shown in table 1.5. The concentration of inorganic phosphorus in the plasma of fasting adults is normally between 0·8 and 1·4 mmol/l (2·5–4·5 mg/100 ml). Higher values are found in children (p. 40).

Phosphorus is present in all animal and vegetable cells so that dietary phosphorus deficiency does not occur in man. A clinical syndrome of phosphorus depletion is recognised in patients with phosphate-losing renal tubular disorders and in patients taking excessive doses of phosphate-binding antacids such as aluminium

TABLE 1.5. State of phosphorus in human plasma (based on data collected by Marshall & Nordin 1971).

		Concentrations in mmol/l
Organic phosphorus		
Lipid phosphorus		2·58
Other organic phosphorus		0·19
Total organic phosphorus		2·78
Inorganic phosphorus		
Diffusible phosphorus		0·87
HPO_4^{--}	0·44	
$NaHPO_4^{-}$	0·26	
$H_2PO_4^{-}$	0·10	
$CaHPO_4$	0·04	
$MgHPO_4$	0·02	
Protein bound		0·22
Total inorganic phosphorus		1·12
Total plasma phosphorus		3·88

hydroxide (p. 210). About two thirds of the dietary phosphorus is absorbed in the intestine; an active transport mechanism is involved and depends on the presence of sodium (Harrison & Harrison 1963).

The diffusible fraction of the plasma phosphorus is filtered by the glomeruli and normally more than 80% is reabsorbed in the proximal tubule (p. 50). There is no evidence of tubular secretion. The homeostasis of phosphate is principally controlled by parathyroid hormone and calcitonin in their action on phosphate reabsorption and in a steady state the kidneys excrete what the gut absorbs (Fourman & Royer 1968).

Chapter 2: Some Clinical Features of Metabolic Bone Disease

Jackson (1967) tells the story of a girl of 21 who complained of weakness, lassitude and anorexia. The medical clinic sent her to the psychiatric department as 'neurotic'. As she also had amenorrhoea she was sent to a gynaecologist who at first thought that she was pregnant. Later she developed a painful swelling of the hip. After radiological diagnosis the pathologists and the orthopaedic surgeons agreed that the 'osteoclastoma' should be curetted. When the bone lesions became multiple, the surgeons presented her as 'an interesting bone case' and a student, who recently had heard a lecture on the subject, made the correct diagnosis of hyperparathyroidism. The serum calcium was 3·8 mmol/liter (15 mg/100 ml).

This story serves as a reminder that many of the disorders of calcium metabolism are accompanied by vague or indefinite symptoms such as lassitude, weakness, paraesthesiae or bone pains. Patients with hyperparathyroidism, hypoparathyroidism or osteomalacia are all too easily thought neurotic or given the unhelpful label of 'rheumatism'. For these reasons the patient in whom a diagnosis is made probably owes a greater debt to the clinician who first suspects a disorder of calcium metabolism than to the specialist who confirms it. In the clinical assessment of the patient with suspected metabolic bone disease there is every reason for a comprehensive history and clinical examination: relevant information may be found in any system and specific questions related to the kidney or the gastro-intestinal tract are needed for particular patients. However there are certain clinical features which are particularly valuable as pointers to a possible diagnosis of metabolic bone disease.

Bone pains

Bone pains are an almost constant feature of adult patients with osteomalacia (Morgan et al 1970) or of children with rickets. In osteomalacia the pain is more often in the limbs than in the trunk and is usually worse at night. The pain seldom improves spontaneously. In contrast, patients with symptoms due to 'osteoporosis' are more likely to have back pain in episodes which have an acute onset and spontaneous improvement. Each episode presumably represents a crush fracture of a vertebra.

Bone pain is found in a few patients with hyperparathyroidism even in the absence of radiological abnormalities (Fourman & Royer 1968). A constant local pain may, however, be a clue to the presence of a giant-cell tumour.

In Paget's disease bone pain occurs only in a minority of the patients. Indeed, in a disorder which has an incidence of up to three per cent of the middle-aged or elderly (Collins 1966) it is remarkable how few have symptoms of any kind.

Bone pain is a feature of many other disorders notably primary bone tumours, osteomyelitis and multiple myeloma. It is sometimes found in leukaemia and in secondary tumours although some bone metastases are quite symptomless until a fracture occurs. Some patients have difficulty in distinguishing bone pain from joint pain and disorders of the joints should be included in the differential diagnosis. In addition joint disorders are an occasional complication of metabolic bone diseases such as hyperparathyroidism (p. 89).

Fractures

Fractures after minor trauma are a feature of 'osteoporosis'. Recently it has become clear that there is a universal loss of bone with age, especially in females. For each patient with thin bones and fractures there are many with equally thin bones and no fractures (Newton-John & Morgan 1970). Fractures are sometimes the presenting feature of juvenile osteoporosis and of the accelerated bone loss which occurs, for example, in liver disease and Cushing's syndrome.

Fractures after minor trauma complicate metastatic bone disease, multiple myeloma, osteomalacia, Paget's disease, hyperparathyroidism, osteopetrosis and osteogenesis imperfecta. In children the 'battered-baby syndrome' has to be considered (Kempe 1971, Cameron 1972); in Denver, for instance, 25 per cent of all fractures seen in the first two years of life are due to this.

Muscular weakness

Muscular weakness, especially a weakness of the proximal muscles may be the presenting complaint in osteomalacia, and in hyperparathyroidism (Smith & Stern 1967). The patients particularly note difficulty in climbing stairs, in getting up out of bed or out of a chair and in walking. They show a characteristic 'waddling' gait.

Muscular weakness is a feature of vitamin D deficiency in other species; affected sheep, for example, have more difficulty in moving downhill than uphill and so congregate near the tops of hills (Nisbet et al 1970).

Deformity

Deformity may result from multiple fractures as in osteogenesis imperfecta or from bone softening as in osteomalacia and rickets. Some of the characteristic deformities of rickets are shown in fig. 2.1. The deformities of Paget's disease are well known. One particularly important type of deformity is change in the bodily proportions.

Abnormalities of the bodily proportions. Leonardo da Vinci was one of the earliest artists to take an interest in proportions (McMurrich 1930). He observed that the distance between the finger-tips with arms outstretched was equal to that between the crown and heel. The pubic symphysis accurately bisects the latter distance. Although Leonardo da Vinci only observed the proportions in males, they seem to apply equally to females aged less than 50 (Dequeker 1972). These measurements should be made on recumbent patients as standing height is unreliable (Brown & Wigzell 1964).

In clinical medicine reduction in the upper segment occurs with disorders of the spinal column. Elderly ladies with crush fractures and wedging of the thoracic vertebrae have reduced upper segments as do some patients with untreated hyperparathyroidism or osteomalacia. Reduction in the lower segment is found with long-standing growth defects. Figure 2.2 shows a woman found to have coeliac disease and osteomalacia in adult life. In childhood her growth had been poor and this is indicated by her very short legs. A similar reduction in the lower segment is sometimes found in congenital heart disease (Livesley 1971). Anomalies of the proportions are found in a number of inherited diseases. Thus a low upper segment/lower segment ratio is commonly found in Marfan's syndrome, homocystinuria and mucopolysaccharidosis IV (Morquio-Brailsford syndrome). A high ratio is found in familial hypophosphataemia, in achondroplasia and in dysplasia epiphysialis multiplex and similar disorders (Sharrard 1971).

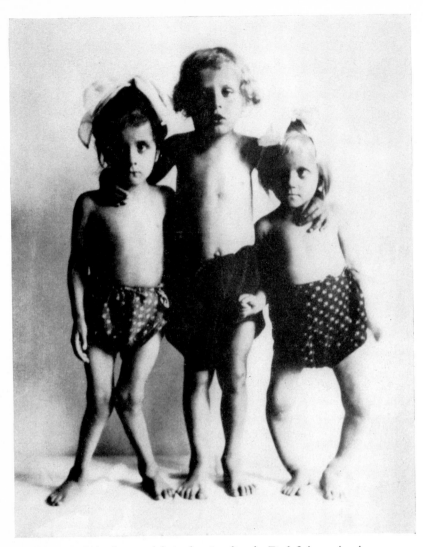

FIGURE 2.1. Severe rickets due to vitamin D deficiency in six-year old children. These appearances, familiar to previous generations, are now so uncommon in developed countries that they are not always promptly recognised. *Courtesy Wellcome Museum of Medical Science.*

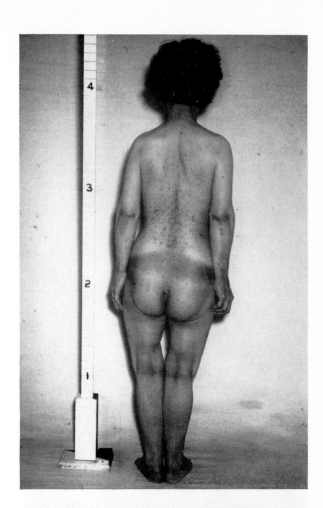

FIGURE 2.2. Abnormal proportions in a woman aged 58 who was found in adult life to have osteomalacia and coeliac disease.

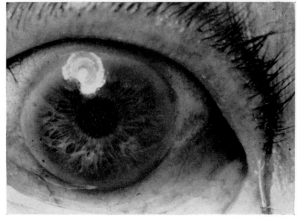

FIGURE 2.3. Eye to show corneal calcification in a patient with primary hyperparathyroidism. The calcification is most marked at the lateral margin of the cornea. The white area above the pupil is an artefact from the lighting.

Calcification of the cornea

This is easily missed unless it is looked for. In some patients it is not seen except on slit lamp examination. Calcification of the cornea must be distinguished from the corneal arcus ('arcus senilis'). Calcification is found in the most superficial parts of the cornea and is more marked in the lateral and medial areas (fig. 2.3): it is usually continuous with the scleral margin and has a granular appearance. An arcus, on the other hand, is completely circular or may be limited to the superior and inferior areas. The arcus is separated from the sclera by a clear margin of cornea. Corneal calcification is found in patients with hypercalcaemia of any cause and in a normocalcaemic patient suggests previous hypercalcaemia. It is also occasionally found in patients who have had previous iridocyclitis as part of Still's disease (Smiley et al 1957).

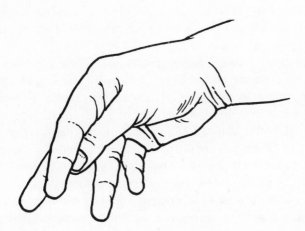

FIGURE 2.4. Hand in tetany.

Tetany

Tetany consists of muscular spasms affecting the hands (fig. 2.4) and the feet. Infants with tetany may have generalised convulsions or spasm of the laryngeal muscles causing a high pitched crowing sound and respiratory difficulty (laryngismus stridulus). Although such dramatic symptoms of motor nerve excitability may be the acute reason for the patient's presentation, symptoms of sensory nerve excitability, especially paraesthesiae ('pins and needles') and vague muscle pains, often happen first. A good account of the history of tetany, together with Trousseau's classic description, is given by Fourman and Royer (1968).

There are a number of standard tests designed to provoke muscle spasm in patients with latent tetany (Hoffman 1958, Schaaf & Payne 1966). In Trousseau's test a sphygmomanometer cuff on the arm is inflated to more than the systolic blood pressure for no more than four minutes. In a positive test the hand goes into tetanic spasm usually within two minutes. Positive results requiring more than two minutes are sometimes found in normal people. Another test sometimes called the Trousseau-von Bonsdorf test, involves a period of severe hyperventilation at the conclusion of a Trousseau test. This is a more sensitive test of latent tetany but is also more liable to false positive results. To elicit Chvostek's sign, tap over the facial nerve in the parotid area. A positive result is indicated by twitching of the muscles at the angle of the mouth. This test, too, has limited value as positive results are found in about 25% of normal people. False negative results are occasionally found in patients with other evidence of latent tetany. False negative results in all these tests are found in patients on anticonvulsant drugs, especially the hydantoins; these drugs may also prevent tetany in patients with severe hypocalcaemia.

Tetany is most commonly caused by a fall in the plasma ionised calcium below 1·1 mmol/l (Fanconi & Rose 1958). If the plasma proteins and blood pH are normal this corresponds to a total plasma calcium of about 1·8 mmol/l. Thus any disorder which causes hypocalcaemia (such as hypoparathyroidism or osteomalacia) or alkalosis (such as overbreathing or persistent vomiting) can cause tetany. In renal failure tetany is uncommon although the serum calcium may be very low. This protection is usually attributed to the metabolic acidosis which the patients also have; indeed in these patients tetany may be precipitated by intravenous sodium bicarbonate. There is some evidence which suggests that the rate of fall in serum ionised calcium is as important as the actual concentration; there appears to be some adaptation. Much rarer causes of tetany include hyperkalaemia and, strangely, tetany has also been described during recovery from hypokalaemia (Fourman 1954). Tetany has been associated with hypomagnesaemia but this abnormality seldom occurs without hypocalcaemia or a low plasma ionised calcium. Similarly cattle with hypomagnesaemic tetany (grass tetany) also have hypo-

calcaemia (Hall & Reynolds 1972). It is still not clear whether hypomagnesaemia by itself can cause tetany (Zimmet 1968). A few patients
have tetany which cannot be explained.

In the differential diagnosis of tetany the history usually provides
the most valuable information. Overbreathing is probably the most
common single cause of tetany and the symptom is relieved by
rebreathing. If there are no other clues in the history, (such as thyroid
surgery, vomiting or bone pains), estimation of the serum calcium
and of acid-base status will provide leads for further investigation.

Clinical features of particular disorders and of hypercalcaemia
and hypocalcaemia are considered later.

Chapter 3: The Investigation of Metabolic Bone Disease

A large number of chemical and other investigations are used in the study of patients with suspected metabolic bone disease. Radiology and some specialised tests with a limited application are discussed in subsequent chapters; this chapter is concerned with tests relevant to many disorders.

BLOOD CHEMISTRY

There is a circadian rhythm in the concentrations of many substances in blood and urine; some are also affected by meals. For the greatest precision therefore, blood and urine samples for analysis should be taken at a regular time of day; my practice is to take samples from fasting subjects between 8 a.m. and 9 a.m.

Serum calcium
It is important for the clinician to be aware of the method used by his laboratory for the estimation of serum calcium. Most large laboratories use either atomic absorption spectrophotometry (Pybus et al 1970) or the Technicon Auto-Analyser. With both methods good precision is obtainable and both give a normal range of about 2·2–2·6 mmol/l (8·8–10·4 mg/100 ml). Many other methods are used (Bold 1970) and it is important for each laboratory to determine its own normal range. Some reports of normocalcaemic hyperpara-thyroidism (p. 101) arose from a misunderstanding of the normal range for serum calcium. With good methods and careful analytical work, a narrow normal range for total serum calcium is obtained so that minor but clinically significant hypercalcaemia may be detected (Yendt & Gagné 1968, Baume et al 1969, Davies et al 1971). The normal range for total serum calcium does not vary significantly with age or sex (Werner et al 1970).

The accuracy of measurements of the serum calcium can be affected in a number of different ways. The effect of meals is controversial but is probably small and inconsistent. There is a small fall in serum calcium between midnight and 6 a.m.; this cannot only be the result of recumbency and haemodilution because there is a rise in plasma parathyroid hormone levels at the same time (Wills 1970b, Jubiz et al 1972). Technical factors may be important. Proteins precipitate from plasma on storage and take calcium with them; serum is preferable if there is to be any delay in the analysis. Apparent serum calcium values are greatly increased after contact with cork stoppers (Smith et al 1965) or wooden orange-sticks (Zarembski 1972).

Other errors arise from the manner in which the blood sample is obtained. Spuriously high serum calcium values result from venous stasis and are the consequence of ultrafiltration of the plasma *in vivo*. In taking blood for serum calcium estimation a tourniquet should be avoided; if venepuncture is otherwise difficult the blood should be taken quickly after the application of the tourniquet: ultrafiltration is a function of time as well as pressure. Ultrafiltration also underlies the less well known effect of posture on serum calcium. Serum calcium values are up to 0·25 mmol/l (1·0 mg/100 ml) higher in ambulant than in recumbent patients (fig. 3.1). This factor needs to be considered when comparing patients' results with a normal range obtained from ambulant subjects.

The serum calcium errors due to ultrafiltration, and the apparently low serum calcium values associated with hypoproteinaemia, may be allowed for either by 'correcting' the serum calcium for the serum protein content or by direct measurement of serum ionised or ultrafiltrable calcium.

The 'corrected serum calcium' Just under half of the serum calcium is bound to protein (table 1.3 page 10). Most of this is bound to albumin (fig. 3.2) and this binding is influenced by pH. At a low pH, albumin has a lower affinity for calcium perhaps because of competition by hydrogen ions for the binding sites (Sachs & Bourdeau 1971, Pedersen 1972, Lindgärde 1972). However changes in pH within the clinical range of values make only small differences to the proportion of calcium which is ionised (Wills & Lewin 1971, Lindgärde 1972). Many formulae and nomograms have been advocated for the correction of serum calcium results. The serum albumin, the total

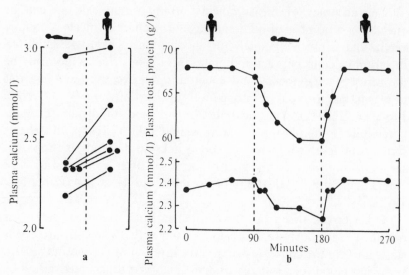

FIGURE 3.1. Changes in plasma calcium with posture.
(a) Changes in plasma calcium in six subjects reported by Stoker and
Wynn (1966). The first column gives the results after at least one hour
of recumbency and the second column after fifteen minutes upright.
(b) Changes in plasma calcium and plasma proteins in a normal man
aged 41 (Smeenk & van den Brand 1965).

protein, the serum albumin and globulin separately, and the specific
gravity have all been used for this purpose. It is difficult to know
which of the formulae to advise for use in practice but it is reasonable
to choose one based on serum albumin measured by modern analytical
techniques. The formula devised by Orrell (1971) adjusts all serum
calcium results to a serum albumin concentration of 34 g/l. For every
1 g/l by which the serum albumin exceeds or falls short of this figure,
0·018 mmol/l (0·072 mg/100 ml) is subtracted or added from the
observed value for total serum calcium. One result of applying a
formula such as this should be a narrowing of the normal range for
serum calcium and a greater ease of identification of marginally
abnormal patients. It should be emphasised that it is important for
each laboratory to determine its own normal range for corrected
serum calcium. This depends on the choice of methods for both
albumin and calcium.

Ionised calcium At one time the only method available for ionised
calcium was a bioassay using an isolated frog heart. More recently

colourimetric calcium assays on serum or ultrafiltrates have been used for ionised calcium (Rose 1972, Putman 1972) but the development of a calcium ion-selective electrode represents a major advance in this measurement (Raman 1970a, Radde et al 1971, Hansen & Theodorsen 1971, Fuchs & Paschen 1972). The use of the calcium electrode ideally calls for fresh blood samples and requires considerable technical expertise. Nevertheless the calcium electrode is likely

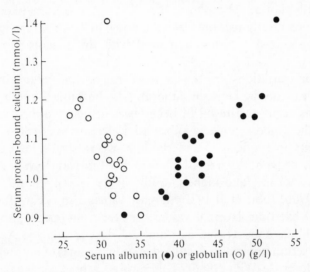

FIGURE 3.2. Relationship between serum albumin and the protein-bound fraction of the serum calcium (●) in twenty normal subjects studied by Raman (1971). A positive correlation is seen which is not found for the relationship between serum globulins and protein-bound calcium (○) in the same subjects.

to become a valuable tool for research and clinical work in specialised centres. In most patients with disorders of the parathyroids, the total serum calcium reflects the ionised serum calcium, but there are a few patients with hyperparathyroidism who have abnormalities only in the ionised fraction (Transbøl et al 1970a).

Ultrafiltrable (diffusible) calcium The determination of plasma ultrafiltrable calcium has become simpler recently with technical advances in ultrafiltration membranes (Farese et al 1970, Bergman & Isaksson 1971, Rose 1972, Putman 1972). The difference between the ionised and the ultrafiltrable calcium concentrations represents the complexed calcium. This is difficult to measure with any confidence as the accuracy is limited by the errors of both the other measurements. Measurements of complexed calcium have no recognised place in diagnosis.

Serum inorganic phosphorus

The serum inorganic phosphorus in adults is normally between 0·8 and 1·5 mmol/l (2·5–4·8 mg/100 ml). Whole serum contains much organically bound phosphorus (p. 29): while 'serum phosphorus' is therefore strictly incorrect as an abbreviation for serum inorganic phosphorus, it is a term often used with this meaning in clinical practice.

Minor variations in the normal range for serum inorganic phosphorus occur between laboratories but much more serious variations occur as a result of haemolysis or delay in the centrifugation of the blood sample; a substantial increase may result from as little as an hour's delay (Vanderlinde & Kowalski 1971). The serum inorganic phosphorus has a circadian rhythm with lowest values in the early morning and highest results in the afternoon and evening (Wills 1970b, Jubiz et al 1972). Higher values also occur after meals and after exertion. Normal values for serum inorganic phosphorus vary with age and sex (fig. 3.3) and are high in infancy. A detailed study of serum phosphorus values between the ages of six and twenty was made by de Wijn (1966). This showed a brief secondary rise at puberty.

Hypophosphataemia At all ages the plasma inorganic phosphorus is principally controlled by the renal tubules (Corvilain & Abramow 1972). Thus a low serum inorganic phosphorus is found in patients with hyperparathyroidism, vitamin D deficiency, hypokalaemia (Anderson et al 1969, Vianna 1971) and other congenital or acquired defects of phosphate reabsorption (chapter 12). Hypophosphataemia also occurs during intravenous therapy with carbohydrate-containing fluids, particularly with total parenteral nutrition ('intravenous hyperalimentation') with phosphorus-free fluids (Betro & Pain 1972, Dudrick et al 1972). Hypophosphataemia is sometimes found in patients who are vomiting or starving but nutritional deficiency of phosphorus is unknown. Phosphorus depletion does occur after oral treatment with phosphate binding antacids such as aluminium hydroxide (p. 210).

A bone disorder resembling osteomalacia or rickets is one consequence of prolonged phosphorus depletion (chapter 12). Acute hypophosphataemia leads particularly to disorders of the red cells, associated with a marked reduction in organic phosphates notably adenosine triphosphate and 2,3-diphosphoglycerate. Acute haemolytic anaemia has been described (Jacob & Amsden 1971).

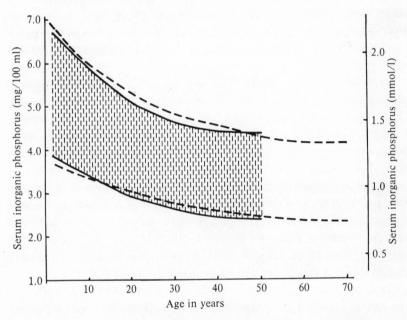

FIGURE 3.3. Normal values for serum inorganic phosphorus at different ages (data of Greenberg et al 1960). The interrupted lines outline the 2½ standard-deviation limits (99% limits) for males while the solid lines with vertical shading indicate the corresponding range for females. There were too few females aged over 50 to allow valid conclusions about that group.

Hyperphosphataemia The most common cause of a high serum inorganic phosphorus is renal insufficiency. Rarer causes include hypoparathyroidism, excessive phosphate intake in milk, metastatic carcinoma in bone, hyperthyroidism, haemolysis, blood transfusion, and muscle damage in malignant hyperpyrexia (Pollock & Watson 1971, Betro & Pain 1972).

Serum alkaline phosphatase (ALP)

The alkaline phosphatases (EC 3.1.3.1) of the serum are a group of enzymes derived from the liver, bone, kidney, gut and placenta. Their function is unknown except that bone alkaline phosphatase may be a pyrophosphatase (Russell & Fleisch 1970). Kaplan (1972) has provided a useful review of the clinical aspects of alkaline phosphatase.

Blood for alkaline phosphatase estimation should ideally be taken from fasting subjects because a rise of up to 25% is found after meals in some patients of blood groups O and B (Langman et al 1966). Lipaemic serum may give high values for serum ALP with some methods.

Normal range in adults The normal range of serum alkaline phosphatase in adults is usually quoted as 3–13 King-Armstrong Units (KAU)/100 ml, 1·0–4·0 Bodansky Units, 0·8–3·0 Bessey-Lowry Units, 2–8 Buch & Buch Units or 20–85 international units. There are several other systems of units for serum ALP measurement and this variety is quite unsatisfactory. The definition even of 'international units' varies from one set of assay conditions to another. Conversion factors for some pairs of methods have been determined (Deren et al 1964); these are subject to error not least because different methods respond differently to the various iso-enzymes. For these reasons it is important that each laboratory should quote a normal range appropriate to its own method.

In a normal population the results for serum ALP measurements are not distributed in a statistically normal manner, but approximately in a log-normal manner. For this reason values for serum ALP between 13 and 18 KAU/100 ml (85–120 international units) are sometimes found in people with no evidence of disease. Values greater than these usually indicate disease, particularly of liver and bone, but are also found in growing children and in normal pregnancy.

Normal range in children Although there have been several attempts to provide one there is still no satisfactory normal range for serum ALP in children. In children as in adults the values for serum ALP have a log-normal rather than a normal statistical distribution. This is clear from careful studies of infants aged under one year (Asanti et al 1966), of children aged from one to three years (Stephen & Stephenson 1971) and of adolescents (Round 1972). Unfortunately most of the studies of serum ALP in the full age range of normal children fail to recognise this and the improper use of statistical methods appropriate to gaussian distributions leads to an underestimate of the upper limit of the normal range. Further errors were introduced in some studies by the use of Hoffman's procedure for determining normal ranges from mixed hospital results (Belfield & Goldberg 1971). That this, too, is not valid for non-gaussian distributions was emphasised by Elveback et al (1970) and Prescott et al (1973).

In order to provide some guidelines for the use of alkaline phosphatase measurements in children figures 3.4 and 3.5 has been drawn from the data of Clark and Beck (1950). The results shown here indicate, as do Stephens and Stephenson (1971), the danger of attempting to diagnose rickets on the basis of alkaline phosphatase

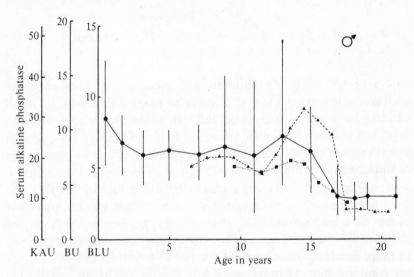

FIGURE 3.4. Serum alkaline phosphatase values in normal males at different ages: KAU = King-Armstrong Units, BU = Bodansky Units, BLU = Bessey-Lowry Units.

— ● — ● —   Mean and range from Clark and Beck (1950) (original data: Bessey-Lowry units.)

– ▲ — ▲ –   Mean from de Wijn (1966) (original data: Bodansky units).

... ■ ...... ■ ...   Mean from Round (1972) (original data: King-Armstrong units).

The conversion factors used for drawing the vertical axes were those of Deren et al (1964).

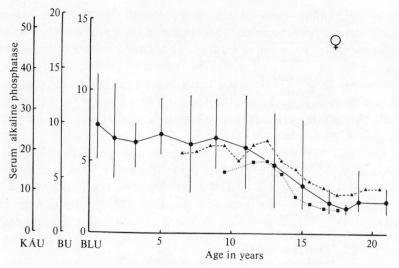

FIGURE 3.5. Serum alkaline phosphatase values in normal females at different ages. Symbols and conversion factors as in figure 3.4.

values alone; while few children with rickets have alkaline phosphatase values lower than 31 King-Armstrong Units, many normal children have results in excess of this value. The figures also show the brief but substantial rise in serum ALP at the time of the pubertal growth-spurt in boys. Because of all these difficulties the serum 5′ nucleotidase is a more valuable test than serum ALP in children with suspected hepatobiliary disease (Belfield & Goldberg 1971).

High serum alkaline phosphatase Table 3.1 outlines the principal causes of a high serum ALP. Disorders of the liver or the bone are the most frequent and most of the bone disorders listed are described in more detail in other parts of the book. Intestinal or renal causes for a high serum ALP are much less common. The placental ALP rises during the progress of normal pregnancy and falls gradually to normal in the first few weeks of the puerperium (Pirani et al 1972). A high serum ALP is sometimes derived from neoplastic tissue and this is known as the Regan isoenzyme after a patient of that name with bronchial carcinoma. This isoenzyme resembles the placental isoenzyme and is found in between 10% and 20% of patients with carcinomas of the bronchi, breast, genito-urinary tract and gastro-intestinal tract (Laurence & Neville 1972).

The determination of the source of alkaline phosphatase In most

TABLE 3.1. Causes of a high serum alkaline phosphatase.

Liver alkaline phosphatase

Biliary obstruction
Cholestasis of other causes (e.g. drugs)
Metastatic tumour in liver
Cirrhosis (portal, postnecrotic and primary biliary cirrhosis)
Virus infections, including infectious hepatitis, mono-
    nucleosis, cytomegalovirus infections
Alcoholism
Congestive heart failure
After pulmonary embolism

Bone alkaline phosphatase

Normal children
Fracture healing
Metastatic tumour in bone (some cases)
Rickets and osteomalacia
Hyperparathyroidism (some cases)
Osteogenic sarcoma
Uraemic osteodystrophy (some cases)
Paget's disease of bone
Hereditary hyperphosphatasia

Intestinal alkaline phosphatase

Some normal people after meals
Intestinal strangulation and infarction
A few patients with malabsorption (Dent et al 1968)

Renal alkaline phosphatase

Renal carcinoma (rarely)

Placental alkaline phosphatase

Normal pregnancy

Tumour alkaline phosphatase

---

cases the likely source of a high serum ALP is indicated by the clinical features and other investigations. In the patient with an unexplained illness and a high serum ALP various methods have been used for determining the source of the ALP (Kaplan 1972). These include ALP separation by electrophoresis, determination of the heat-stability of the ALP and the use of inhibitors with a specificity for a particular isoenzyme. Electrophoresis has been carried out on starch-gel and on polyacrylamide gel; while intestinal alkaline phosphatase is readily demonstrated it is seldom easy to distinguish clearly between the liver and bone isoenzymes in sera (Winkelmann et al 1972). Heat inactivation is a more valuable method: after heating serum to 56°C for 15 minutes, the activity of bone ALP is reduced to a greater extent than liver ALP while placental ALP is very little affected. Bone and liver isoenzymes are denatured by urea to a greater extent than the other isoenzymes while inhibition by phenylalanine is particularly a feature of the intestinal and placental alkaline phosphatases.

None of these tests discriminate completely between liver and bone alkaline phosphatase and the most satisfactory method for this is the use of the serum 5′ nucleotidase (EC 3.1.3.5) (Hill & Sammons 1967, Belfield & Goldberg 1969). This enzyme is an alkaline phosphatase which promotes the hydrolysis of nucleoside monophosphates. Its activity in the serum is increased in most patients with liver disease and a high serum ALP, while very few patients with bone disorders have an increased serum 5-nucleotidase. Other serum enzymes can also be helpful in the distinction between patients with bone and liver ALP elevations in the serum. One of the most promising is the serum gamma-glutamyl transpeptidase (Lum & Gambino 1972.)

A low serum alkaline phosphatase It is difficult to define the lower limit of the normal range, but low values for serum ALP are found in hypophosphatasia (p. 266) and in some patients with vitamin D poisoning. Children who are not growing for any reason have lower values than would be expected for their age.

Serum acid phosphatase

Many different acid phosphatases circulate in the serum; prostatic acid phosphatase and red-cell acid phosphatase each have more than one fraction (Posen 1970). Some acid phosphatase in the serum is derived from the bone, principally from osteoclasts, and an increase in the total serum acid phosphatase has been noted on occasion in hyperparathyroidism and in Paget's disease of bone (Woodard & Marcove 1969, Woodhouse 1972).

Serum parathyroid hormone

Radioimmunoassay has provided a method for the estimation of parathryoid hormone (PTH) in serum or plasma. At present antisera have been prepared with bovine parathyroid hormone and, while these cross-react with circulating human parathyroid hormone, this cross-reaction is not complete. This limits the specificity of the assays so that most laboratories still find that as many as one third of patients with undoubted hyperparathyroidism have apparently normal levels of PTH in the serum (Potts et al 1971b, Purnell et al 1971, O'Riordan et al 1972). Antisera which were more specific for human circulating PTH have been made from time to time (Reiss & Canterbury 1971, Arnaud et al 1973) and are likely to become more readily available after the structure of human PTH has been determined. Apart from hyperparathyroidism, high serum concentrations of PTH are found in renal osteodystrophy, in pseudohypoparathyroidism and in some patients with osteomalacia or rickets (Melick & Martin 1971, Arnaud et al 1972). High serum concentrations of immunoassayable PTH are also noted in pseudohyperparathyroidism but the PTH-like substance in the serum of these patients differs in a number of respects from ordinary human PTH (Riggs et al 1971b).

Serum calcitonin

Both bioassays and radioimmunoassays have been described for serum calcitonin (Deftos 1971, Raisz et al 1972b). By neither method can the calcitonin in normal serum be detected with confidence even after calcium infusion. Calcitonin has not yet been demonstrated in the peripheral blood of patients with hypercalcaemia. Most patients with medullary carcinoma of the thyroid (p. 217) have measurable calcitonin in the serum and most of these patients have a substantial rise in the concentration of calcitonin in the serum after calcium infusion (Deftos et al 1971, Raisz et al 1972b). Many patients with the Zollinger-Ellison syndrome also have raised levels of calcitonin in the plasma (Sizemore et al 1973). The main clinical role for serum calcitonin estimations at present is the confirmation of the diagnosis of medullary carcinoma and the detection of early cases in families with the familial form of the disease.

URINE CHEMISTRY AND CLEARANCES

Calcium excretion

Acid should be added to urine collected for calcium estimation; calcium phosphates otherwise precipitate out. Calcium excretion by

the kidney has a circadian rhythm with a maximum during the day
and a minimum at night. Meals are the principal cause of the day
time excess and fasting subjects have a natural rhythm in which the
maximum calcium excretion is in the early morning (Ede et al 1972).
Measurements both of the excretion of calcium in 24 hours and of
renal tubular calcium handling are used in the investigation of
patients with metabolic bone disease.

24 hour urine calcium excretion The normal range for calcium
excretion in 24 hours has been controversial particularly because the
results in most series do not fit a gaussian distribution. In the study
of Hodgkinson and Pyrah (1958) 90% of the men excreted less than
7·5 mmol calcium per day while 90% of the women excreted less
than 6·3 mmol. These figures were therefore taken as the upper
limits of the normal ranges. More recently Davis et al (1970) studied
normal subjects on a free diet outside hospital; 95% of the men
excreted less than 10 mmol calcium daily while 95% of the women
excreted less than 8·5 mmol daily. Robertson and Morgan (1972)
in a group of normal men showed that the upper 70% of the values
approximated to a gaussian distribution with a mean of 5·5 mmol/day.
The mean plus two standard deviations was 10·7 mmol/day (430
mg/day). Their statistical techniques need to be applied to different
age and sex groups; in the meantime caution is needed before regarding a man with a calcium excretion of less than 10·7 mmol/day as
abnormal. It is even more difficult to define a lower limit to the
normal range for daily calcium excretion but it is reasonable to view
with suspicion values lower than 2·5 mmol/day (100 mg/day).

The urinary excretion of calcium varies with age and sex. Results
are generally lower in females than in males and in both sexes calcium
excretion falls after the age of 60 (Bulusu et al 1970, Davis et al
1970). Dietary calcium affects urinary calcium excretion only to a
small extent and the change in calcium excretion with age probably.
reflects changes in intestinal calcium absorption (Davis et al 1970).
The urinary excretion of calcium is no greater in hard-water areas
than in soft-water areas (Dauncey & Widdowson 1972). A calcium
intake in divided doses increases the urine calcium to a greater
extent than the same calcium intake in a single dose (Phang et al
1968). Total starvation does not depress the urine calcium: indeed
the calcium excretion rises in therapeutic starvation (Garnett et al
1970).

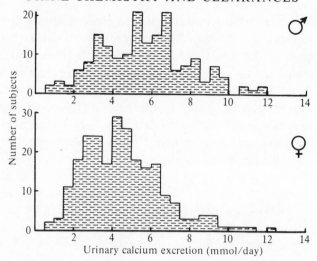

FIGURE 3.6. Urinary excretion of calcium in 178 males and 240 females between the ages of 20 and 69 studied by Bulusu et al (1970) and Davis et al (1970). These were normal subjects or medical out-patients with minor complaints and all the specimens were collected outside hospital. The two series used had similar mean values both for males and for females.

Disorders associated with a high calcium excretion in the urine are listed on page 133. A low calcium excretion is associated with rickets, osteomalacia and hypoparathyroidism. In both groups of disorders there is a substantial overlap with the normal range, however that is defined. The measurement of calcium excretion is, therefore of limited value in diagnosis.

Tests of renal tubular reabsorption of calcium There is no good evidence of a tubular maximum (Tm) for calcium reabsorption; the apparent Tm increases as the filtered load of calcium increases (Shaw 1971). However at any filtered load, the proportion of the calcium which is reabsorbed varies with factors such as sodium excretion or the concentrations of parathyroid hormone or calcitonin. In clinical practice tests of calcium reabsorption are useful in the differential diagnosis of hypercalcaemia and also perhaps in the identification of hypoparathyroidism. In general calcium reabsorption is high in hyperparathyroidism but low in hypoparathyroidism and in non-parathyroid hypercalcaemia (fig. 4.5, p. 68).

The results of such tests have been expressed in two different ways: as the percent tubular reabsorption of calcium (TRCa %) (Transbøl et al 1970a) and as the calcium excretion in mg per 100 ml of glomerular filtrate (Peacock et al 1969). The calculation of TRCa % requires measurement of the serum ultrafiltrable calcium (UFCa) and the 24 hour calcium excretion; this fact alone limits its availability to a few centres. However Transbøl et al also calculated a 'TRCa %' from the total serum calcium. Although this has no physiological meaning it does discriminate almost as well as TRCa % between patients with hyperparathyroidism and patients with other hypercalcaemias. TRCa % is calculated as follows:

$$\text{TRCa } \% = \left(1 - \frac{\text{Excreted calcium}}{\text{Filtered calcium}}\right) \times 100$$

$$= \left(1 - \frac{\text{Ca}_u \times \text{Cr}_p}{\text{UFCa} \times \text{Cr}_u}\right) \times 100$$

where Ca_u is urine calcium concentration (in a 24 hour sample), Cr_p is plasma creatinine concentration and Cr_u is urine creatinine concentration. These calculations assume that the creatinine clearance measures the glomerular filtration rate. 'TRCa %' is calculated in the same way except that total serum calcium is used instead of UFCa. This investigation is best carried out with a diet of average or low calcium content and is of little value when the renal function is poor.

Phosphorus excretion

The daily excretion of inorganic phosphorus in the urine depends almost entirely on the diet and its measurement contributes nothing to the investigation of patients with metabolic bone disease.

Information of clinical value can be obtained from tests of the renal tubular reabsorption of phosphorus. Phosphorus is reabsorbed in the proximal convoluted tubule and there is no evidence of tubular secretion (Brunette 1972). Unlike calcium there is a tubular maximum for phosphate reabsorption (TmP) (fig. 3.7). In normal people TmP varies with the glomerular filtration rate (GFR) and the ratio TmP/GFR or 'theoretical renal phosphorus threshold' is the most useful investigation of renal tubular phosphate handling (Bijvoet 1969). TmP/GFR can be determined by careful simultaneous measurements of serum and urine phosphorus during a phosphate infusion

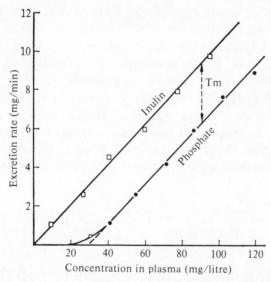

FIGURE 3.7. The relationship between excretion rate and concentration in plasma for inulin (□) and for phosphate (●) during intravenous infusion. The data for inulin should be multiplied by 10. The
extrapolated line through the phosphate data intersects the x-axis at a
point equal to TmP/GFR, in this case 30 mg/litre. (From Bijvoet
(1969) by permission).

(Bijvoet 1969, Stamp & Stacey 1970). This can be a laborious procedure for both patient and staff, so that it is not a test which can
be widely used or used repeatedly to follow the effect of treatment.
Bijvoet et al (1969) have however devised a method for predicting
TmP/GFR from estimations of phosphorus and creatinine in fasting
samples of serum and urine. Their nomogram, based on 100 phosphate infusion studies, is shown in figure 3.8. From this diagram
values for TmP/GFR may be determined. The results, predicted
TmP/GFR (or θ), agree reasonably well with TmP/GFR measured by
phosphate infusion, particularly if two or three observations are made
(fig. 3.9).

Many other indices of the renal tubular reabsorption of phosphorus have been advocated in the past (Bijvoet et al 1969). Some
are still widely used especially the proportion of the filtered phosphate which is reabsorbed (% TRP); this is computed in a manner
analogous to TRCa %. The disadvantage of this index and of many

others, is that it is greatly influenced by variations in the filtered load of phosphorus and thus by variations in dietary phosphorus. The percentage TRP is also reduced in chronic renal failure; TmP/GFR is affected by renal failure to a smaller extent and is valid in patients with a GFR of more than 40 ml/min (Bijvoet & Morgan 1971, Popovtzer et al 1972). There seems no justification for the continued use of indices other than predicted TmP/GFR.

TmP/GFR is higher in normal children than in adults and high values are also found in most patients with hypoparathyroidism, hyperthyroidism or active acromegaly (Bijvoet et al 1969, Corvilain &

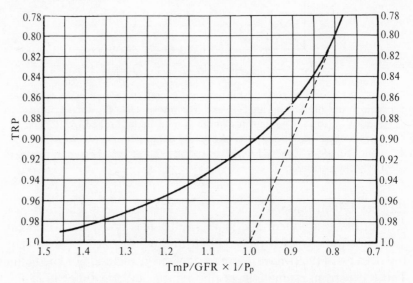

FIGURE 3.8. A nomogram for the prediction of TmP/GFR from simultaneous measurements of the concentration of phosphorus and creatinine in urine and serum from fasting patients. A figure for the rate of flow of urine is not needed. TRP is first determined as follows:

$$TRP = 1 - \frac{\text{Excreted phosphate}}{\text{Filtered phosphate}} = 1 - \frac{P_u \times Cr_p}{P_p \times Cr_u}$$

where P_p is plasma inorganic phosphorus, P_u is urine inorganic phosphorus, Cr_p is plasma creatinine and Cr_u is urine creatinine. When TRP is less than 0·80, TmP/GFR = TRP × P_p. When TRP is more than 0·80, TmP/GFR × $1/P_p$ is read from the nomogram and multiplied by P_p to give TmP/GFR. (From Bijvoet & Morgan 1971 by permission).

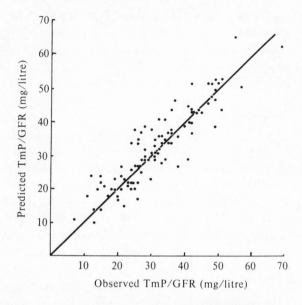

FIGURE 3.9. The relationship between TmP/GFR predicted from the nomogram in figure 3.8 and TmP/GFR measured by phosphate infusion in 100 subjects (from Bijvoet et al 1969 by permission).

Abramow 1972). Low values are found in many patients with hyper-parathyroidism or osteomalacia (Bijvoet et al 1969, Dent & Stamp 1970). In osteomalacia changes in TmP/GFR are often the earliest chemical evidence of response to treatment with vitamin D.

Urinary inorganic pyrophosphate

Pyrophosphate $(PO_3-O-PO_3)^{4-}$ is a normal constituent of plasma and urine (p. 7). The urine inorganic pyrophosphate is almost entirely endogenous and not derived from dietary pyrophosphate which is destroyed in the gut. Measurements of urine pyrophosphate are difficult and most patients with metabolic bone disease have normal values. High values are found in some patients with hyper-thyroidism and low values in patients with hypophosphatasia (Russell 1965, Russell & Hodgkinson 1969, Russell et al 1969). Increases in plasma and urine pyrophosphate have been reported in some patients with osteogenesis imperfecta and pyrophosphate assay has been suggested as a test for unaffected carriers of this genetic abnormality

(Solomons & Styner 1969, Hathaway et al 1972). Other workers have not so far been able to confirm these results and the clinical value of urinary pyrophosphate estimations must be regarded as controversial (Russell et al 1971).

Urinary hydroxyproline

Collagen turnover can be studied by the measurement of the urinary excretion of hydroxyproline as this amino-acid is found in significant amounts only in collagen. As the bone contains 55–60% of the total body collagen, disorders of bone are the principal causes of increases in urinary hydroxyproline. Such increases are associated both with increased bone destruction and with increased bone formation although in most disorders these two processes usually change together. These components may be separated to some extent because the non-dialysable urinary hydroxyproline, which is bound in poly-peptides and is about 10% of the total, is derived from collagen synthesis. The dialysable urinary hydroxyproline is derived from collagen breakdown and from the diet (Haddad et al 1970a, Krane et al 1970).

In adults, the total hydroxyproline excretion is between 100 and 380 μmol/24 hours (13–50 mg/24 hours) in most series. High values are found in normal children, in whom there is a substantial increase at the time of the pubertal growth spurt (table 3.2). High values are found with the breakdown of collagen during prolonged fasting (Ball et al 1972) and occasionally with disorders affecting extra-skeletal collagen such as severe psoriasis or after extensive burns. An increased urinary hydroxyproline excretion is more frequently found in bone disorders notably Paget's disease of bone but also in some patients with hyperthyroidism, hyperparathyroidism, osteo-malacia or neoplastic metastases in bone (Birkenhäger 1970).

Low values for hydroxyproline excretion are found in children with poor growth as in pituitary dwarfism and in malnutrition includ-ing kwashiorkor (Whitehead 1965).

Some authors advise that hydroxyproline excretion results should be expressed in relation to surface area. This correction does not eliminate the need to allow for the effect of age nor does it reduce the variance of results from normal subjects. Indeed in young children the variance is actually increased by this manoeuvre (Anderson et al

TABLE 3.2. Total hydroxyproline excretion in urine (μmol/day) in normal subjects at different ages. Detailed figures for the first month of life are given by Klein and Teree (1966).

Children (Kivirikko & Laitinen 1965)

Age (years)	Mean	Standard deviation
0–1	288	78
1–5	257	66
5–8	390	62
8–11	517	134

Adolescents (Zorab 1969)

Age (years)	Boys Mean	Boys S.D.	Girls Mean	Girls S.D.
11–12	523	248	417	211
12–13	595	224	527	230
13–14	710	335	390	197
14–15	839	366	290	135
15–16	812	317	237	98
16–17	619	244	242	101
17–19	420	183	207	111

Adults

Mean	Standard deviation	Reference
237	88	Ravenni et al 1962
224	70	Anderson et al 1965

1965, Kivirikko & Laitinen 1965). When collecting urine for hydroxyproline assay, the patient should avoid gelatine-rich foods such as ice-cream, jelly (jello) and soups made with bone stock. Observation of this rule reduces the total hydroxyproline of normal subjects within the normal range above, and an even more severe restriction of dietary hydroxyproline intake narrows the normal range still further (Haddad et al 1970a). Despite these precautions it is not easy to define the place of urinary hydroxyproline estimation in the investigation of metabolic bone disease; it is a relatively insensitive test in most conditions. Perhaps it is most useful for assessing the response of patients with Paget's disease of bone to various drugs.

SPECIALISED CHEMICAL INVESTIGATIONS

Balance studies

In the past careful balance studies have contributed much to our knowledge of normal and abnormal calcium metabolism. These studies are extremely expensive and unless very carefully carried out can be quite misleading (Isaksson & Sjögren 1967, Fourman & Royer 1968). Balance studies still have a part to play in research but have no place in the routine investigation of patients with suspected metabolic bone disease.

Tests of intestinal calcium absorption

Net absorption of calcium can be determined by balance studies, but simpler and cheaper methods for determining calcium absorption involve the use of radioactive isotopes of calcium, ^{45}Ca and ^{47}Ca. Most of these tests provide a measure of the one-way flux of calcium from lumen to blood, as the re-secretion of labelled calcium is small (Rose et al 1965). Various techniques have been advocated. The calcium isotope has been administered in water to fasting subjects or, a little more realistically, in milk in an ordinary diet. Subsequent measurements have included measurements of the stool radioactivity (Rose et al 1965, Bullamore 1970), of plasma radioactivity (Nordin et al 1968) and of retention of radioactive calcium by whole-body counting (Sjoberg & Nilsson 1970) or counting a forearm in a large volume liquid scintillation counter (Wills et al 1970). Methods involving plasma radioactivity measurements have the disadvantage that the blood levels found depend on isotope uptake by bone as much as on isotope absorption by the gut. In general methods involving stool counting are the most practical and most directly relevant to intestinal absorption.

The various techniques lead to similar conclusions. Calcium absorption falls off with increasing age (Bullamore et al 1970) and low values are found in patients with intestinal disease and vitamin D deficiency. High values are found in hyperparathyroidism and in some stone-formers with hypercalciuria (Pak et al 1972b). Calcium absorption is greatly influenced by the dietary calcium and one result can only be compared with another if it was obtained with a similar dietary content of calcium (Spencer et al 1969).

Kinetic studies

Studies with calcium isotopes on bone accretion and resorption have been valuable in research into the pathophysiology of the various disorders but are too elaborate to have a place in routine clinical investigation (Harris & Heaney 1969 & 1970, Reeve & Veall 1972). Perhaps the most promising technique for the future is measurement of total body calcium after neutron activation. Although this technique still has limited accuracy it may be particularly useful in comparing patients before and after a course of treatment. It is likely to become available only in specialised centres (Fremlin 1972, Nelp et al 1972).

TREPHINE BIOPSY OF BONE

This investigation is probably not as widely used as it should be. The technique is simple and seldom causes the patient much discomfort. Patients who have had both tests say that a trephine biopsy from the iliac crest is less unpleasant than a sternal marrow aspiration.

Indications and contra-indications

Bone biopsy is indicated in the differential diagnosis of hypercalcaemia, in the diagnosis of osteomalacia, in the assessment of uraemic osteodystrophy and in the differential diagnosis of obscure osteosclerotic lesions. Bone biopsy has no place in the 'diagnosis' of osteoporosis and is unnecessary in the hypercalcaemic patient with subperiosteal erosions or the patient with convincing pseudofractures as evidence of osteomalacia. In my experience the only patients who developed wound infections were those with sepsis elsewhere and I regard sepsis somewhere as a contra-indication to biopsy. Thrombocytopaenia is not a contra-indication to bone biopsy: excessive bruising is unusual.

Technique

A variety of methods have been advocated including both percutaneous techniques and open operations. In the procedure described here, specimens are obtained from the iliac crest with the 5 mm trephine (fig. 3.10) of Williams and Nicholson (1963). The 8 mm trephine is not recommended.

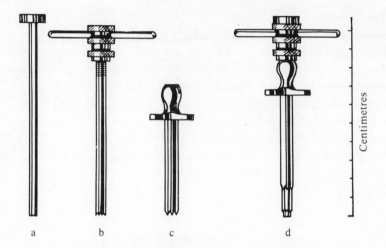

FIGURE 3.10. Williams-Nicholson trephine. The stillette (a) has been modified by the removal of the centre pin. The trephine (b) and the outer toothed tube (c) are shown in the assembled instrument (d). (Courtesy of Editor, *British Journal of Hospital Medicine*.)

After premedication the patient lies on his back at the edge of the bed or, better, on a firm couch or trolley. Right-handed operators find it slightly easier to use the left iliac crest, but it is a kindness to avoid the side on which the patient usually sleeps. Under local analgesia (Lignocaine 2%) and with full aseptic precautions, a 2 cm incision is made in the skin over the iliac crest, 2–3 cm posterior to the anterior superior spine (fig. 3.11). The periosteum, which may need further local analgesia, is incised and deflected. The outer toothed tube of the trephine is held firmly on the iliac crest and the inner tube is then rotated firmly with the other hand until an adequate specimen has been obtained. The trephine is removed by rocking it with a circular movement and then taking it out at an angle. The bone sample is expelled with the stillette. After the wound has been sutured and dressed, the patient lies on the operated side for half an hour to ensure haemostasis. The specimen should be fixed in buffered formalin.

This technique differs from that of Williams and Nicholson (1963) only in that, to avoid undue distortion of the specimen the centre pin of the stillette is not used. Other procedures have been described (Bordier et al 1964, Burkhardt 1971, Dragoo & Irwin 1972); they appear satisfactory but I have no experience of their use. Bordier's technique produces a transiliac sample with two cortical bone samples and a small specimen of trabecular bone which is said to be more representative than that obtained by iliac crest biopsy. Transiliac biopsy is a more substantial surgical procedure and it is doubtful whether it is justified even for specialised quantitative histological techniques (Bordier & Tun Chot 1972). Other authors advocate the use of the posterior iliac crest, but there is one case report of dangerous bleeding after blind biopsy at this site (McNutt & Fudenberg 1972).

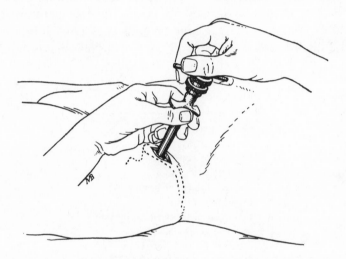

FIGURE 3.11. Bone biopsy: operative technique. In the interests of clarity the gloves and drapes are not shown. (Courtesy of Editor, *British Journal of Hospital Medicine*.)

Complications

In a personal series of 300 biopsies wound infection has occurred twice. On both occasions the patients had sepsis elsewhere at the time but the infection at the biopsy site responded rapidly to treatment with tetracycline. Bruising, sometimes extending widely over the abdominal wall, was not an infrequent complication before the value of having the patient lie on the operated side was appreciated. A few patients complain of discomfort at the biopsy site; this responds to simple analgesics and seldom persists for more than two days.

Interpretation

The characteristic histological features of the various disorders are described elsewhere in the book; textbooks of bone pathology such as those by Collins (1966) and Woods (1972) are also valuable. The specimen should be sent to a pathologist who is equipped to make undecalcified as well as decalcified sections. Decalcified sections are valuable for demonstrating the cellular abnormalities, such as the excess of osteoclasts in hyperparathyroidism and uraemic osteodystrophy or the malignant cells of metastatic bone disease.

Undecalcified sections are valuable for demonstrating uncalcified bone matrix known as osteoid. It is not always appreciated that osteoid is present in normal bone (Woods et al 1968, Johnson et al 1971a, Ellis & Peart 1972, Raina 1972). For this reason it is important

TABLE 3.3. Causes of excessive osteoid.

Osteomalacia and rickets
Renal osteodystrophy
Phosphate depletion
Chronic acidosis
Paget's disease of bone
Hyperthyroidism
Fibrogenesis imperfecta ossium
'Axial osteomalacia'
Chronic fluoride intoxication
Diphosphonate therapy

to measure the amount of osteoid and as bone surfaces are often cut obliquely, measurement of the width of the seams is the least satisfactory method. Much more satisfactory are measurements of width in terms of the number of birefringent laminae seen in polarised light, of the extent of osteoid on the bone surfaces and of the area of osteoid relative to the area of bone. These measurements discriminate well between patients with osteomalacia and normal subjects. In osteomalacia the iliac crest appears to be representative of trabecular bone in other parts of the skeleton with respect to the proportion of osteoid (Woods et al 1968).

An excess of osteoid occurs in disorders other than osteomalacia (table 3.3). In Paget's disease excessive osteoid is sometimes found in parts of the bone without the characteristic histological features of the disease (Paterson et al 1968). As these patients have an abnormal serum alkaline phosphatase and may have bone pains, it can be difficult to distinguish them from patients with osteomalacia.

DIETARY ASSESSMENT

There are occasions when it is important to have an assessment of a patient's dietary intake of vitamin D. Very occasionally the assessment of vitamin A or vitamin C intake may be relevant but it is doubtful whether the assessment of dietary calcium is ever helpful in diagnosis (Walker 1972a).

In the assessment of dietary intake the retrospective dietary history of Burke (1947) is widely used, together with standard tables such as those of McCance and Widdowson (1960). This interview method has been criticised because, when the results are compared with those from seven-day records, a poor correlation is found in individuals. The two methods agree better when groups of people are compared (Young et al 1952, 1953). The retrospective dietary history has some inherent advantages in that it does not create an artificial situation and in that it should reflect long term food habits. Burke herself indicated one of the defects of the dietary history: the fact that figures are produced may give a quite unjustified impression of the accuracy of the results. An additional source of imprecision applies to estimates of vitamin D intake. The vitamin D content of eggs and dairy products varies with the conditions under which the hens and cows are kept. Free-range hens in summer have more vitamin D in their eggs than hens kept indoors. However hens fed on a mash rich in vitamin D have eggs with a very high vitamin D content.

Despite these limitations the retrospective dietary history certainly has a place in comparisons between groups of patients. As vitamin D is found only in a limited number of foodstuffs, retrospective dietary histories for vitamin D intake have some value even in the individual, provided they are made by experienced dieticians who are not aware of the suggested diagnosis, provided they are interpreted with caution and provided enquiries are also made about exposure to sunlight.

Chapter 4: Hypercalcaemia: Differential Diagnosis, Clinical Features and Treatment

Hypercalcaemia has many causes (table 4.1) but in a survey of 25,847 consecutive clinic patients Boonstra and Jackson (1965) found that the most common were hyperparathyroidism and malignant disease. The disorders listed produce hypercalcaemia by several different mechanisms including increased bone resorption, increased intestinal absorption and renal retention of calcium; in some disorders such as hyperparathyroidism several factors contribute to the hypercalcaemia. Each disorder causing hypercalcaemia is considered in later chapters.

TABLE 4.1. Causes of hypercalcaemia. The figures in brackets represent the number of patients with each disorder found in the survey of Boonstra and Jackson (1965).

Primary hyperparathyroidism	(31)
Malignant disease*, reticulosis and myeloma	(19)
Vitamin D excess	(5)
Milk-alkali syndrome	(4)
Hyperthyroidism	(2)

Uncommon causes of hypercalcaemia

Sarcoidosis
Idiopathic hypercalcaemia of infancy
Paget's disease (only if very active or after immobilisation)
Tertiary hyperparathyroidism
Adrenal insufficiency (Addison's disease or hypopituitarism)
Vitamin A poisoning
Immobilisation

* Including pseudohyperparathyroidism.

DIFFERENTIAL DIAGNOSIS

In many patients found to have hypercalcaemia the cause can be determined from the clinical features or radiological studies. In other patients however additional investigations are needed to make a diagnosis.

Serum parathyroid hormone

This measurement has many limitations at present and is not widely available. The specificity of the antisera for the circulating form of parathyroid hormone varies greatly and most laboratories still find a substantial overlap in serum parathyroid hormone results between normal subjects and patients with hyperparathyroidism. A few laboratories have antisera which are more specific and which appear to distinguish completely between normal sera and sera from patients with hyperparathyroidism (Reiss & Canterbury 1971, O'Riordan et al 1972, Arnaud et al 1973).

With current methods a raised value for serum parathyroid hormone in a hypercalcaemic patient strongly supports the diagnosis of hyperparathyroidism. It is likely that specific methods for the estimation of circulating human parathyroid hormone will become more widely available in the near future; this will then be a most valuable test in the differential diagnosis of hypercalcaemia.

Steroid suppression tests

When corticosteroids are administered to patients with hypercalcaemia the serum calcium falls to normal or near-normal values in sarcoidosis and vitamin D poisoning and in most patients with malignant disease, but remains elevated in hyperparathyroidism (fig. 4.1). There are important exceptions to these rules which are described below.

Procedure (Dent & Watson 1968) Before treatment is started at least two base-line measurements of the serum calcium should be made, and these, with those done subsequently should be taken with minimal stasis at the same time each day. Hydrocortisone (40 mg eight-hourly by mouth) is given for ten days after which the dose is reduced slowly over the next few days to avoid problems from adrenal suppression. The serum calcium is measured on alternate days. It is

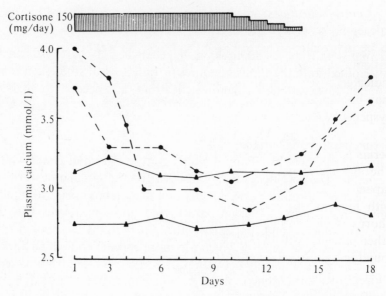

FIGURE 4.1. Steroid suppression tests in four patients with hypercalcaemia. In the two patients with primary hyperparathyroidism (▲) there was no change in the serum calcium whereas there was a prompt fall in the serum calcium in the two patients (●) with hypercalcaemia due to bone metastases from breast carcinoma. From Wills (1973a) by permission.

important to measure the serum albumen concentration on these samples and to allow for this in interpreting the results; the serum albumen frequently falls on steroids, with an expansion of the plasma volume.

Interpretation A fall in serum calcium into the normal range is seen in patients with idiopathic hypercalcaemia, with vitamin D poisoning, with sarcoidosis, with myeloma and with leukaemia. Most patients with carcinoma show a fall in serum calcium but in some, notably those with advanced cancer, there is no change (Thomas et al 1958b, Thalassinos & Joplin 1970, Ashkar et al 1971). Patients with hyperparathyroidism very seldom respond to steroids, but exceptions have been reported, notably in patients with osteitis fibrosa (Dent & Watson 1968, Gamble 1970). I have seen an apparent 'response' to steroids in a patient with hyperparathyroidism who developed pneumonia.

Contra-indications In some centres, every patient with hyper-calcaemia has a steroid suppression test as a routine. This practice is to be deprecated. The test is unnecessary as well as misleading in patients with osteitis fibrosa. In addition the steroid test is contra-indicated when steroids themselves are contra-indicated. The test may be dangerous in patients with an infection or patients with the dyspepsia which is sometimes a feature of hyperparathyroidism.

Serum phosphorus and TmP/GFR

The fasting serum phosphorus reflects the tubular reabsorptive capacity for phosphate and is low in less than half of patients with hyperparathyroidism (fig. 4.2). However a low serum phosphorus is also found in pseudohyperparathyroidism and rarely in other patients with hypercalcaemia. A normal serum phosphorus is found in a substantial minority of patients with hyperparathyroidism, especially if there is renal impairment. For these reasons, while a low value supports the diagnosis of hyperparathyroidism, a normal value does not exclude it.

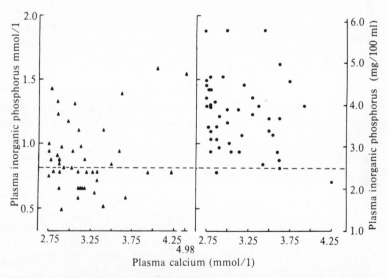

FIGURE 4.2. Plasma inorganic phosphorus concentrations in relation to the plasma calcium in 44 patients with primary hyperparathyroidism (▲) and 44 patients with hypercalcaemia of other causes (●). From Wills (1973a) by permission.

Measurements of the renal tubular handling of phosphorus (p. 50) are also of limited value in the differential diagnosis of hypercalcaemia. Like serum phosphorus none of these measurements discriminate completely between normal subjects and patients with hyperparathyroidism (Thomas et al 1959, Wills & McGowan 1964, Nordin & Bulusu 1968, Transbøl et al 1970a).

Plasma chloride and acid-base status

Many patients with hyperparathyroidism have a high or high-normal plasma chloride and a mild metabolic acidosis. Patients with hypercalcaemia with other causes generally have a low or low normal plasma chloride level and a mild metabolic alkalosis. Provided that a patient has no other reason to have an acid-base disturbance, measurement of the plasma chloride and capillary blood pH makes a valuable contribution to the diagnosis of hypercalcaemia. Figures 4.3 and 4.4 show the results obtained by Wills (1971b).

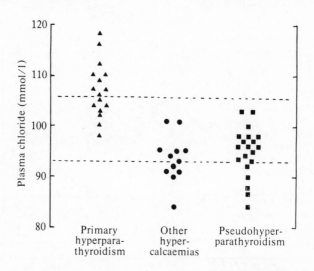

FIGURE 4.3. Plasma chloride levels in sixteen patients with primary hyperparathyroidism (▲), twenty patients with pseudohyperparathyroidism (■) and twelve patients with hypercalcaemia of other causes (●). Data of, or collected by, Wills (1971b). The horizontal dashed lines indicate the 2 SD limits for twelve normal subjects studied by the same author.

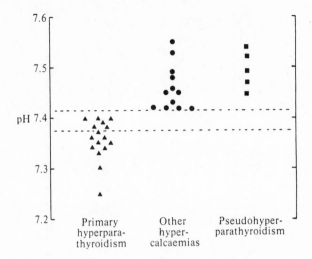

FIGURE 4.4. Arterial or arterialised venous blood pH in primary hyperparathyroidism (▲), pseudohyperparathyroidism (■) and other hypercalcaemias (●). Data of Wills (1971b).

The reason for the acidosis of hyperparathyroidism is not yet entirely clear. Parathyroid hormone appears to have a direct action on the renal tubule limiting the reabsorption of bicarbonate (Muldowney et al 1971, Siddiqui & Wilson 1972). The alkalosis of patients with hypercalcaemia of other causes is presumably the result of the suppression of circulating parathyroid hormone levels; alkalosis is also found in hypoparathyroidism (Barzel 1969). It is remarkable that with these tests pseudohyperparathyroidism of malignant disease does not behave like primary hyperparathyroidism; the recent evidence that the hypercalcaemic agent in these patients is not necessarily parathyroid hormone or even a peptide may provide a clue to the reason for this.

Urinary calcium excretion
Although most patients with hypercalcaemia have hypercalciuria, this is less often true of hyperparathyroidism than of hypercalcaemia of other causes (p. 99). In hyperparathyroidism there is increased renal tubular reabsorption of calcium and tests which reflect this are valuable in determining the cause of the hypercalcaemia (fig. 4.5).

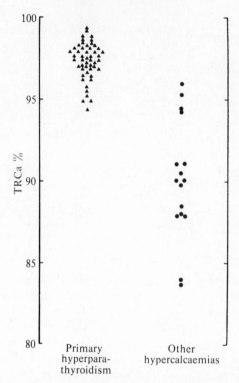

FIGURE 4.5. Tubular reabsorption of calcium (TRCa %) in 49 patients with primary hyperparathyroidism (▲) and 16 patients with hypercalcaemia of other causes (●). Data of Transbøl et al (1970a).

Other investigations

The urinary excretion of 3′,5′-cyclic adenosine monophosphate (cyclic AMP) is higher in hyperparathyroidism than in patients with other hypercalcaemias; when methods for cyclic AMP are more widely available this may become useful in the differential diagnosis of hypercalcaemia (Neelon et al 1973).

Multivariate analysis based on estimations of plasma bicarbonate, chloride, phosphorus, urea and alkaline phosphatase has given promising results in patients with hypercalcaemia (Fraser et al 1971a).

Patients with obscure hypercalcaemia should have a radiograph of the hands to seek for evidence of hyperparathyroid bone disease. If there is no evidence of osteitis fibrosa, and the diagnosis is still in doubt, a bone biopsy should be done to seek histological evidence of hyperparathyroidism (p. 86).

CLINICAL FEATURES

Hypercalcaemia of any cause may give rise to general symptoms of fatigue, malaise, thirst and polyuria (Fourman & Leeson 1959). Other common symptoms include anorexia, nausea and vomiting, and often constipation.

Neurological and psychiatric changes These are best known in hyperparathyroidism but are also found in hypercalcaemia with other causes (Karpati & Frame 1964, Streeto 1969). Some patients complain of weakness and muscle pains; others have a wide variety of neurological symptoms, including ataxia and visual symptoms. The mental changes include depression, irritability or inability to concentrate. These changes usually improve with treatment of the hypercalcaemia; they probably have an organic basis as a striking increase in the protein content of the cerebro-spinal fluid has been observed in hypercalcaemia (Krawitt & Bloomer 1965).

Renal changes The polyuria of hypercalcaemia is probably related to changes in the distal tubule. There is a large volume of hypotonic urine, which is not reduced by anti-diuretic hormone so that the condition resembles nephrogenic diabetes insipidus. The mechanism is not entirely clear but there is histological evidence of deposition of calcium around the distal tubules. The tubules fail to maintain the high parenchymal sodium content in the renal medulla (Eigler et al 1962, Porter & Wells 1964, Bank & Aynedjian 1965).

The glomerular filtration rate is reduced in many patients with hypercalcaemia whatever the cause. If the hypercalcaemia is not unduly prolonged this change is reversible.

Renal stones do occur in patients with hypercalcaemia of any cause but despite the severe hypercalciuria, they are curiously uncommon in disorders other than hyperparathyroidism.

Acute pancreatitis This is well recognised as a complication of hyperparathyroidism (p. 85) but it is also described in patients with hypercalcaemia due to vitamin D poisoning (Leeson & Fourman 1966b), multiple myeloma (Meltzer et al 1962) and pseudohyperparathyroidism due to carcinoma of the lung (Gault & Kinsella 1965).

Acute hypercalcaemia Extreme hypercalcaemia, whatever the cause, is associated with dehydration, confusion, coma and death in anuria. In adults survival is unusual with serum calcium levels of 5 mmol/l or more although children have survived despite brief periods at higher levels. The symptoms of acute hypercalcaemia are best exemplified by those of acute hyperparathyroidism (p. 107).

Metastatic calcification This gives rise to few clinical symptoms other than those consequent on renal damage. Corneal calcification (p. 33) is worth seeking; some patients with hypercalcaemia develop an acute red eye. Deafness due to calcification in the ear drums has been described in hyperparathyroidism (Bellin & Gershwin 1935) and in vitamin D poisoning (Harris 1969).

Electrocardiogram and electroencephalogram

In hypercalcaemia changes may be seen in both the electrocardiogram and the electroencephalogram. The ECG changes include a short QT interval and sometimes a prolonged PR interval. The T waves are flattened in lead 1 and in leads 2 and 3 widened with disappearance of the isoelectric part of the ST segment (Yu 1952, Muggia & Heinemann 1970a).

EEG abnormalities, especially bursts of high-voltage slow waves, have been described in hypercalcaemia but the proportion of patients affected is controversial (Etheridge & Grabow 1971). The same abnormality is found in several other conditions including uraemia, hypoxia, hypoglycaemia and water intoxication (Swash & Rowan 1972).

PATHOLOGY

Patients with hypercalcaemia have histological evidence of metastatic calcification less often than patients with renal failure but deposits in the lungs, kidneys, skin, blood vessels, heart and stomach are described (Mulligan 1947, Gayler & Brogdon 1965, Hemet & Chleq 1973). The renal changes are important. Within 24 hours of the induction of experimental hypercalcaemia there are degenerative changes in the ascending loop of Henle, the distal tubules and the collecting ducts. Electron microscopy shows that there is destruction of mitochondria. Hypercalcaemia of long-standing is associated with calcification in and around the tubular cell and in the lumen. There is patchy atrophy and regeneration in the collecting ducts (Hamburger et al 1968). An account of the renal changes in hyperparathyroidism is given on page 90.

The parathyroid glands would be expected to appear atrophic in patients with hypercalcaemia; in practice it is difficult to recognise this by light microscopy. Characteristic changes are seen with the electron microscope (Altenähr 1972).

TREATMENT

The treatment of hypercalcaemia is ordinarily that of the underlying disorder but treatment of the cause is not always practical. The hypercalcaemia of malignant disease can be particularly troublesome and the hypercalcaemia of vitamin D intoxication may persist for some months after the vitamin is withdrawn. In both examples treatment of the hypercalcaemia is indicated for the relief of symptoms and the protection of the kidney. In other cases, severe hypercalcaemia is a life-threatening emergency which needs urgent attention.

Some authors recommend a low calcium diet as part of the management of patients with hypercalcaemia. While the avoidance of excess calcium in the diet is reasonable, it is doubtful whether (apart from infantile hypercalcaemia) a low calcium diet contributes enough to justify the effort. All but the mildest cases of hypercalcaemia tend to be dehydrated and some may be potassium depleted; intravenous therapy with saline, and added potassium if needed, should be given. Other therapeutic measures are available for a direct attack on the hypercalcaemia; none is ideal but their indications and limitations are discussed in the sections which follow.

Phosphate

Intravenous and oral therapy with phosphate is the most widely studied method for the control of hypercalcaemia. Oral phosphate is given as a mixture of phosphates to have a neutral pH. Suitable preparations are now available commercially (p. 285). The initial dose is 1–3 grams (of phosphorus) per day according to the patient's size. The serum calcium should be checked daily at first and the dose adjusted appropriately to give a maintenance dose which is the minimum consistent with control of the serum calcium. Oral phosphate therapy is effective in the management of hypercalcaemia of malignant disease and myeloma (Goldsmith & Ingbar 1966, Goldsmith et al 1968a, Thalassinos & Joplin 1968), in hyperparathyroidism (Dent 1962, Goldsmith & Ingbar 1966, Eisenberg 1968), and in vitamin D poisoning (Goldsmith & Ingbar 1966).

Intravenous phosphate therapy is used in the management of acute hypercalcaemia, especially in the patient who is vomiting or in coma. The formulation of Goldsmith and Ingbar (1966) calls for a $0.1M$ solution containing in one litre 81 mmol (11·50 grams) of Na_2HPO_4 and 19 mmol (2·59 grams) of KH_2PO_4. Such a solution should have a pH of 7·4 and one litre will provide 3·1 grams of phosphorus, 162 mmol of sodium and 19 mmol of potassium. In the first instance 500 ml of this should be given slowly over at least eight hours and the patient should be carefully observed. To reduce the possibility of hypocalcaemia, measurements should be made during and after the infusion if possible; failing that, electrocardiographic recordings are helpful. The infusion may be repeated after twenty-four hours but should not be repeated if there is evidence of a rising blood urea, oliguria or an elevated serum phosphorus more than twenty-four hours after the infusion (Fulmer et al 1972). Intravenous phosphate therapy is very effective in reducing the serum calcium and may lead to a rapid improvement in the very ill patient with severe hypercalcaemia. It should however be replaced by oral therapy as soon as possible; it is probably safer to undertreat than to overtreat.

Side-effects Oral phosphate has few reported side effects. Some patients develop diarrhoea but this is usually temporary and may be relieved by the omission of one or two doses. More serious is the possibility of extraskeletal calcification. Dudley and Blackburn (1970) observed patients treated with oral neutral phosphate for from 9 to 87 months. Six out of nine patients had conjuctival calcification demonstrated by slit-lamp examination, five had radiological evidence of extraskeletal calcification, and two had progressive renal impairment. Other authors (Thalassinos & Joplin 1968, Kistler & Neubauer 1970) found no evidence of extraskeletal calcification which was not likely to have been present before treatment. Furthermore in most patients renal function improves with phosphate therapy and it seems likely that treatment with phosphate is less damaging to the kidney than the hypercalcaemia itself. One of Professor Dent's patients with hyperparathyroidism has now had oral phosphate therapy for 13 years with only a very slow deterioration in renal function (Stamp 1971).

Hypocalcaemia is seldom seen with careful oral phosphate therapy but a combination of calcitonin and oral phosphate has caused hypocalcaemia (Parsons et al 1970). A rise in the serum phosphorus occurs in some of the patients, particularly those with malignant disease who have a high serum phosphorus before tretament. These are probably the patients in whom caution is indicated to avoid extraskeletal calcification if treatment has to be prolonged.

Intravenous phosphate therapy has been associated with more serious side effects (Suki et al 1970). There are case reports of hypotension, massive extraskeletal deposition of calcium, acute oliguric renal failure and death. Some of these cases have been patients in whom excessive doses have been used and hypocalcaemia has been caused. In addition some of the patients with untoward side effects were already dangerously ill with the hypercalcaemia or with the neoplastic disease itself. Most workers have used cautious phosphate infusions without difficulty (Stamp 1971, Fulmer et al 1972).

Mode of action The mode of action of phosphate therapy is not well understood. The excretion of calcium in the urine decreases and it is thought that calcium phosphate salts are deposited in soft tissue and bone (Hebert et al 1966). Studies on rats and rabbits have suggested that extensive and damaging soft tissue calcification may occur with oral phosphate therapy (Spaulding & Walser 1970, Jowsey & Balasubramaniam 1972). However man appears to be different and there is little evidence of soft tissue calcification in most of the patients subsequently coming to autopsy. There is fair evidence of deposition of calcium and phosphate in bone even in patients with myeloma (Goldsmith et al 1968a). Furthermore there is now chemical and kinetic evidence that even in rats the principal site of the calcium deposition is the bone (Feinblatt et al 1970, Haddad & Avioli 1970).

Sodium sulphate

Intravenous infusions of sodium chloride and sodium sulphate both reduce the serum calcium in patients with hypercalcaemia but sodium sulphate appears to be the more effective (Chakmakjian & Bethune 1966). Either salt causes increased sodium excretion which itself increases urine calcium output but sodium sulphate therapy is additionally effective because unreabsorbable calcium sulphate complexes are formed in the urine.

Practical details of sodium sulphate therapy are given by Walser (1970) who regarded sulphate as the method of choice for the management of severe hypercalcaemia.

Side effects Sodium sulphate therapy appears to be remarkably safe. Nausea occurs in a few patients especially if the infusion is rapid. Sodium overload has been described (Heckman & Walsh 1967) and sodium sulphate is clearly contraindicated in patients with renal failure or poor cardiac reserve. Hypokalaemia is often seen but may be prevented by the addition of a small proportion of potassium sulphate to the intravenous fluid. Hypomagnesaemia is also possible.

Frusemide (furosemide)
Frusemide and ethacrynic acid promote calcium excretion as well as sodium excretion. If large intravenous doses of frusemide are given, and the sodium, potassium and water losses replaced, this becomes a method for lowering the serum calcium although not all patients respond and a normal serum calcium is not achieved in all those who do (Suki et al 1970, Humbert et al 1972, Baguet et al 1972). This treatment is probably contraindicated in renal failure and as very large volumes of intravenous fluid are needed careful monitoring of fluid, sodium, potassium and magnesium balances is needed. A bed scale is valuable if available.

There seems little place for this form of therapy: it is not uniformly effective; its control requires constant attention which may be impractical in some emergencies; its effectiveness diminishes after a few days (Toft & Roin 1971) so that it is unlikely to be of any value in longer-term management.

Chelating agents
Sodium ethylene diamine tetra-acetate (sodium edetate, sodium EDTA) is a chelating agent with a powerful avidity for calcium and heavy metals. Given intravenously it binds calcium and the calcium-EDTA complexes are excreted in the urine. Disadvantages of this method are that it must be given intravenously, that each infusion has a transient effect and that its control calls for estimation of the

serum calcium fraction not bound to EDTA. The appropriate com-
pleximetric methods for calcium estimation are not widely available.
In addition there have been reports (Dudley et al 1955) of renal damage after EDTA therapy and this method has fallen into disuse.

Corticosteroids

In several studies steroid therapy has been thought to be of value in
the management of hypercalcaemia of all causes other than hyperparathyroidism. It is of course effective in the rare hypercalcaemia of
adrenal insufficiency and a good response to large doses (hydrocortisone 120 mg daily in divided doses) is usually seen with vitamin
D poisoning, sarcoidosis and the milk-alkali syndrome. In vitamin D
poisoning, corticosteroids probably act by reducing the excessive
intestinal calcium absorption without interacting directly with vitamin
D (Favus 1970). Prednisone in a short course has been effective in
hypercalcaemia due to immobilisation (Lawrence et al 1973). In the
much more common problem of hypercalcaemia in malignancy its
value is more controversial. Perhaps 50% of these patients respond to
steroids but a larger proportion of patients with myeloma or breast
cancer respond. In pseudohyperparathyroidism no more than 20%
of patients respond to steroids (Kessinger et al 1972). In those malignant disorders which do respond, the steroids are effective by reducing
bone resorption, perhaps by a direct action on the tumour (Lazor &
Rosenberg 1964, Muirhead 1967).

Phosphate seems to be more consistently effective in the hypercalcaemia of malignant disease (Thalassinos & Joplin 1968 & 1970,
Fulmer et al 1972). Even when steroids are effective, they are slow
in action and take several days to give a worthwhile reduction in the
serum calcium. The dangers of long-term steroid therapy are well
known. For these reasons steroid therapy probably has at most a
small role in the present-day management of vitamin D poisoning,
sarcoidosis and perhaps immobilisation hypercalcaemia.

Mithramycin

Mithramycin is an antibiotic with cytotoxic activity; like actino-
mycin D it appears to act by the inhibition of RNA synthesis (Yarbro
et al 1966). When used in neoplastic disease hypocalcaemia has been
noted and, more recently, the place of mithramycin in the management
of hypercalcaemia has been explored. In most patients with severe

hypercalcaemia due to malignant disease a single intravenous injection of mithramycin (25 g per kilogram) is followed by a gradual fall in serum calcium toward normal values over 48 hours (Perlia et al 1970, Slayton et al 1971, Elias & Evans 1972, Elias et al 1972). At the same time there is a fall in the serum phosphorus level and in the urinary calcium excretion. Mithramycin has also been effective in reducing the serum calcium in a few patients with hyperparathyroidism (Perlia et al 1970, Singer et al 1970). The hypocalcaemic action of mithramycin probably results from an inhibition of bone resorption possibly by antagonism to the action of vitamin D.

Side effects The larger doses of mithramycin used in anti-tumour therapy have been associated with nausea and vomiting, with haematological disorders, with liver and renal tubular damage and with skin changes. Much smaller does are used in the management of hypercalcaemia and so far side-effects from these doses appear to be uncommon. Of 69 patients studied by Slayton et al (1971) one had liver damage and another thrombocytopaenia and bleeding.

Calcitonin

Calcitonin has recently become available commercially for the treatment of painful Paget's disease of bone and also for the management of hypercalcaemia. Earlier studies indicated that intramuscular calcitonin may be effective in lowering serum calcium levels in some patients with hypercalcaemia.

Some patients with hyperparathyroidism have had a worthwhile response to calcitonin (West et al 1971, Hesch et al 1971) but normal values are seldom achieved. Other patients have shown very modest responses to calcitonin (Sørensen et al 1970, Cochran et al 1970, Hill et al 1972). In the hypercalcaemia of vitamin D intoxication a good, though slow, response to calcitonin was found in three patients by Buckle et al (1972) although saline infusions may also have contributed to the improvement. Of two patients with vitamin D poisoning and hypercalcaemia studied by West et al (1971) one, a child, appeared to respond while an adult appeared to have gained no advantage from calcitonin. Objective assessment of the value of calcitonin in vitamin D poisoning is difficult as there may be great variations between patients in the rate at which the serum calcium falls after stopping the vitamin D. In the hypercalcaemia of malignant disease a partial or complete response was noted in most of the patients studied by

Silva and Becker (1973). In two patients with thyrotoxic hyper-calcaemia, calcitonin may have contributed to an improvement in the serum calcium although normal values were not achieved and other therapy was used in addition (Buckle et al 1969, Sørensen et al 1970).

Most workers have used a dose of 4–8 MRC units/kg per day by intramuscular injection although Silva and Becker gave 8 MRC units/kg every 6 hours. There is so far no good evidence that the intravenous route has any advantage over intramuscular therapy. Calcitonin is probably inappropriate in the long-term treatment of hypercalcaemia as it must be given parenterally and as resistance to its action, possibly due to antibody development, has been described (Singer et al 1972, Dubé et al 1973).

Side effects Calcitonin appears to have few side effects although nausea and vomiting may occur with higher doses. There is a possi-bility of a reaction to the foreign material and an intradermal test should be done especially in patients with a history of allergy. Hypocalcaemia has not been described as a result of treatment with calcitonin alone.

Mode of action In some studies the response to calcitonin seemed to be better related to the bone turnover rate than to the degree of hypercalcaemia, and it seems likely that the main action of calcitonin is an inhibition of bone resorption (Haddad & Avioli 1970). In addi-tion there may be a small diminution of renal tubular reabsorption of calcium as an increase in calcium excretion is noted in some (but not all) patients (Cochran et al 1970, Sørensen et al 1970).

Oestrogens

Oestrogens inhibit parathormone-induced bone resorption (Atkins et al 1972) and may have a place in the medical management of some postmenopausal women with mild hyperparathyroidism. Gallagher and Nordin (1972) obtained a modest reduction in the serum calcium (though not into the normal range) in a group of these patients.

In one patient with intractable hypercalcaemia from parathyroid carcinoma, stilboestrol diphosphate was effective in reducing the serum calcium when other measures had failed (Sigurdsson et al 1973).

While oestrogen therapy may be valuable in some patients with breast cancer and hypercalcaemia, in others oestrogens may precipi-tate hypercalcaemia (Muirhead 1967, Muggia & Heinemann 1970b).

Cellulose phosphate

This is a resin of cellulose to which phosphate is attached with ether linkages. It binds calcium in the intestine and so reduces its absorption. Reports of its use in hypercalcaemia are limited to two cases who had a modest reduction in serum calcium (Pak et al 1968). The only side effect noted was hypomagnesaemia.

Dialysis

There are very few case reports of the use of dialysis in the control of hypercalcaemia and even in those there is no unanimity about its value. Haemodialysis has been used in a hypercalcaemic emergency as a means of buying time (Eisenberg & Gotch 1968). Peritoneal dialysis with calcium-free solutions has been effective in a case of vitamin D poisoning (Nolph et al 1971).

CHOICE OF METHODS FOR THE CONTROL OF HYPERCALCAEMIA

In most cases oral phosphate therapy is the method of choice. It is effective and appears to be reasonably safe. In patients who are vomiting or unconscious intravenous phosphate should be used but the treatment needs to be carefully monitored as described earlier. The patient should be changed to phosphate by mouth as soon as it is practical. Renal failure is not a contraindication to phosphate therapy but the potassium salt may need to be replaced by sodium in the infusion.

In sarcoid hypercalcaemia steroid therapy is probably the method of choice. In vitamin D poisoning and immobilisation hypercalcaemia, there is no information on the relative merits of steroid therapy and phosphate which are both effective. However I feel that oral phosphate is probably preferable to long-term steroid therapy. Apart from these three disorders steroid therapy is seldom indicated. Sodium sulphate is of doubtful value because it is less effective than phosphate, because it must be given intravenously and because large volumes of fluid are needed. Frusemide, too, is not uniformly effective in controlling hypercalcaemia and its use requires very elaborate monitoring. Diaylysis has been tried too seldom to allow any opinion on its value.

In hypercalcaemia resistant to phosphate therapy the only drugs likely to be effective are mithramycin and possibly stilboestrol.

Chapter 5: Hyperparathyroidism

An association between a bizarre bone disease and the parathyroid glands was first established nearly fifty years ago. The interesting stories of the early patients have been described by Fourman and Royer (1968) and by Albright (1970).

INCIDENCE

The true prevalence of hyperparathyroidism in the general population is not known but the introduction of routine biochemical screening with automatic analysers has indicated an incidence of about 1 in 1,000 in a clinic population. For example, Boonstra and Jackson (1971) found fifty cases among 50,330 patients attending a general diagnostic clinic. Few of these patients had any symptoms which would have suggested hyperparathyroidism. In early reports the disorder was thought to be rare as only the patients with bone disease were included. In 1934 Albright and others recognised that many more patients had renal problems than had gross bone disease. The advent of biochemical screening has led to the recognition of still more patients.

The proportion of patients with parathyroid adenomas in unselected autopsies has varied from 0 to $7 \cdot 6\%$ in different series. Alveryd (1968) found that the highest incidence ($12 \cdot 3\%$) was in the age group 70–79 years; many of these patients however also had advanced renal disease.

Sex and age incidence
In almost all series females predominate over males in a ratio of between 3 to 1 and 2 to 1. This was true both in the early days when most patients had bone disease (Norris 1947) and today when many patients have only minor symptoms (Boonstra & Jackson 1971). The preponderance of females is the result of a particularly high incidence among post-menopausal women (Muller 1969).

79

Primary hyperparathyroidism has been found at all ages from birth (p. 109) to 92 (Davidson et al 1971). The greatest incidence is in the third, fourth, fifth and sixth decades (Pyrah et al 1966).

Familial incidence

Hyperparathyroidism may occur in more than one member of a family (Pyrah et al 1966, Burden 1971). Families are described with hyperparathyroidism in parents and children as well as families with cases in several siblings. Hillman et al (1964) described neonatal hyperparathyroidism in two siblings whose parents were first cousins. In most cases of familial hyperparathyroidism primary chief-cell hyperplasia is the disorder responsible, although in one family oxyphil adenomas were common (Marsden et al 1971). Some patients with familial hyperparathyroidism represent examples of multiple endocrine neoplasia type 1 (p. 94, Jackson & Boonstra 1967).

Hyperparathyroidism is described sufficiently often in families to justify a check of the serum calcium on the immediate relatives of patients.

PATHOLOGY OF PARATHYROID GLANDS

The normal parathyroid gland has two main types of secretory cell: chief-cells which are the most numerous and oxyphil cells which are characterised by acidophil granules in the cytoplasm. Evidence for the presence of parathyroid hormone in the cytoplasm of chief-cells has been obtained by immunofluorescence studies (Hargis et al 1964). Oxyphil cells are not seen in childhood and their function is not known. In addition there are fat cells and bands of fibrous tissue dividing the glands into cords. An overactive gland may have a normal size when the fat cells have been replaced by secretory cells. The fat cells are scarce in childhood and in malnourished subjects.

Water-clear cells are not seen in normal human parathyroid glands but are of importance as the cell of one type of hyperplasia. The curious appearance of these large cells is due to the presence of vacuoles whose function is unknown (Altenähr 1972).

The main pathological disorders associated with hyperparathyroidism are hyperplasia (chief cell or water-clear cell), adenomas (mostly chief cell in type) and carcinoma. Table 5.1 shows the

TABLE 5.1. Causes of hyperparathyroidism in 343 cases (Cope 1966)

Cause	Number of cases	
Neoplasia		
Single adenoma	263	(77%)
Double adenoma	13	(4%)
Carcinoma	15	(4%)
Hyperplasia		
Water-clear cell	15	(4%)
Chief cell	37	(11%)

proportions of these in one series. Recent accounts of the pathology and electron microscopy of these lesions have been given by Hoehn et al (1969), Faccini (1970), Roth (1971), Altenähr (1972) and Thiele et al (1973).

Adenoma
The benign adenoma was the earliest disorder described as a cause of hyperparathyroidism and it is still the most common in all series. To the naked eye the gland may not be greatly enlarged but it is a reddish brown colour unlike the normal glands which are often yellowish brown because of their fat content. The lower glands are more often affected than the upper.

Histologically the adenoma usually occupies the whole of the gland, leaving only a rim of normal tissue. In most adenomas the principal cell-type is the chief cell but mixed-cell adenomas include water-clear cells, oxyphil cells or both. The development of an autonomous adenoma in a patient with secondary hyperparathyroidism ('tertiary hyperparathyroidism') is now well recognised. These are usually chief cell adenomas and at exploration the other glands sometimes show evidence of hyperplasia. Less well recognised is the possibility than an adenoma (and in one case a carcinoma) could be superimposed on a primary hyperplasia (Kramer 1970).

Oxyphil adenomas are uncommon and only a minority of the recognised cases are associated with hyperparathyroidism (Selzman & Fechner 1967).

Haemorrhage into an adenoma occurs occasionally and may cause acute hyperparathyroidism (Chodack et al 1965). Infarction of an adenoma has also been described in a few patients who have had a spontaneous remission of their hyperparathyroidism (Wills 1971a). In one case the infarction was accompanied by a transient acute hypercalcaemia (Howard et al 1953). Multiple adenomas are described in many series; Black (1969) suggested that some of these cases were really examples of chief cell hyperplasia.

Primary chief-cell hyperplasia (nodular hyperplasia)

This has only been recognised recently as a cause of hyperparathyroidism (Cope et al 1958) but is now identified increasingly frequently. In one recent series (Haff & Ballinger 1971) this disorder was the pathological cause of hyperparathyroidism in 31 out of 74 cases. Other series describe it less often but it is still an important cause of hyperparathyroidism. Its particular importance lies in the difficulty of distinguishing between chief cell hyperplasia and adenoma, especially by frozen section. The difference is important because of the difference in the surgical management of the two disorders.

In primary chief cell hyperplasia all the glands are enlarged, though often to different sizes, and show a nodular appearance. Microscopically there is a variation in the predominant cell type from area to area; there may be nodules composed principally of water-clear cells or oxyphil cells. For this reason examination of a small part of a gland by frozen section may give appearances indistinguishable from those of an adenoma. There are usually fewer fat cells than in normal glands and unlike adenomas there is seldom a compressed rim of normal tissue. Intrafollicular amyloid is found in some cases, particularly those associated with multiple endocrine neoplasia (Leedham & Pollock 1970). The abnormalities of chief cell hyperplasia may be more obvious on electron microscopy (Black 1969).

Primary water-clear cell hyperplasia

This accounts for between 5% and 10% of the cases of hyperparathyroidism, The glands are all enlarged but unequally so, the upper glands usually being larger than the lower. They are lobulated and a striking chocolate brown or mahogany colour. They may be recognised by the surgeon because of 'pseudopodia', projections extending into the tissues of the neck.

Histologically the glands consist entirely or almost entirely of large water-clear cells with sometimes a few smaller cells of a transitional type. There is little connective tissue or fat and the cells are arranged in an acinar pattern; the overall appearance is not unlike that of a renal carcinoma.

Parathyroid cysts

Parathyroid cysts are uncommon, some sixty cases having been reported. The great majority of these are symptomless, but a few cases have had hyperparathyroidism; these may represent patients with cystic degeneration of an adenoma (Rogers et al 1969, Howell 1972). Parathyroid cysts are rarely found in the mediastinum (Thacker et al 1971).

Parathyroid carcinoma is considered on page 111.

CLINICAL AND PATHOLOGICAL FEATURES

The only feature typical of hyperparathyroidism is the fact that it is so frequently atypical. However the important clinical features are related to the hypercalcaemia itself or to the renal consequences or to the bone disease. The modes of presentation of hyperparathyroidism are shown in table 5.2. The marked decrease in the proportion of patients with bone disease and the increase in recent years in the numbers of patients with nonspecific symptoms is clearly shown. Many of the patients presenting with renal or bone complications also admit to more general symptoms on enquiry.

At one time it was thought that patients with hyperparathyroidism could have either bone disease or renal disease but seldom both. The two groups were mutually almost exclusive and it was even suggested that two different hormones could have been involved. Now patients with a 'bone' presentation and osteitis fibrosa often in fact have severe renal damage (Hellström & Ivemark 1962) while patients with other symptoms have histological evidence of bone disorder more often than would be suspected by radiology. Nonetheless the variety of manifestations of hyperparathyroidism still needs explanation. One factor explored by Lloyd (1968) was the role of the parathyroid lesion itself. He noted that bone disease was generally associated with

TABLE 5.2. Presenting features of hyperparathyroidism in two series of patients. Series 1
(Cope 1960) consists of 230 patients identified
before 1960. Series 2 covers 116 patients
identified after 1960 (Epstein et al 1970,
Vasconez et al 1970, Hillegas & Evans 1971).

Presentation	Series 1 (Percent)	Series 2 (Percent)
Bone disease	27	10
Renal stones or urinary infection	57	57
Peptic ulcer	8	7
Pancreatitis	2	3
Fatigue and other constitutional symptoms	2	10
Hypertension	1	1
Mental disorders	1	2
CNS disorders	1	—
Hypercalcaemic crisis (without bone disease)	—	1
Gout	—	1
Infant with tetany	—	2
Serendipity	1	8

the large, rapidly growing tumour; while renal lithiasis was associated
with less active, but chronic, hyperparathyroidism. Patients with
bone disease certainly tend to have very high concentrations of parathyroid hormone in the blood (O'Riordan et al 1972). Another
possible factor is the inhibitor of the growth of calcium oxalate
cysrals demonstrated in the urine by Dent and Sutor (1971). Patients
with stones of nephrocalcinosis were those with absent or reduced
quantities of the inhibitor, while those with normal amounts of the
inhibitor were spared, irrespective of the degree of hypercalciuria.

CLINICAL FEATURES RELATED TO THE HYPERCALCAEMIA

Many patients with hyperparathyroidism have general symptoms
including muscular weakness, lassitude, thirst and polyuria, and
anorexia and nausea. These symptoms are probably related to the
hypercalcaemia, but, in a few patients, may be the consequence of

renal failure. The thirst and polyuria may be sufficiently severe to suggest the diagnosis of diabetes insipidus (p. 91). Hypertension is present in about half the patients. The muscular weakness may be demonstrable objectively (p. 90). Corneal calcification (p. 33) is found in about a quarter of patients with hyperparathyroidism (Watson 1972). Calcification in the ear drums has been described as a cause of deafness (Bellin & Gershwin 1935). Calcification of the cutaneous blood vessels may lead to trophic changes and patches of gangrene (Winkelmann & Keating 1970).

Psychiatric changes

Hyperparathyroidism may present with a psychiatric disorder which varies from minor depression or irritability to frank psychosis or catatonic stupor. Not a few patients have been described as 'cussed' or 'truculent' and they may be quite uncooperative about their treatment. These symptoms improve with relief of the hyperparathyroidism (Karpati & Frame 1964, Hockaday et al 1966, Flanagan et al 1970). The reason for the psychiatric disturbance in hyperparathyroidism is not clear but the likeliest factor is the hypercalcaemia itself. Mental changes have been described in other disorders associated with hypercalcaemia.

Pancreatic disorders

Both acute and chronic pancreatitis have been described too often in hyperparathyroidism to be coincidental (Pyrah et al 1966). Possible explanations include the formation of pancreatic calculi or the premature conversion of trypsinogen to trypsin favoured by the high concentration of calcium in the pancreatic juice. In addition acute hypercalcaemia stimulates enzyme secretion by the pancreas in man (Goebell et al 1972). The pancreatitis may be a consequence of the hypercalcaemia because there are a few case reports (p. 69) of pancreatitis in hypercalcaemia with other causes. Acute pancreatitis can cause a fall in the serum calcium (p. 144); in hyperparathyroidism this occasionally means that the patient is normocalcaemic during the acute attack.

Sub-acute and chronic pancreatitis may be a cause of recurrent abdominal pain in patients with hyperparathyroidism. The symptoms cease after parathyroidectomy. In some of these cases the diagnosis may be suggested by finding radiological evidence of pancreatic calcification or calculi. In one recent personal case, a man of 42, hyperparathyroidism had led to recurrent bouts of abdominal pain for ten years. At least one of these attacks was caused by pancreatitis as may have been the others; by the time he was investigated he had permanent pancreatic damage with malabsorption and diabetes mellitus.

BONE CHANGES

Bone pain is an uncommon symptom in hyperparathyroidism. One patient complained of a 'jarring pain' in the legs. He felt that there was 'no padding between the bones of the feet, ankles, knees and hips'. Running was particularly painful (Barnhart 1967). If a giant-cell tumour is present pain is more likely, may be localised and associated with local swelling. There is a case-report of a 58 year old woman with a strategically placed giant-cell tumour which caused spinal-cord compression (Shaw & Davies 1968). The bone resorption at the finger ends occasionally leads to shortening of the distal phalanges and a 'pseudo-clubbing'.

Pathology

The classical disorder of the bone in hyperparathyroidism is known as osteitis fibrosa. Although there is no suggestion of inflammation this term is widely used. An older name, von Recklinghausen's disease of bone, is falling into disuse. Reviews: Collins (1966), Pyrah et al (1966).

Osteitis fibrosa is most obvious in parts of the skeleton where normal bone turnover is most active. Thus the trabecular bone of the vertebrae, the phalanges, the ends of the long bones, and parts of the skull show the most obvious changes although it is likely that the whole skeleton is affected. The bone shows increased activity by fibroblasts with deposition of excessive fibrous tissue in the marrow and increased numbers of osteoclasts mostly lying in lacunae on bone surfaces undergoing resorption. Osteoblasts are also active and areas of bone regeneration, particularly isolated fragments or trabeculae of coarse woven bone, may be surrounded by plump osteoblasts. A moderate excess of uncalcified osteoid is often found (Olah 1973). In some areas bone resorption and bone regeneration may be seen in close proximity to each other. The overall result is usually progressive loss of bone especially from compact bone.

Hitherto there has been a clear distinction, among patients with hyperparathyroidism, between the few with radiologically evident bone disease and an abnormal serum alkaline phosphatase value, and those presenting with renal disease. However it is now clear, both from conventional histology and from micro-radiography, that the bone changes of hyperparathyroidism are found more often than the radiological signs would suggest (Byers & Smith 1971, Meunier et al 1972). Osteoclasts may not be the only cells responsible for bone resorption in hyperparathyroidism; evidence of osteolysis by osteocytes has been put forward by Bordier et al (1973b). Detection of this change appears to provide an even more sensitive test for hyperparathyroidism.

Two forms of cystic change in the bone are found in hyperparathyroidism. The more common cysts are of any size or shape and may be single or multiple. They contain mucus or brown fluid and probably result from haemorrhage or necrosis. Less common are giant-cell tumours or 'brown tumours', which appear cystic by x-ray and may in fact contain a cystic area. The tumours contain principally osteoclasts within a stroma of spindle-cells. Mitotic figures are seen in each type of cell. Histologically the tumour may be indistinguishable from osteoclastomas not associated with hyperparathyroidism. However, giant-cell tumours in the shafts of long bones or in the ribs, mandible or clavicle are more likely to be associated with hyperparathyroidism especially if they are multiple.

Giant-cell tumours heal slowly after parathyroidectomy to give a fibrous tissue mass. In the jaw, healing may be so slow that local surgery is sometimes needed for cosmetic reasons (Kennett & Pollick 1971). In the occasional patient with giant-cell tumours in the jaw whose hyperparathyroidism is not amenable to surgery, local excision may also contribute to the patient's comfort (Buckerfield 1971).

One case of fibrosarcoma superimposed on osteitis fibrosa has been described by Lee et al (1955). It presented soon after the successful removal of a parathyroid adenoma and was rapidly fatal.

Radiology
Radiologically evident bone changes are found in between 10% and 20% of patients with hyperparathyroidism in recent series. The main changes include subperiosteal erosions, bone cysts and, more

rarely, widespread demineralisation, sometimes with patchy osteo-sclerosis. Generalised demineralisation of the skeleton is only found in patients with longstanding disease and is now seldom seen. It is non-specific and difficult to detect reliably unless it is severe. The results of bone demineralisation: fractures, deformity and loss of stature are also seldom seen.

Much more common, and more useful to the clinician, are sub-periosteal erosions. These are best seen in the phalanges but may also be detected at the outer ends of the clavicles, in the ulna, in the femoral neck and on the upper surfaces of the ribs. They consist of small areas of bone resorption under the periosteum so that the edge of the cortex has a crenellated or lace-like appearance (fig. 5.1). Any phalanx may be affected but the middle phalanges are said to show subperiosteal erosions most frequently. The erosions are usually on the radial aspect. In the distal phalanges, especially in the thumb, the erosions may lead to extensive destruction and shortening but bone resorption at this site is by no means unique to hyperpara-thyroidism (Greenfield 1969: page 304). The erosions at the ends of the clavicles are fairly useful as they may be seen on a routine chest radiograph; rheumatoid arthritis may cause similar appearances at this site. After hyperparathyroidism has been corrected the erosions heal.

Skull Various changes in the skull have been described and include a mottled appearance and areas of bone resorption. Resorption from the inner table gives the skull a fenestrated appearance, the 'pepper-pot skull' (fig. 5.2). Similar appearances have been described occasionally in Cushing's syndrome and Paget's disease.

Lamina dura The lamina dura is the cortical bone of the tooth socket. It disappears in many cases of hyperparathyroidism with bone disease, and reforms after parathyroidectomy (Vender et al 1971). Hyperparathyroid patients without subperiosteal erosions scarcely ever lose the lamina dura. Loss of the lamina dura does occur in some patients with other conditions such as Paget's disease, fibrous dysplasia, osteomalacia, hyperphosphatasia, Cushing's syn-drome, dental sepsis and of course the edentulous (Greenfield 1969, Burwood 1972). The demonstration of an absent lamina dura is more of an undertaking than hand x-rays and in general this investiga-tion has little additional value.

Cysts and tumours It is difficult to distinguish radiologically

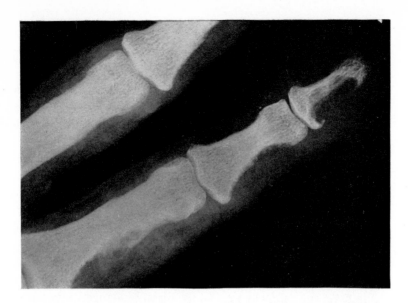

FIGURE 5.1. Subperiosteal erosions in phalanges of the hand in primary hyperparathyroidism.

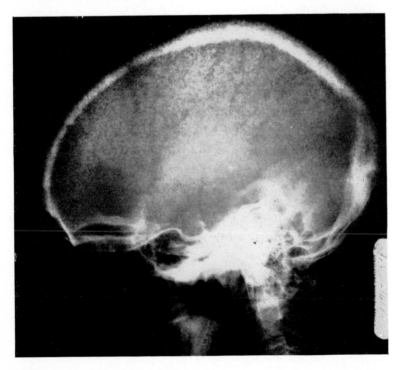

FIGURE 5.2. Multiple translucencies in the skull (pepper-pot skull) in a woman with hyperparathyroidism (courtesy of Dr. T. C. K. Marr).

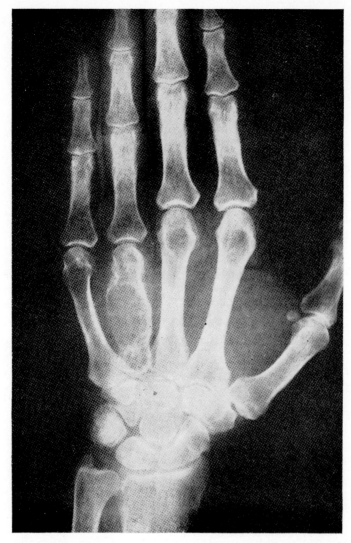

FIGURE 5.3. Solitary osteoclastoma of a metacarpal in a woman later found to have hyperparathyroidism (Fourman & Royer 1968).

between the cysts and giant-cell tumours of hyperparathyroidism and either may resemble unrelated bone lesions such as simple cysts, secondary neoplasms, including secondary parathyroid carcinoma, and myeloma. Most patients with cysts and giant-cell tumours also have other radiological evidence of hyperparathyroidism. Giant-cell tumours are usually multilocular; the overlying cortex may be thin and expanded (fig. 5.3). After parathyroidectomy these cysts slowly heal but in some an area of bone sclerosis or a thick walled translucency may persist for many years.

Bone sclerosis Bone sclerosis is a common feature of uraemic osteodystrophy with secondary hyperparathyroidism but is also occasionally found in small areas of bone in primary hyperparathyroidism (Doyle 1966, Eugenidis et al 1972).

Bone radiology in the diagnosis of hyperparathyroidism All patients in whom hyperparathyroidism is suspected should have a radiograph of the hands. If subperiosteal erosions are found, this is very valuable evidence in favour of hyperparathyroidism. In patients with a normal serum alkaline phosphatase value it is doubtful whether there is any point in doing any additional x-rays.

JOINT DISORDERS

Three forms of arthropathy have been described in hyperparathyroidism. First a mechanical arthritis may be secondary to subchondral fractures or erosions which are part of the bone disease. This disorder may mimic rheumatoid arthritis but it can often be distinguished by the presence of osteitis fibrosa. The disorder may lead on to osteoarthritis (Bywaters et al 1963, Ryckewaert et al 1966, Lipson & Williams 1968, Gravelle 1970). Secondly patients may develop pseudo-gout (synonyms: crystal synovitis, pyrophosphate arthropathy, chondrocalcinosis). In chronic cases calcification of the hyaline cartilage may be seen radiologically. If an effusion is present and especially in acute episodes, calcium pyrophosphate crystals may be aspirated. Acute pseudo-gout sometimes follows parathyroidectomy (Bilezikian et al 1973). Thirdly true gout may occur as a consequence of the hyperuricaemia often found in hyperparathyroidism (Scott et al 1964). This too may cause calcification in cartilage (Dodds & Steinbach 1966) and a synovitis with both uric acid and calcium pyrophosphate crystals is described (Grahame et al 1971).

Two cases of hyperparathyroidism presented as a result of avulsion of tendons from bones (Preston & Adicoff 1962, Preston 1972). In the earlier report a 33 year old man was attempting to push his car out of the snow when both knees 'gave out' and he was found to have avulsed both quadriceps tendons and the left triceps tendon from bone which was the site of osteitis fibrosa.

Muscle Changes

Muscular weakness and wasting may be detected on clinical examination, usually in the patient with fairly severe hyperparathyroidism and bone disease. The muscles most severely affected are the proximal muscles of the legs so that the patients have difficulty climbing stairs. Histology and electron microscopy of the muscle show morphological changes which are nonspecific and their pathogenesis is not clear (Smith & Stern 1967, Cholod et al 1970).

Renal Complications

Renal damage represents the most serious complication of hyperparathyroidism and results particularly from calcification; other factors in some cases are pyelonephritis or an impacted calculus. Calcification is found particularly in the medulla and pyramids and is seen much more frequently by microscopy than by radiology. In the early case the main damage is to the distal tubules and to a smaller extent the loops of Henle and the collecting ducts. The calcification is both extracellular and intracellular and may lead to a fibrosis of the interstitial tissue. This in turn leads to the obstruction and loss of some nephrons, and to a secondary pyelonephritis. The eventual result is small fibrotic kidneys associated with uraemia and hypertension. A full account of the renal pathology in both human and experimental hyperparathyroidism has been given by Pyrah et al (1966). Similar pathological changes are found in patients with hypercalcaemia or hypercalciuria of other causes.

Radiology

Many authors limit the use of the term nephrocalcinosis to radiologically evident calcification; this is a little arbitrary as tomography may reveal calcification which is otherwise undetectable. There are many causes of nephrocalcinosis and in the majority of cases where the cause is hyperparathyroidism there are diffuse bilateral opacities of varying size usually involving the medulla more than the cortex (Hamburger et al 1968). In a smaller proportion there are masses of calcium scattered irregularly throughout the renal parenchyma and in a smaller number still the calcification is so fine and uniform as to give a 'spontaneous renogram'.

Clinical consequences

Renal calculi Albright et al (1934) first noted that hyperparathyroidism should be sought among patients with renal calculi and it is likely that between 3% and 10% of patients with recurrent renal calculi have hyperparathyroidism. The exact proportion varies between different series probably as a result of real variations between the populations studied. In hyperparathyroidism the stones are usually composed of calcium oxalate or apatites or mixtures of these, but uric acid stones also occur with an increased frequency in hyperparathyroidism (Frank et al 1970).

In a patient with renal calculi and hyperparathyroidism, the parathyroid surgery should be done first because of the danger of precipitating acute hyperparathyroidism (p. 107).

Renal tubular defects Renal tubular damage is probably the earliest detectable pathological change in hyperparathyroidism, and polyuria and polydipsia are sometimes the earliest symptoms. In some patients the volume of hypotonic urine is so large that diabetes insipidus may be considered. Objective evidence of a defect in urine concentrating ability can be obtained by determining the maximum urine osmolality after a period of water deprivation. Thirst is a well-recognised symptom of hyperparathyroidism. It seems to be out of proportion to the polyuria and is relieved by parathyroidectomy (Fourman & Leeson 1959).

Other renal tubular defects in hyperparathyroidism have characteristic chemical consequences. There is often a defect in bicarbonate reabsorption (Muldowney et al 1971, Siddiqui & Wilson 1972) leading to a metabolic acidosis. There are defects in phosphate reabsorption (p. 65) in calcium excretion (p. 67), in amino-acid reabsorption (Cusworth et al 1972) and in the tubular handling of uric acid, leading in some cases to clinical gout. The tubular reabsorption capacity for glucose (TmG/GFR) is sometimes increased in hyperparathyroidism; this is not a sufficiently consistent finding to be helpful in diagnosis (Aurell et al 1971).

Pyelonephritis Urinary infection occurs fairly often in hyper-parathyroidism. In the series of Britton et al (1971), for example, 25 out of 81 patients were affected at the time of parathyroidectomy.

Hypertension It is difficult to give figures for the incidence of hypertension in hyperparathyroidism as the definition of hypertension is arbitrary. However figures of 49% (Hellström & Ivemark 1962), 28% (Pyrah et al 1966), 40% (Ohlsson 1970) and 20% (Rosenthal & Roy 1972) have been suggested. Conversely Rosenthal and Roy (1972) found seven patients with hyperparathyroidism among 900 presenting with hypertension. It seems clear therefore that hypertension is a real feature of hyperparathyroidism and contributes to its mortality: of 21 patients collected by Hellström et al (1958) five died of cerebral haemorrhage and three of cardiac failure. Parathyroidectomy corrects the hypertension in about half of the affected patients but some patients may develop hypertension for the first time after surgery.

The pathogenesis of the hypertension is not yet clear. Most authors regard the renal damage as the most likely factor but, in addition, the hypercalcaemia itself may contribute (Madhavan et al 1970, Weidmann et al 1972).

Renal failure Uraemia is a major cause of death in patients with untreated hyperparathyroidism. A low glomerular filtration rate is particularly associated with those patients with skeletal changes or nephrocalcinosis. It is less often seen in patients with renal calculi alone (Hellström & Ivemark 1962). Various factors contribute to renal failure: nephrocalcinosis with inflammatory changes and loss of nephrons, pyelonephritis, hypertension and, rarely, impaction of a calculus. Although in some patients the renal failure progresses after parathyroidectomy, in general there is a modest improvement (p. 105).

DISEASES ASSOCIATED WITH PRIMARY HYPERPARATHYROIDISM

Peptic ulcer

The relationship between hyperparathyroidism and peptic ulcer has been controversial. However it now seems likely that there is an

increased incidence of peptic ulcer among patients with hyperparathyroidism (Pyrah et al 1966, Ellis & Nicoloff 1968, Black 1971a).
In various series the incidence of peptic ulcer in hyperparathyroidism
has been between 10% and 25% thus not greatly in excess of the
incidence of peptic ulcer in the general population. Among 300
patients with peptic ulcers, Frame and Haubrich (1960) found four
with hyperparathyroidism, an incidence much in excess of that of
hyperparathyroidism in the general population.

A few of the patients with both disorders have multiple endocrine
adenomatosis (see below) which may be associated with peptic
ulceration whether or not the Zollinger-Ellison syndrome is included.
When these patients are excluded, patients with peptic ulcer and
hyperparathyroidism mostly have duodenal ulcers which are often
severe and may be familial. Treatment with antacids may worsen the
symptoms. Relief of the hyperparathyroidism often leads to healing
of the ulcer. Surgery for the ulcer in the presence of unrecognised
hyperparathyroidism may lead to acute hypercalcaemia.

If there is a relationship between hyperparathyroidism and peptic
ulcer what is its mechanism? In hypoparathyroidism the output of
gastric acid is often low and returns to normal when the serum calcium
becomes normal. In studies on volunteers, intravenous infusions of
calcium led to an increase in serum gastrin and in gastric acid output
(Reeder et al 1970, Ottenjann 1971). Although studies of gastric acid
secretion in primary hyperparathyroidism have yielded conflicting
results it is now clear that many of these patients have a high plasma
gastrin and a high basal acid output (Kelly 1970, Christiansen &
Aagaard 1972a, Dent et al 1972). Another suggestion has turned on
the gastric secretion of calcium. In the resting stomach the output of
calcium in the gastric juice is moderately increased in hyperparathyroidism compared with controls but this difference disappears after
stimulation. There was a difference between the calcium secretion in
gastric juice before and after parathyroidectomy in patients with
hyperparathyroidism so that calcium is unlikely to be an important
factor (Christiansen & Aagaard 1971, 1972b). Yet another possibility,
supported by experimental work with rats, is that a tendency to
develop ulcers results from defective secretion of gastric mucus in
hyperparathyroidism (Kelly 1970). In conclusion, although increased
acid secretion seems the most likely cause of peptic ulcer in hyperparathyroidism other factors may also be important.

Multiple endocrine neoplasia

Two syndromes of multiple endocrine neoplasia are described; hyperparathyroidism may be a component of either. In the commoner type 1 syndrome (formerly multiple endocrine adenomatosis or the pluriglandular syndrome) the other components may include pituitary tumours (especially acidophil adenomas, acidophil hyperplasia and chromophobe adenomas), pancreatic tumours (both insulin-producing and gastrin-producing) and, less commonly, tumours or hyperplasia in adrenal cortex or thyroid although these seldom cause clinical symptoms (Ballard et al 1964, Craven et al 1972). The disorder is associated with a very high incidence of peptic ulcer even in those patients without a Zollinger-Ellison tumour, and appears to be inherited as an autosomal dominant (Wermer 1963). The nature of the disorder is not clear; that an auto-immune process may be a factor is suggested by a family study with multiple endocrine adenomatosis in a mother and auto-immune Addison's disease in four of her children (Mershon & Deitrich 1966). Table 5.3 shows the main features in 85 cases collected by Ballard et al (1964).

In this syndrome the most common parathyroid disorder is chief-cell hyperplasia but adenomas and clear-cell hyperplasia are also described. The hyperparathyroidism appears to be fairly benign with relatively little renal damage and bone disease is rare. Of 33

TABLE 5.3. Components of syndrome of multiple endocrine neoplasia type 1 in 85 cases

	No. of cases	percent
Hyperparathyroidism	74	87
Pancreatic tumours	69	81
Pituitary tumours or hyperplasia	55	65
Peptic ulcer	49	58
Adrenal cortical adenoma or hyperplasia (but only two cases of Cushings syndrome and one of aldosteronism)	31	36
Thyroid disorders (but hyperthyroidism only in 2 cases)	15	18
Diarrhoea	11	13
Steatorrhoea	4	5
Bronchial carcinoid	1	1

patients who have died of the syndrome, peptic ulcer was responsible for 16 and hypoglycaemia for 6. However a patient with a Zollinger-Ellison syndrome and hyperparathyroidism should have the latter treated first; this reduces the excess gastrin secretion and relieves the symptoms in some cases (Turbey & Passaro 1972).

Hypercalcaemia in the Zollinger-Ellison syndrome is not necessarily due to hyperparathyroidism as in some cases it is relieved by removing the pancreatic tumour (Sircus et al 1970).

In multiple endocrine neoplasia type 2 (formerly Sipple's syndrome), hyperparathyroidism may be part of a familial syndrome of which the other components are phaeochromocytoma, medullary cell carcinoma of thyroid, neurofibromatosis and, less commonly, Cushing's syndrome (Paloyan et al 1970, Kaplan et al 1970, Keynes & Till 1971, MacGillivray & Anderson 1971, Keiser et al 1973). This disorder appears to be quite distinct from multiple endocrine neoplasia type 1, and as in the latter, the hyperparathyroidism is seldom severe. The usual histological change is chief-cell hyperplasia and it is not yet clear whether the hyperparathyroidism associated with this syndrome is a part of the disorder or is secondary to high circulating concentrations of calcitonin from the medullary cell carcinoma or from elsewhere. There is a single report of a patient with a parathyroid adenoma and phaeochromocytoma but without a thyroid carcinoma (Keene & Correa 1971).

Hypercalcaemia may be found in familial phaeochromocytoma without evidence of parathyroid overactivity, and may be relieved by adrenalectomy (Swinton et al 1972).

Malignant neoplasms

In patients with parathyroid adenomas there appears to be an increased incidence of malignant neoplasms, especially those of the thyroid, gastro-intestinal tract, genito-urinary tract and the breast (Kaplan et al 1971).

Asthma

There is a suggestion of an association between asthma and hyperparathyroidism. Relief of the hyperparathyroidism may lead to an improvement in the asthma (Åberg et al 1972a).

Cerebrovascular disease

Strokes occur in elderly patients with hyperparathyroidism but it is not yet clear whether the two disorders are causally related or coincidental (Boström & Alveryd 1972). Hypertension (p. 92) could be a factor.

Diabetes mellitus

A possible association between hyperparathyroidism and diabetes mellitus is suggested by a 54% incidence of diabetes in one series of 31 patients with hyperparathyroidism (Irvin et al 1972).

Gallstones

An increased incidence of gallstones among patients with hyperparathyroidism has been suggested by Selle et al (1972).

CLINICAL CHEMISTRY

The principal chemical changes include a raised serum calcium in almost all patients at some time, a low serum inorganic phosphorus in many and, in a minority, an increased serum activity of alkaline phosphatase. In addition many patients have a mild metabolic acidosis and there are often changes detectable in the renal tubular handling of calcium and phosphorus.

Blood chemistry

Calcium An abnormal serum calcium is the most valuable single clue to the presence of hyperparathyroidism and is the result of (i) increased intestinal absorption of calcium (Avioli et al 1965), (ii) increased bone turnover, especially resorption (Harris & Heaney 1969 or 1970) and (iii) increased renal tubular reabsorption of calcium (Peacock et al 1969, Transbøl et al 1970a). These factors contribute in varying degrees to the hypercalcaemia of different cases.

The total serum calcium may be normal from time to time in some patients and the problems associated with the very small number of patients with prolonged periods of normocalcaemia are discussed later (p. 101). In addition there appears to be an excessive day-to-day variation in serum calcium values in patients with hyperparathyroidism (Drach & King 1970). For these reasons the serum calcium should be estimated on several occasions in patients in whom hyper-parathyroidism is suspected. Many patients with undoubted hyper-parathyroidism have serum calcium results which are only very slightly outwith with normal range (Hodgkinson & Edwards 1963, Parfitt et al 1964, Yendt & Gagné 1968). For this reason great care is needed both in the collection of samples and in the analyses (p. 36).

In view of this estimates of the serum ionised or ultrafiltrable calcium levels should have advantages over estimates of the serum total calcium in the diagnosis of hyperparathyroidism. Indeed a few patients with hyperparathyroidism have been described in whom the ionised but not the total serum calcium was increased (Fanconi & Rose 1958, Transbøl et al 1970a, Bergman & Hagberg 1972). This implies a change in the binding of calcium to protein, possibly as a result of the metabolic acidosis. Until recently the methods have been so difficult that they have been confined to a few centres. Even there the poor precision of the results compared with that for total calcium estimation meant there was little advantage in estimating ultra-filtrable or ionised calcium. However there have been recent advances in techniques and it is now clear that both ultrafiltrable and ionised calcium estimations are superior to estimations of total calcium in the diagnosis of hyperparathyroidism (Transbøl et al 1970b). Where possible these measurements should be made; the techniques still require experience and technical expertise and in their absence the mainstay of diagnosis will continue to be careful assays of serum total calcium interpreted in relation to the serum proteins (p. 37).

Inorganic phosphorus A low serum inorganic phosphorus is found in about half of the patients with primary hyperparathyroidism and in many of the rest the result is near the lower limit of the normal range (fig. 4.2, p. 65). The low serum phosphorus is the result of diminished tubular reabsorption of phosphate (see below). High normal or high values for serum phosphorus may be found in patients with severe renal impairment.

Alkaline phosphatase Increased activity of alkaline phosphatase in the serum is found in about 20% of patients with primary hyper-parathyroidism and correlates fairly well with radiological evidence of osteitis fibrosa (Dent & Harper 1962, Pyrah et al 1966, Epstein et al 1970).

Chloride and pH In 1964 Wills and McGowan noted that many

patients with hyperparathyroidism had a high serum chloride. Subsequent work has demonstrated that this is a feature of the mild metabolic acidosis which frequently accompanies hyperparathyroidism (p. 66). Provided that a patient has no other reason to have an acid-base disorder, estimation of the plasma chloride, or better the capillary blood pH, may make a valuable contribution to the differential diagnosis of hypercalcaemia (p. 66).

Magnesium A low serum magnesium is found in a minority of patients with hyperparathyroidism. Patients with the highest values of serum calcium are most likely to have this abnormality which is probably caused by renal losses of magnesium (Sutton 1970, King & Stanbury 1970).

Uric acid An increase in the serum uric acid is found in most patients with hyperparathyroidism and may lead to clinical gout. The abnormality is caused by increased reabsorption of uric acid in the renal tubule (Scott et al 1964, Jackson & Harris 1965).

Parathyroid hormone In the present state of techniques for the assay of plasma PTH an elevated value provides good evidence in favour of hyperparathyroidism while a normal value does not exclude it (p. 63). Plasma levels of PTH can be depressed by calcium infusion or increased by EDTA infusion in hyperparathyroidism caused both by hyperplasia and by adenoma. The hyperparathyroidism cannot therefore be regarded as autonomous (Murray et al 1972).

Urine chemistry and clearances
Urine calcium It has long been recognised that in hyperparathyroidism the urinary excretion of calcium is not increased as much as might be expected from the serum calcium. For example, of 49 patients reported by Transbøl et al (1970a), 25 had a calcium excretion of less than 7·5 mmol/day and 14 excreted less than 5 mmol/day. The mean for the whole group was 7·5 mmol/day compared with a mean of 13·4 mmol/day in a group of patients with hypercalcaemia of other causes. The difference between the two groups was significant but, in each, the range of results was very wide (fig. 5.4). Thus in a patient with hypercalcaemia a calcium excretion of less than 6 mmol/day provides some support for a diagnosis of hyperparathyroidism whereas a result greater than 6 mmol/day contributes nothing. Low calcium excretion is particularly found in patients with advanced renal damage (Hellström & Ivemark 1962).

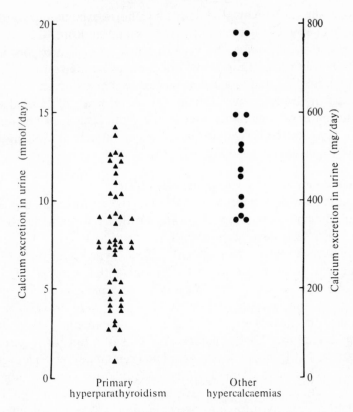

FIGURE 5.4. Urinary excretion of calcium in 49 patients with primary hyperparathyroidism (▲) and 16 patients with hypercalcaemia of other causes (●). Data of Transbøl et al (1970a).

Indices of the tubular handling of calcium have provided a more precise method for using these differences in diagnosis. These are described on pages 49 and 67.

Urine phosphorus In hyperparathyroidism most patients have evidence of decreased tubular reabsorption of phosphorus which is best demonstrated by determining the ratio TmP/GFR (p. 50). The daily excretion of phosphorus depends on the diet and is not usually changed in hyperparathyroidism because a new steady state is reached with a lower serum phosphorus value. In a few patients the daily phosphorus excretion is increased because of bone destruction but this increase is very small compared with the total. For these reasons measurement of daily phosphorus excretion has nothing to contribute to the diagnosis of hyperparathyroidism.

Urine hydroxyproline The urinary excretion of hydroxyproline is generally abnormal in the patients who have an elevated serum alkaline phosphatase and radiological evidence of bone disease. However increased hydroxyproline excretion in the absence of bone disease and normal excretion in its presence have both been described (Smith 1967). It is doubtful whether this investigation contributes anything to the diagnosis of hyperparathyroidism.

Special chemical tests for hyperparathyroidism

The patients with a marginal elevation of the serum calcium present special difficulties in diagnosis and for this reason a number of provocative tests have been devised.

Calcium infusion test In normal subjects hypercalcaemia induced by calcium infusion causes an inhibition of the secretion of parathyroid hormone (PTH) and thus a fall in phosphate excretion by the kidney. In hyperparathyroidism PTH secretion is probably autonomous and calcium infusion causes a much smaller fall in phosphorus excretion. This has formed the basis of a test for hyperparathyroidism but in many series there has been an appreciable overlap between the results from hyperparathyroid and control subjects. Recently Pak et al (1972a) have re-examined this test and have obtained a very encouraging discrimination between their controls and their patients (half of whom had normal or marginal serum calcium results). They felt that changes in phosphorus excretion during the first 12 hours after infusion might be affected by factors other than parathyroid hormone secretion and demonstrated that good discrimination was obtained by comparing the second 12 hour period with the corresponding period on a previous control day. This revised test appears to be very promising and merits further assessment.

Phosphorus deprivation tests Phosphorus deprivation tests are used in the hope of making the chemical abnormalities of hyperparathyroidism more apparent. In particular it is claimed that phosphorus deprivation, with a low phosphorus diet and administration of aluminium hydroxide, causes unequivocal hypercalcaemia in patients with hyperparathyroidism. This appears to be true of some patients (Eisenberg 1968) but the specificity of the test is not yet clear.

In a refinement of this test, Adams et al (1970b) used four days of phosphorus deprivation followed by four days in which a thiazide diuretic is given in addition. This modified test produced unequivocal hypercalcaemia in some patients who were later found to have abnormal parathyroid glands. These studies must be interpreted with some caution as all those patients initially had serum calcium values which were outside a conventional normal range. In addition the specificity of these changes in serum calcium is not yet proved. The test may have a place in the diagnosis of patients with marginal serum calcium results.

The venous compression test Krull et al (1969) claimed that venous compression of the arm with rhythmic fist clenching produced a much greater rise in the local serum calcium in hyperparathyroidism than in normal controls or patients with hypercalcaemia of other causes. Unfortunately these results have not been confirmed by other workers (Greig et al 1970, Buxton et al 1970).

The hydrocortisone suppression test for distinguishing hyperparathyroidism from hypercalcaemia of other causes is described on page 63.

Normocalcaemic Primary Hyperparathyroidism

The diagnosis of primary hyperparathyroidism classically depends on the demonstration of a high serum calcium. However during the past twenty years there have been case reports of patients, especially those with parathyroid hyperplasia, with a normal serum calcium and in recent series as many as 20% of hyperparathyroid patients have been normocalcaemic (Grimelius et al 1973). The subject has been well reviewed by Wills (1971a). Some of the case reports represent patients in whom the serum calcium was elevated only intermittently (Johnson & Conn 1969) and other reports result from a misunderstanding of the normal range for serum calcium. However there remain a few cases of undoubted normocalcaemic hyperparathyroidism including some with osteitis fibrosa (Frame et al 1970, Heath & Wills 1971).

The factors which contribute to a lack of hypercalcaemia are not known for every case but a few are patients who also had vitamin D deficiency. Thus two normocalcaemic patients of Woodhouse et al (1971b) and one hypocalcaemic patient of Keynes and Caird (1970) only developed hypercalcaemia after treatment with vitamin D. While it is possible that these patients could really be patients with 'tertiary hyperparathyroidism', it is also possible that in the presence of vitamin D deficiency parathyroid hormone is ineffective because it cannot promote the production of 1,25-dihydroxycholecalciferol by the kidney (p. 25).

MANAGEMENT

Hitherto it has been orthodox teaching that all patients with primary hyperparathyroidism should be treated surgically in the first instance. Thus 'because of the risk of progressive renal damage, operation should not be delayed once the diagnosis has been made' (Fourman & Royer, 1968). In view of the greatly increased number of patients discovered as a result of multiphasic screening, many of them symptomless, this view is beginning to be questioned (Bakke 1970, Gough et al 1971, Harrison 1973). The operation is not without risk and we know very little of the natural history of untreated mild hyperparathyroidism. Purnell et al (1971) have undertaken a prospective study of this problem. Their early results indicated that most of the symptomless patients, with a serum calcium less than 2·75 mmol/l (11 mg/100 ml) and no demonstrable bone or renal disease, did well without surgery.

The best advice which can be given at present is probably as follows: patients should be treated surgically if they have a marked increase in the serum calcium (more than 2·75 mmol/l) or have evidence of bone disease, renal impairment, renal stones or gastrointestinal complications, or if for any reason regular follow-up is likely to be difficult. Other patients may be followed without surgery but with regular determinations of their serum chemistry and renal function. In this group surgery would be reserved for the patients with evidence of deterioration.

Preoperative measures

Some patients may be dehydrated as a result of polyuria or vomiting; this should be corrected before operation. Patients with severe hypercalcaemia may need urgent reduction of the serum calcium with phosphate. Laryngoscopy to check for the function of the recurrent laryngeal nerves is worthwhile in patients who have had previous neck surgery. The anaesthetist should be aware of the danger of cardiac arhythmias in hypercalcaemic patients particularly any who are also on digitalis (Smith & Petruscak 1972).

Localisation of the parathyroid tumour Occasionally the adenoma may be felt in the neck but even in patients with hyperparathyroidism a palpable lump is more likely to be a thyroid nodule than a para-thyroid adenoma (Wang et al 1970). An exception is parathyroid carcinoma (p. 111) which is often palpable. Parathyroid adenomas are sometimes calcifed (Arnstein et al 1971, Polga & Balikian 1971) and some adenomas may cause deformity in a barium swallow (Clark & Taylor 1972). Mediastinal parathyroid tumours are occasionally visible on a chest radiograph (Salgado et al 1971).

A variety of special methods have been proposed for the localisation of abnormal parathyroids. Arteriography of the thyro-cervical trunk has been helpful in some cases (Safrit et al 1970, McGarity et al 1971, Rossi et al 1971). The presence of a tumour is indicated more often by displacement of the inferior thyroid artery, or a branch, than by a tumour blush. This test is of limited value and should only be undertaken by experienced operators as there is some danger to the cerebral circulation (Irvin et al 1972, Dubost 1973).

Methionine labelled with 75-selenium (a γ-emitter) is taken up by cells involved in protein synthesis. This includes the thyroid and parathyroid. If the thyroid has been suppressed, the scan can be used to localise an overactive parathyroid (Potchen et al 1967). In practice this test has not proved as valuable as had been hoped (Keeling & Todd-Pokropek 1969, Di Giulio & Morales 1969). Recently thermo-graphy has given encouraging results in a few patients (Samuels et al 1972).

In vivo staining of the parathyroid glands with toluidine blue dye has been advocated for assisting the surgeon at the time of operation (Di Giulio & Lindenauer 1970, Singleton & Allums 1970, Skjoldborg & Nielsen 1971). This substance is, however, rather toxic and the staining of the glands is often inconsistent (Ackerman & Winer 1971). Methylene blue has also been used; it may be less toxic (Dudley 1971).

Perhaps the most promising technique is measurement of serum parathyroid hormone levels in blood obtained by selective venous catherisation (Davies et al 1973b, Wells et al 1973). This technique is difficult and is likely to be limited to a few centres for some time, but for patients with a previous unsuccessful neck exploration this may have great advantages.

Operative procedure

Details of the operative procedure are given by Keynes (1961), Gordan and Goldman (1970), Blalock (1971), Romanus et al (1973) and Adie and Taylor (1973). It is important that a search should be made for all four glands even though on occasion there may be more or less than four. Facilities for frozen section examination are very important for identifying parathyroid tissue, but are of limited value for distinguishing between adenoma and hyperplasia. The finding of one adenoma is not an indication for stopping the dissection; all four glands should be identified. Adenomas may be multiple or a patient may have both an adenoma in one gland and hyperplasia in others (Rubens et al 1969, Haff et al 1970, Kramer 1970). In addition it is difficult to distinguish adenoma from primary chief-cell hyperplasia in a single gland. If four glands cannot be found Haff and colleagues recommend a subtotal thyroidectomy and removal of the cervical and upper mediastinal fat pads.

Mediastinal parathyroid adenomas are found in from 1% to 4% of the patients and some of these can be removed through the cervical incision, especially if a vascular pedicle running into the mediastinum is seen. A formal sternum-splitting operation is usually done separately after the patient has been re-admitted and the diagnosis of continuing hyperparathyroidism confirmed (Black 1971b).

Very occasionally a parathyroid adenoma may be found within the thyroid gland (Vellar et al 1973).

Postoperative care

The general management is similar to that appropriate after thyroidectomy. There should be a careful watch for hypocalcaemia and in a few cases there is transient or permanent hypoparathyroidism. This may be suggested clinically by the onset of depression. True permanent hypoparathyroidism will be an indication for long-term treatment with vitamin D but more patients have a temporary hypoparathyroidism and the diagnosis should be reviewed after a few months. If possible the dose of vitamin D should be reduced progressively and the patient carefully followed without treatment.

If patients with bone disease, usually those with an elevated serum alkaline phosphatase activity preoperatively, much more severe symptoms may develop. Hypocalcaemia occurs early in the post-operative period with tetany and sometimes severe psychiatric disturbance (Vincent et al 1962). It is ascribed to the avidity of the healing bones for calcium, the 'hungry bone syndrome'. In severe cases tetany may lead on to convulsions and fractures (Davies & Friedman 1966). Substantial amounts of calcium orally or intravenously may be needed and oral calcium supplements should be continued for several months. Patients whose hypocalcaemia persists for more than two weeks should also receive vitamin D or dihydrotachysterol for a short period (Dent 1962). Purnell et al (1971) have suggested that, in future, serum parathyroid hormone levels will be of value in distinguishing hypocalcaemia due to hungry bones from that due to hypoparathyroidism.

It is possible that magnesium deficiency contributes to the post-operative symptoms in some patients with bone disease (King & Stanbury 1970). It is reasonable to give short-term magnesium supplements to any patient with hypomagnesaemia.

Prognosis after surgery
The majority of patients become normocalcaemic after surgery; the incidence of 'failed' operations (with persistent or recurrent hypercalcaemia) varies between 1 in 4 and 1 in 15 in different series (Clark & Taylor 1972). In most of these patients further surgery reveals persisting parathyroid tissue in the neck or mediastinum and it is this group in which techniques for localisation of the tumour are particularly indicated. Rare causes of recurrent hypercalcaemia are active metastases from a parathyroid carcinoma (Melvin & Castleman 1971) and coincidental vitamin D intoxication (Haff & Ballinger 1971).

The main motive for surgery is the prevention of continuing renal impairment due to nephrocalcinosis. Studies of the renal function after surgery have not demonstrated marked improvements: in the majority of the patients of Purnell et al (1971) there was no change in creatinine clearance. In the series of Ohlsson (1970) of 73 patients followed for three to nine years after surgery there was, overall, a modest improvement in inulin clearance both in those with and those without abnormal values preoperatively (table 5.4). Continuing deterioration in glomerular filtration rate is found in a few patients

(Purnell et al 1971, Britton et al 1971). Of 21 patients with treated hyperparathyroidism who died subsequently, the cause of death was renal failure in no less than eleven (Hellström et al 1958). This deterioration may be due to recurring urinary tract infection or to continuing hypertension. After surgery renal stones already present diminish in number and new stone formation is almost prevented. The renal concentrating power also improves in most patients although half have some persisting impairment (Ohlsson 1970).

TABLE 5.4. Inulin clearance before operation and at least two years after parathyroidectomy in 73 patients with primary hyperparathyroidism (data of Ohlsson (1970) reproduced by permission).

Preoperative inulin clearance (ml/min)	Number of patients	Average preoperative inulin clearance (ml/min)	Average increase in clearance (ml/min)
16–40	9	29	7
41–60	13	52	2
61–80	24	72	5
more than 80	27	93	6

Of the other clinical consequences of hyperparathyroidism, hypertension is relieved in about half of the patients affected but some 20% of patients may first develop hypertension postoperatively (Hellström et al 1958). In some but not all patients with peptic ulcers parathyroidectomy appears to lead to an improvement in the ulcer (Pyrah et al 1966).

Patients with a good response to surgery should be followed up for an appreciable period: perhaps five years. This will detect recurrent hyperparathyroidism and also provide an opportunity to review renal function and check for urinary infection and hypertension.

Medical management

In most series there are a few patients who have persistent hyperparathyroidism after adequate and sometimes repeated surgery. In addition there are a few patients who refuse surgery. Both groups should be treated medically and oral phosphate is probably the treatment of choice (p. 71). Dent (1962) has described a patient with hyperparathyroidism and bone disease whose symptoms and bio-chemical abnormalities improved markedly on disodium hydrogen phosphate in a dose of 10–15 g (equivalent to 2·2–3·2 g elemental phosphorus) daily. Details of this treatment and of other methods for the management of hypercalcaemia are given in the preceding chapter.

SPECIAL FORMS OF HYPERPARATHYROIDISM

ACUTE HYPERPARATHYROIDISM

Acute hyperparathyroidism, sometimes called parathyroid intoxica-tion, in an uncommon but dangerous emergency (Breidahl & Hamilton 1970, Kaminski & Willman 1972, Johansson et al 1973). The attack is sometimes precipitated by minor surgery and may first be detected in a patient with an unexpectedly stormy postoperative course after any type of surgery (Heimann & Nilsson 1970). Because of this a patient who has hyperparathyroidism but also requires surgery for something else, such as a renal stone, should ordinarily have the parathyroidectomy first.

The symptoms of acute hyperparathyroidism result from the very high and usually rising plasma calcium. Patients are severely ill and complain of muscular weakness, nausea, vomiting, fatigue and abdominal pain. Some patients are admitted in a coma and high fever may be found in some. Table 5.5 shows the main symptoms in 65 reported cases. It is seen that, in these patients, symptoms related to the bones or the urinary tract are seen much less often than non-specific symptoms.

The main physical signs include dehydration, hypotonia, hyper-tension, tachycardia and fever. An unusually high proportion of these patients have a palpable neck mass (20 out of 65). Pancreatitis is a fairly common complication of acute hyperparathyroidism and may be the presenting feature. Renal vein thrombosis may occur (Pringle & Smith 1964). In patients who die calcification is found in many tissues including the myocardium, heart valves, lungs and kidneys (Thomas et al 1958a).

The condition is rapidly fatal if untreated but among patients who have early surgery 80% survive. The patients should be rehydrated and the plasma calcium level should be brought down before urgent surgery is undertaken. Intravenous phosphate (p. 72) is probably the treatment of choice provided that its dangers are recognised and the patient is carefully monitored (Fulmer et al 1972).

TABLE 5.5. Principal symptoms in 65 reported patients with acute hyperparathyroidism (Lemann & Donatelli 1964, Pringle & Smith 1964, Payne & Fitchett 1965, Chodack et al 1965, Clunie et al 1967, Breidahl & Hamilton 1970, Heimann & Nilsson 1970).

Symptom	Number of cases
Nausea and vomiting	48
Muscular weakness	43
Fatigue and lethargy	38
Weight loss	34
Confusion	31
Bone pain	28
Abdominal pain	26
Polyuria	23
Constipation	21
Polydipsia	13
Coma	12
Renal colic	12

HYPERPARATHYROIDISM IN PREGNANCY

Among reported cases of hyperparathyroidism in pregnancy there is a 50% incidence of abortion, stillbirth, neonatal death or other problems in the infant (Ludwig 1962, Johnstone et al 1972). Hyperparathyroidism may reveal itself in pregnancy, either because of the maternal symptoms (which are not masked by the pregnancy), or by the detection of hypocalcaemia in the infant (Hartenstein & Gardener 1966, Ertel et al 1969, Bronsky et al 1970). In the mother the usual history of renal stones, polydipsia or bone pain is found in some cases and in one case the diagnosis was made because of an attack of acute pancreatitis six hours postpartum. In the majority of cases however, the mother has no clear symptoms and the disorder is detected because of tetany or convulsions in the infant who is found to have hypocalcaemia, hyperphosphataemia and sometimes hypo-magnesaemia. In most cases the hypocalcaemia in the infant improves after a few days; in a few there is permanent hypoparathyroidism. The symptoms may be made worse or be detected for the first time when the feeds are changed to cow's milk which has a phosphate content substantially higher than that in human milk. It seems likely that the disorder in the infants is caused by the excessive plasma calcium in the mother, rather than by the excessive circulating para-thyroid hormone (Fairney & Weir 1970).

Treatment If hyperparathyroidism is detected during the preg-nancy, parathyroid surgery should not be deferred. The hypocalcae-mia in the infant is relieved with calcium and a low phosphate feed, for a few days or weeks. In infants with permanent hypopara-thyroidism vitamin D will be needed.

PRIMARY HYPERPARATHYROIDISM IN INFANTS AND CHILDREN

Hyperparathyroidism, usually the result of primary hyperplasia, has been described in young infants and may be familial (Mühlethaler et al 1967, Goldbloom et al 1972). The patients may present with hypotonia (curiously with brisk reflexes), poor feeding, constipation and respiratory problems. Some cases have been discovered at autopsy in infants who have died suddenly. Most patients have had severe hypercalcaemia (one surviving patient had a serum calcium of 6·75 mmol/l) and most also had serum phosphate values below the normal range for their age. Many of the patients had marked de-mineralisation of the skeleton; some also had pathological fractures or subperiosteal erosions and appearances similar to those of rickets have been found (Fretheim & Gardborg 1965). Early diagnosis and surgery offers the only chance of survival. Parathyroid hyperplasia has also been described in newborn infants of mothers with hypo-parathyroidism (Landing & Kamoshita 1970) but few had hyper-calcaemia; the disorder should perhaps be regarded as a form of secondary hyperparathyroidism. It resolves spontaneously in the patients who survive.

Primary hyperparathyroidism is recognised in older children whose symptoms, like those in adults, may be very vague and non-specific.

Both boys and girls may be affected and most have a parathyroid adenoma rather than hyperplasia. Bone disease appears to be more common than renal lithiasis at this age (Bjernulf et al 1970). Radiological appearances of the bone may resemble those of late rickets but patches of osteosclerosis are sometimes seen (Rajasuriya et al 1964, Lloyd et al 1965, Lomnitz et al 1966).

SECONDARY HYPERPARATHYROIDISM

The parathyroid glands respond to hypocalcaemia of any cause and evidence of secondary hyperparathyroidism is found in many patients with rickets, osteomalacia or renal failure and in chronic fluoride poisoning (Teotia & Teotia 1973). These patients have low or normal values for the serum calcium. There may be radiological evidence of parathyroid overactivity, especially subperiosteal erosions, but giant-cell tumours are rare. Bone histology demonstrates hyperparathyroid changes more frequently and also reflects the underlying disorder. The parathyroid glands are similar in microscopical and ultrastructural appearances to those of primary chief-cell hyperplasia, but the cells are more uniform (Altenähr 1972). Oxyphil cells are found especially in the hyperplasia of renal failure (Christie 1967). Recently good evidence has been obtained of the high plasma content of immunoreactive parathyroid hormone in rickets and in renal osteodystrophy.

In general the condition remits when the primary disorder is treated; the special problems in the management of the bone disease of renal failure are discussed in chapter 11.

TERTIARY HYPERPARATHYROIDISM

The term tertiary hyperparathyroidism was suggested by St. Goar in 1962 to describe patients with secondary hyperparathyroidism who develop an autonomous parathyroid adenoma. The condition usually follows secondary hyperparathyroidism due to malabsorption or renal failure (Davies et al 1968) and is characterised by hypercalcaemia. The other chemical tests reflect the underlying disorder and bone biopsy may provide evidence of this too with, for example, osteoid seams wider than would be expected with hyperparathyroidism alone. Tertiary hyperparathyroidism does not respond to treatment of the underlying disorder; indeed hypercalcaemia may first become evident while osteomalacia is being treated with vitamin D. Where possible the condition should be treated by parathyroidectomy. Tertiary hyperparathyroidism is an increasing problem in patients with renal failure treated with regular dialysis (chapter 11).

PARATHYROID CARCINOMA

Carcinoma is the cause of hyperparathyroidism in between 0·5% and 3% of the cases in different series (Pyrah et al 1966). Although it is likely that there are a few parathyroid carcinomas which do not cause hyperparathyroidism, the great majority are functional and present with hyperparathyroidism (Holmes et al 1969, Schanz & Castleman 1973, Murie et al 1973).

The diagnosis of parathyroid carcinoma may be suggested preoperatively by the finding of a cervical mass which is present in 30%–50% of cases. Unexplained unilateral vocal cord paralysis accompanying hypercalcaemia also suggests the diagnosis. Hypercalcaemia recurring more than three months after the removal of an 'adenoma' may be due to carcinoma, as multiple adenomas usually cause persistent rather than recurrent hypercalcaemia. In patients with carcinoma the hypercalcaemia is often severe with marked general symptoms. Bone disease, often with bone pain, was present in 40 of the 54 patients reviewed by Gale and Owens 1972.

At operation the surgeon should be suspicious of a tumour which is unusually large or hard or is accompanied by a fibrous reaction. Because of the fibrous reaction carcinomas are often greyish white in colour unlike other parathyroid tumours. Histologically they are difficult to identify with confidence. Unless there is obvious infiltration into adjacent tissues or frequent mitoses, parathyroid carcinoma can resemble a benign adenoma. In an adenoma there may be variations in nuclear size and shape and even tumour cells lying within blood vessels so that these features by themselves do not justify the diagnosis of carcinoma. The carcinoma often has more dense fibrous tissue both around it and within it but this too is not diagnostic. For these reasons the differentiation between adenoma and carcinoma by frozen section can be very unreliable. It is possible that electron microscopy has a place in the identification of carcinoma (Faccini 1970).

The tumours in these patients grow slowly, spreading by local invasion and metastasising relatively late. Metastases are found most commonly in the cervical lymph nodes, the lung and more rarely in liver, bone, pancreas and adrenals. There is a propensity for local implantation at an operation site. Death is more often due to hyperparathyroidism (pancreatitis, renal damage or intractable hypercalcaemia) than to the spread of the tumour (Holmes et al 1969, Walls et al 1972). The five year survival is about 50% and the ten year survival about 13%.

Wide resection of the tumour is the most valuable form of treatment. This may entail removal of the adjacent thyroid, and any skeletal muscle related to the tumour. A recurrent laryngeal nerve may have to be sacrificed and a dissection of the lymph nodes on the same side is indicated. If the hyperparathyroidism recurs, repeated resections may be valuable and the removal of a functioning metastasis has been helpful on occasion (Davies et al 1973a). Radiotherapy does not contribute much even to the palliative managment of the tumour. In patients with intractable hypercalcaemia useful relief may be had with oral phosphate. If this fails mithramycin should be used; this drug is very effective in reducing the serum calcium to normal and acts directly on the bone resorption rather than on the tumour (Singer et al 1970, Melvin & Castleman 1971). In a single case where mithramycin, too, failed, stilboestrol diphosphate was effective (Sigurdsson et al 1973).

PSEUDOHYPERPARATHYROIDISM

Pseudohyperparathyroidism is a term introduced to describe patients with the chemical and often clinical features of hyperparathyroidism associated with a tumour without metastases to bone. This interesting condition is considered more fully in chapter 6.

HYPO-HYPERPARATHYROIDISM

This term was applied by Costello and Dent (1963) to a patient with hypocalcaemia and radiological evidence of osteitis fibrosa. This rare disorder is described on page 164.

Chapter 6: Other Causes of Hypercalcaemia

HYPERCALCAEMIA IN MALIGNANT DISEASE

Malignant disease is one of the most important causes of hyper-calcaemia, and about ten percent of patients with neoplasia experi-ence hypercalcaemia at some time in their illness. In most patients the hypercalcaemia is associated with osteolytic metastases. In a smaller number the tumour produces a substance with parathyroid hormone-like activity (pseudo-hyperparathyroidism). In a few patients the hypercalcaemia has a cause unrelated to the malignancy, as in the instances of primary hyperparathyroidism reported in patients with carcinomas of the breast and other tissues (Katz et al 1970, Kaplan et al 1971).

In a patient with malignant disease, hypercalcaemia may be the cause of the presenting symptoms. In the more advanced case the symptoms of hypercalcaemia can dominate the clinical picture. Un-treated hypercalcaemia may be the cause of death in a patient whose malignancy is not particularly advanced. In such patients it is im-portant to recognise and treat the hypercalcaemia (p. 71) but in patients with advanced or terminal carcinoma, the ethics of treating the hypercalcaemia are debatable (Freedman & Jurkowitz 1971). The general subject of calcium metabolism and hypercalcaemia in malig-nant disease has been reviewed by Szymendera (1970), Muggia and Heinemann (1970a) and Kessinger et al (1972).

HYPERCALCAEMIA ASSOCIATED WITH BONE METASTASES

Most patients with radiological evidence of skeletal metastases have hypercalciuria but relatively few have hypercalcaemia. There is poor correlation between the apparent extent of the metastatic neoplasm and the severity of the distrubance in calcium metabolism (Galasko & Burn 1971).

The clinical features of patients who do become hypercalcaemic are those of the hypercalcaemia as well as those of the underlying disease (Warwick et al 1961). The acute onset of hypercalcaemia in a patient who was previously well should raise the suspicion of an occult neoplasm. Bone pain and local bone tenderness are often, but not always, found in these patients and a sudden increase in bone pain is sometimes associated with the onset of hypercalcaemia. In patients with breast cancer hypercalcaemia is sometimes precipitated by the administration of hormones or by oophorectomy (Kessinger et al 1972).

Any degree of hypercalcaemia can be produced by metastatic carcinoma; it is usually associated with marked hypercalciuria. The serum alkaline phosphatase activity is often increased; this is probably a measure of the increased osteoblastic activity associated with many metastases even though osteosclerosis is not radiologically evident. The serum phosphorus is usually normal. In a patient with bone metastases and hypercalcaemia further investigation may be needed to locate the primary neoplasm; the most likely primary tumours are carcinomas of the breast, kidney and lung. Myeloma and leukaemia (see below) enter into the differential diagnosis of osteolytic lesions. Metastases with radiologically obvious osteosclerosis are particularly found with carcinomas of the prostate and breast; they are seldom associated with hypercalcaemia. Bone metastases are frequently found with thyroid carcinoma but seldom cause hypercalcaemia, perhaps because they are slow-growing.

Pathophysiology
The excess calcium in the plasma and urine is derived from the bone and not the diet (Baker 1956, Lee & Lloyd 1971). The metastases themselves are probably the most important factor in this osteolysis but in some patients with breast cancer an osteolytic sterol, produced by the tumour cells, may contribute (Gordan et al 1966, Day et al 1969). Renal retention of calcium may be a factor in some cases. A long period of hypercalciuria could contribute to renal damage which in turn reduces the renal clearance of calcium.

MULTIPLE MYELOMA (PLASMACYTOMA)

Hypercalcaemia is frequently noted in patients with myeloma. At one time it was suggested that an important factor in the increased total serum calcium was increased calcium binding ability of the plasma proteins. Present evidence indicates that although calcium-binding varies more widely in myeloma than in normal subjects, it is seldom greatly increased. The paraproteins have little calcium-binding ability and in many patients the concentration of the other plasma proteins is reduced.

While there are a few patients with a high total serum calcium due to increased calcium binding, in most cases the main factor in the hypercalcaemia is the increased bone dissolution (Szymendera 1970, Lindgärde & Zetterval 1973). The hypercalcaemia improves if the myeloma itself responds to appropriate treatment.

Leukaemia and Hodgkin's Disease

Hypercalcaemia is a rare complication of acute leukaemia (Butler 1970, Stein 1971), chronic myeloid leukaemia (Haskell et al 1971, Steinberg et al 1971) and chronic lymphocytic leukaemia (Galton et al 1970). In all the reported cases there has been evidence of excessive bone destruction; one case had widespread osteolytic lesions and severe hypercalcaemia at a time when the peripheral blood and the marrow were normal (Palva & Salokannel 1972).

Hypercalcaemia is described in Hodgkin's disease and other lymphomas. Most of these patients have evidence of skeletal metastases but a few did not and are likely to have been examples of pseudo-hyperparathyroidism (Plimpton & Gellhorn 1956, Moses & Spencer 1969).

Pseudohyperparathyroidism

Perhaps one fifth of patients with malignant disease and hypercalcaemia have no evidence of metastases in bone. Many of these patients also have a low serum inorganic phosphorus and this syndrome, first described in 1936, has been named pseudohyperparathyroidism or the ectopic PTH syndrome. It is likely that in these cases hypercalcaemia is caused by the elaboration by the tumour of a substance resembling parathyroid hormone (Lafferty 1966, Omenn et al 1969, Kessinger et al 1972).

Squamous cell carcinoma of the lung and carcinoma of the kidney are the most common causes of this syndrome. Rarer causes include oat-cell carcinoma of the lung, pancreatic carcinoma, colonic carcinoma, adrenal carcinoma, parotid carcinoma, hepatoma, reticulum cell sarcoma of spleen and retroperitoneal sarcoma. In these disorders a PTH-like peptide has been identified in the tissue (Kessinger et al 1972, Melick et al 1972). In other cases pseudohyperparathyroidism has been described but a PTH-like substance has not yet been identified: vaginal carcinoma (O'Neill & Mikuta 1970), bladder carcinoma (Svane 1964), gastric carcinoma (Wahl & Röher 1973), ovarian tumours (Rivett & Robinson 1972) and phaeochromocytoma (Swinton et al 1972).

It can be difficult in practice to distinguish between pseudohyperparathyroidism and primary hyperparathyroidism. The serum calcium and phosphorus are similar, the renal tubular handling of calcium is similar (Transbøl et al 1970a) and the bone histology is similar (Meunier et al 1972). There may be differences in the acid-base status in the two conditions (fig. 4.4 p. 67, Wills 1971b) and in the characteristics of the serum parathyroid hormone in radio-immuno-assay (Riggs et al 1971b). Despite these difficulties it is important to make the diagnosis of pseudohyperparathyroidism because it can be relieved by treatment of the tumour and because the tumour which presents in this way is often not disseminated.

While a substance resembling PTH or its prohormone is implicated in many patients with pseudohyperparathyroidism, other substances perhaps including prostaglandins are responsible for some cases (Tashjian et al 1972, Martin et al 1973, Powell et al 1973, Blair et al 1973, Singer et al 1973).

VITAMIN D POISONING

The subject of vitamin D poisoning in man has been well reviewed by Yendt (1970a) who also covered experimental studies in animals. At one time vitamin D was advocated in the management of a wide variety of conditions including rheumatoid arthritis, tuberculosis (especially lupus vulgaris), sarcoidosis, hay fever, asthma and chilblains. There is no evidence that vitamin D has any value in these disorders; this practice has now been abandoned but not before many cases of vitamin D poisoning had been described (Anning et al 1948).

Today vitamin D in large doses is used in the management of hypoparathyroidism and of phosphaturic rickets. In both conditions the control of vitamin D therapy presents problems because the requirements for vitamin D vary greatly, not only from patient to patient, but also in one patient from time to time. One factor contributing to this variability must be the storage of vitamin D within the body so that it acts as a cumulative poison. For example, after episodes of vitamin D poisoning two patients required smaller doses of vitamin D than before (Leeson & Fourman 1966a). Apart from this, vitamin D toxicity has seldom been described with doses of less than 1 mg (40,000 iu) per day.

Vitamin D poisoning is preventable. Patients should not be given pharmacological doses of vitamin D except for hypoparathyroidism, phosphaturic rickets and perhaps renal osteodystrophy. Even in these disorders, patients need careful follow-up with estimations of the serum calcium to prevent hypercalcaemia. The Sulkowitch test should not be used.

The use of vitamin D in public health also provides opportunites for poisoning to occur. In children it has proved difficult to find any level of vitamin D fortification of foods which will consistently prevent both rickets and hypercalcaemia in the community (Seelig 1969, 1970). Recent recommendations that vitamin D should be widely used in the prevention of age-related bone loss in adults could lead to a new increase in the incidence of vitamin D poisoning. These suggestions are based on a supposed contribution of vitamin D deficiency to the bone loss of aging. They fail to recognise that in adults as in children there are great variations in the sensitivity to vitamin D.

Clinical features

Symptoms of vitamin D poisoning have been noted as early as 12 days and as late as 6 years after the start of treatment. The symptoms are in general those of hypercalcaemia (chapter 4) and, unlike hyperparathyroidism, the hypercalcaemia is seldom symptomless.

With hypercalcaemia of other causes, vitamin D poisoning shares the early symptoms of fatigue, malaise, weakness, thirst and polyuria, anorexia, nausea and vomiting. Abdominal pain is particularly prominent in vitamin D poisoning and unlike other hypercalcaemias, diarrhoea often occurs (Chaplin et al 1951). Hypertension has been recorded in some cases (Debré 1948, Debré & Brissaud 1949). In a recent personal case a 74-year-old man who had extensive neck surgery developed vitamin D intoxication and, while hypercalcaemic, a major cerebrovascular accident. Debré (1948) reported two similar cases in children who, afterwards, had permanent mental impairment. While the possibility of coincidence cannot be excluded, these cases provide added reasons for trying to prevent vitamin D poisoning. A normochromic normocytic anaemia is sometimes seen; whether it is a consequence of the vitamin D poisoning or a result of the renal damage is not certain (Gabriel et al 1970).

The late symptoms of vitamin D poisoning include those due to metastatic calcification, nephrocalcinosis and renal failure (Harris 1969, Irnell 1969).

Clinical chemistry

The serum calcium is increased but the degree of hypercalcaemia is variable. All fractions are increased (Anning et al 1948). The hypercalcaemia is caused principally by increased intestinal absorption of calcium and by increased bone resorption (Yendt 1970a). Serum phosphorus levels are generally normal although low values are found occasionally (Howard & Meyer 1948, Lordon et al 1966) perhaps as a result of renal tubular damage; high values are associated with renal failure. Serum alkaline phosphatase activity is usually normal but sometimes low (Powell et al 1948). Despite the renal defects, many cases have a mild metabolic alkalosis with a high plasma bicarbonate and low plasma chloride (Transbøl et al 1970a, Wills 1971b). Less frequent chemical abnormalities include hypokalaemia due to renal tubular damage (Ferris et al 1961) and hypomagnesaemia (Leeson & Fourman 1966a).

The urinary excretion of calcium is almost always increased unless the renal damage is very advanced. One of the earliest signs of renal damage is failure of urinary concentration; this may be detected earlier than changes in the glomerular filtration rate.

Pathological changes

The pathological changes caused by vitamin D excess have been studied much more extensively in experimental animals than in man (Fourman & Royer 1968, Yendt 1970a). In man the principal finding is metastatic calcification which may be extensive or apparently confined to the kidney (Harris 1969, Yendt 1970a). In the bone the changes observed by Bauer and Freyberg (1946) have been interpreted as evidence of wide osteoid seams. In other cases however the bone histology has certainly been normal (Howard & Meyer 1948, Paterson et al 1972). Osteoid seams are found in bone from experimental animals given massive doses of vitamin D; there are also changes in the lipid content of bone which are prevented by the simultaneous administration of large doses of vitamin A (Cruess & Clark 1965, Yendt 1970a).

Radiology

In children dense metaphyseal lines not unlike those of lead poisoning may be found; those in the femoral neck are sometimes noted on a pyelogram done for obscure renal failure (Fanconi & de Chastonay 1950). Generalised osteosclerosis is occasionally found (De Wind 1961). Bone loss is a more difficult change to detect radiologically with confidence but is almost certainly present in severely affected patients with a negative calcium balance (Christensen et al 1951, Holman 1952).

Treatment and prognosis

Withdrawal of vitamin D results in an improvement in the symptoms within a few weeks but hypercalcaemia persisting as long as 14 months has been described (Howard & Meyer 1948). In order to limit the renal damage it is worth shortening the period of hypercalcaemia with phosphate or steroids (chapter 4).

If the disorder is recognised and treated early, renal function improves and may become normal. Metastatic calcification, including that in the eye, gradually resolves. In patients with hypoparathyroidism great caution is needed to prevent the recurrence of hypercalcaemia, even months later, when vitamin D or calcium supplements are started again (Spaulding & Yendt 1964, Leeson & Fourman 1966a).

SARCOIDOSIS

Hypercalcaemia was first noted in patients with sarcoidosis in 1939 by Harrell and Fisher. Even at that time there was a suggestion that the hypercalcaemia was related to an unusual sensitivity to vitamin D; one of their patients developed a serum calcium of 3·55 mmol/l (14·2 mg/100 ml) on a vitamin D intake of 1,000–2,000 units daily. The incidence of hypercalcaemia in sarcoidosis varies greatly between different series from 2%–20% of cases (Goldstein et al 1971); it is more common among patients with severe and widespread sarcoidosis.

In a patient with sarcoidosis other causes of hypercalcaemia should not be omitted from the differential diagnosis. The co-existence of sarcoidosis and hyperparathyroidism is well recognised and may be more than coincidental (Bresnihan 1971, Dawidson & Jameson 1972, Cushard et al 1972a, Åberg et al 1972b).

Pathophysiology

Balance studies have provided evidence of an excessive intestinal absorption of calcium in patients with sarcoid hypercalcaemia (Bell et al 1964). In addition some patients have evidence of increased bone resorption (Bell & Bartter 1967). In these respects the changes found in sarcoidosis resemble those of vitamin D poisoning and there is considerable evidence that some patients with sarcoidosis are intolerant of vitamin D. Even the dose of vitamin D provided by exposure to sunlight may precipitate hypercalcaemia in a patient with sarcoidosis (Scadding et al 1969). The same factor could explain the more frequent occurrence of hypercalcaemia in summer in some studies (Taylor et al 1963, Goldstein et al 1971).

Although only a small proportion of sarcoidosis patients have hypercalcaemia, a much larger proportion have changes in calcium metabolism, as demonstrated by hypercalciuira (Åberg et al 1972b). Furthermore many normocalcaemic patients with sarcoidosis have unmeasurably low concentrations of parathyroid hormone in their serum (Cushard et al 1972a).

Clinical features and investigations

The clinical features of the hypercalcaemia of sarcoidosis are the same as those of hypercalcaemia of other causes. The clinical chemistry is similar to that found in vitamin D intoxication. A minority of patients with sarcoidosis have radiological abnormalities in the bones. These affect particularly the phalanges of hands and feet but other bones may also be involved. The lesions consist of demineralisation with an accentrated trabecular pattern, or 'punched-out' cystic areas or, more rarely, osteosclerotic changes (Greenfield 1969 p. 71, Young & Laman 1972, Lin et al 1973).

Treatment

Hypercalcaemia occurring in a patient with sarcoidosis should be treated with steroids (Scadding 1967). In addition the patient should be advised to avoid undue exposure to sunlight or foods rich in vitamin D. It is difficult to know whether hypercalciuria in a normo-calcaemic patient should be treated but if this is severe or there is a history of renal calculi it would be reasonable to give oral phosphate therapy.

IDIOPATHIC HYPERCALCAEMIA OF INFANTS

This disorder was first described in Britain in 1952 (Lightwood 1952, Payne 1952). In subsequent years many more cases have been reported and two main forms of the disease have been delineated, although there were a few cases with intermediate features. Fraser et al (1966) and Mitchell (1967) have provided valuable reviews of the whole subject; the severe form has been reviewed by Dupont et al (1970).

Incidence

The mild form of infantile hypercalcaemia was found mainly in Great Britain. It was uncommon in the rest of Europe and seldom seen in North America. In Britain between 1953 and 1955 the reported incidence of both forms of infantile hypercalcaemia was 7·2 cases per month, approximately equivalent to one case for every 8,000 births; this was probably an underestimate (British Paediatric Association 1964). Most of these cases were of the mild type. The incidence of this form of hypercalcaemia has since fallen greatly; the reasons for this will be considered later.

The severe form of infantile hypercalcaemia is a very rare disorder which is not limited geographically; the incidence is probably about one case in 150,000 births (Fraser et al 1966). There is no sex pre-ponderance in either form.

Clinical features

Mild form (*Lightwood type*) The symptoms develop suddenly between three and seven months of age in a baby with a normal birth weight and normal progress up to that time. The main problems are anorexia, vomiting and constipation with a failure to thrive. As in other hypercalcaemic disorders, thirst and polyuria may be noted and dehydration is likely to occur. These infants have normal faces and few have cardiac abnormalities; perhaps 10% have systolic murmurs. Hypertension is not uncommon during the period of hypercalcaemia (Coleman 1965).

Severe form (*Fanconi–Schlesinger type*) These infants tend to have low birth-weights and in some the symptoms can be dated back to birth; in others they begin between the third and sixth month of life after a period of apparently normal development. As in the mild form the main symptoms are failure to thrive, with anorexia, vomiting and constipation. Polyuria is common and the child readily becomes dehydrated. In many cases of the severe type there is mental retardation, a characteristic facial appearance and remarkable abnormalities in the cardiovascular system, the bones and the teeth.

The 'elfin face' or 'pekinese face' of infantile hypercalcaemia has been recognised since the early cases (Joseph & Parrott 1958, Dupont et al 1970). In some an odd face has been noted since birth but in most patients it is only recognised after the onset of the hypercalcaemia. In infancy the main features are full sagging cheeks and flabby lips with a prominent upper lip like a 'Cupid's bow'. The forehead is prominent, the bridge of the nose is flat and the chin recedes. There are often epicanthic folds and sometimes a convergent squint. The ears are often pointed, prominent and low-set.

Patients with the severe form of infantile hypercalcaemia frequently have cardiovascular abnormalities. Most patients have a systolic murmur and many have hypertension. In some patients a murmur has been noted some months before the hypercalcaemia developed. The most common anomalies include supravalvular aortic or pulmonary stenosis, coarctation of the aorta and peripheral stenoses in systemic and pulmonary arteries. The electro-cardiogram reflects the ventricular hypertrophy appropriate to the lesion but also shows abnormalities of the T-waves which are broad with a flattened or notched summit (Coleman 1965). The ECG abnormalities persist longer than the hypercalcaemia itself.

Other abnormalities found in these patients include muscular hypotonia, with brisk reflexes and dental abnormalities, particularly absent or small teeth. All have permanent mental retardation but the degree of retardation varies from patient to patient.

Clinical chemistry

During the acute phase the serum calcium is raised to a variable extent, the severe cases having the highest values. Furthermore in a given patient the serum calcium fluctuates widely. Other chemical tests are generally normal apart from those reflecting the renal impairment which is common during the acute phase of the illness. In some patients an increase in serum α_2 globulin has been found (Creery & Neill 1954). A high serum cholesterol has been noted in some children (Forfar et al 1959).

An abnormality of calcium metabolism probably lasts longer than does the hypercalcaemia itself. Barr and Forfar (1969) found that an oral calcium-loading test was abnormal in patients with little or no hypercalcaemia. An abnormal response to an intravenous calcium load lasts even longer (Forbes et al 1972).

Radiology

Bone radiographs are usually normal in the mild form but a few cases have transverse bands of dense bone in the metaphysis similar to those seen in lead poisoning or vitamin D poisoning.

In the severe form there is usually more extensive osteosclerosis in the metaphyses and in the skull where craniosynostosis may occur. A thickening of the lamina dura has been noted and a few patients develop bowing of the long bones.

Pathology

Among patients with the mild form who die the main abnormalities are in the kidney, where there are deposits of calcium, particularly in the outer medulla in relation to the loops of Henle and the collecting ducts (Rhaney & Mitchell 1956).

In the severe form the renal calcification is more extensive and there may be granulomas in the medulla (Lowe et al 1954). The renal pathology of both forms resembles that of vitamin D poisoning (MacDonald 1958). Calcification in other tissues, especially the lungs, is also seen.

Other pathological findings are related to the cardiovascular disorders. In the heart ventricular hypertrophy, calcification of the atrioventricular valves or of the myocardium, and changes in the coronary arteries have been found (Rashkind et al 1961).

Natural history and prognosis

In the mild form a few patients die in the acute episode which untreated lasts from a few months to two years. The great majority survive with no mental or renal impairment, particularly if treated.

The severe form of infantile hypercalcaemia has a poor prognosis. One quarter of the patients die within the first three years, particularly of renal failure. All who survive have mental retardation and some are incapacitated by cardiovascular disorders or renal failure. The hypercalcaemia lasts for up to four years, but even without treatment the serum calcium eventually returns to normal. In the late normocalcaemic phase, the patient is mentally retarded and has persisting cardiovascular and dental abnormalities and radiologically may have areas of increased bone density. The elfin face develops with age in a characteristic manner (Dupont et al 1970). Recently many patients have been described in adolescence or adult life with mental retardation, typical vascular anomalies and an elfin face in whom the diagnosis of previous infantile hypercalcaemia seems reasonable (Warembourg et al 1972).

Treatment

Both forms of the disorder should be treated with a diet containing a minimum of vitamin D and calcium. In practice a low-calcium milk-substitute is available commercially (*Locasol*, Trufood Ltd.) and protein can also be provided from lean meat. Fruit and vegetables contain little calcium. In hard-water areas the use of distilled or deionised water is worthwhile. Vitamin D intake can be reduced further by avoiding exposure to sunlight. The policy of Fraser et al (1966) is to continue the regime for nine months after the serum calcium has become normal. Thereafter they allow a gradual increase in the dietary calcium and vitamin D and the exposure to sunlight, while carefully checking the serum calcium.

Corticosteroid therapy has occasionally been useful in the emergency treatment of acutely hypercalcaemic children and in the management of children whose hypercalcaemia does not respond to dietary measures. The value of long-term steroid therapy in children has to be weighed against its dangers. There are no reports of the use of phosphate in the management of infantile hypercalcaemia; perhaps it should be tried in patients who are difficult to control.

Pathogenesis

The syndrome of infantile hypercalcaemia probably includes several different disorders and it is useful at least to consider the mild form and severe form separately.

Mild form The pathogenesis of this disorder is controversial and most of the argument concerned the role of vitamin D (British Paediatric Association 1964, American Academy of Pediatrics 1967, Yendt 1970a). Infantile hypercalcaemia in the mild form was almost confined to countries where the vitamin D fortification was potentially excessive. It was common in Great Britain at a time when, for various reasons, the intake of vitamin D from all sources could be very large. Intakes exceeding 2,000 units daily were common and some infants had 35,000 units daily. Almost all the affected infants had been fed on cow's milk which has a much higher calcium content than human milk. Thus there was a suggestion that some children were particularly sensitive to a diet containing excessive calcium and vitamin D (although the amounts of vitamin D were not such as were previously thought to cause vitamin D poisoning). In 1957 the extent of vitamin D fortification of foods was substantially reduced and two or three years later the incidence of hypercalcaemia was found to have halved. Much has been made of this apparent delay, but several simple factors could explain it. The incidence of hypercalcaemia was compared with that reported in 1953–1955 when the disease, first identified in 1952, may not have been so readily recognised. In addition, the shelf lives of some of the heavily fortified dried milk preparations could have been longer than the British Paediatric Association anticipated. Thus the epidemiological evidence points to a relationship between hypercalcaemia and vitamin D excess.

Studies on individual patients have been less helpful, but certainly in some there was evidence of an abnormal sensitivity to vitamin D. The vitamin D content of blood and tissues has been measured in a few patients; in none were high values obtained. Taking both types of evidence together it seems very likely that most patients with mild infantile hypercalcaemia have an unusual sensitivity to calcium and vitamin D. The mechanism of this sensitivity may become clearer in the light of our new knowledge of vitamin D metabolism.

Severe form There is little information of value on the pathogenesis of this rare disorder. Epidemiological studies have contributed nothing. The disorder, or at least its physical stigmata, is often present at birth so that an intrauterine origin seems likely. The possibility that maternal overtreatment with vitamin D could contribute to the disorder has been extensively explored, but the evidence is inconclusive. An extreme sensitivity to vitamin D in early infancy is another possibility suggested by the similarity between the cardiovascular lesions and lesions which can be produced with high doses of vitamin D in animals (Seelig 1969). Severe hypercalcaemia has been described in twins, both identical and heterozygous, and in siblings (Manios & Antener 1966, Dupont et al 1970) so that an inborn error of metabolism is a possible explanation. Other possible factors include defects in tryptophane metabolism (Drummond et al 1964) and undiagnosed hyperparathyroidism (Rasmussen et al 1970).

UNCOMMON CAUSES OF HYPERCALCAEMIA

The Milk-Alkali Syndrome

Hypercalcaemia in association with alkali therapy for peptic ulcer was first described by Cope (1935). In 1949 a more severe syndrome including renal failure and ectopic calcification was described in the United States by Burnett et al and named the Milk-Alkali syndrome. In this hypercalcaemia and renal failure result from the excessive consumption of calcium (usually in milk) and alkalis by patients with peptic ulcer (McMillan & Freeman 1965). Cases have been reported in Britain; some were associated with the excessive use of calcium-containing antacids which are available without prescription. Examples of these are *Rennie's Tablets*, *Moorland Tablets* and *Bi-So-Dol* (Fourman & Royer 1968, Riley 1970, Malone & Horn 1971). The pathogenesis of the hypercalcaemia is not entirely clear. There is excessive absorption of calcium in the intestine and no commensurate increase in its excretion by the kidneys. Many patients have evidence of previous renal disease, and renal function is worsened both by the alkalosis and by the hypercalcaemia.

In the severe chronic cases described from the United States hypercalcaemia and renal failure are associated with osteosclerosis and metastatic calcification; these patients consumed as much as one gallon of milk daily. Cases without metastatic calcification are more common and may be associated with an equally severe acute renal failure. The patients have symptoms of hypercalcaemia, especially nausea and polyuria; they also have mental changes of lethargy and disorientation. The serum calcium is increased; the other biochemical abnormalities reflect the renal failure and the alkalosis. Unlike hyper-parathyroidism, the plasma phosphorus is increased but even so, the condition can be difficult to distinguish from hyperparathyroidism with renal failure. The finding of alkalosis (or a low plasma chloride) points towards the milk-alkali syndrome.

Withdrawal of the calcium and alkali leads to a rapid improvement in the hypercalcaemia and renal function. In patients with a short history normal renal function is sometimes regained.

IMMOBILISATION

An increase in bone loss and in urine calcium is commonly seen as a result of immobilisation in normal subjects. Hypercalcaemia itself is uncommon but does occur in patients who also have Paget's disease of bone or malignant disease and some normal adolescents immobilised for fractures (Morgan et al 1968, Hyman et al 1972, Lawrence et al 1973). A minor rise in the serum calcium is not uncommon in fracture patients and in immobilised normal subjects; this is seen more clearly with estimations of the serum ionised calcium (Heath et al 1972a).

THIAZIDE THERAPY

Thiazide diuretics reduce urinary calcium excretion but seldom cause hypercalcaemia except in patients with increased bone resorption. Thus thiazides may precipitate hypercalcaemia in hyperparathyroidism, in idiopathic juvenile osteoporosis, in uraemic osteodystrophy and in hypoparathyroidism treated with vitamin D (Parfitt 1972b, Brickman et al 1972a, Stote et al 1972, Wolf et al 1973).

TUBERCULOSIS

Hypercalcaemia is an unusual finding in tuberculosis and, as in sarcoidosis, appears to be related to an abnormal sensitivity to vitamin D. In the short-term this hypercalcaemia responds to steroids and is relieved by the treatment of the tuberculosis (Shai et al 1972, Sharma et al 1972).

Vitamin A Poisoning

Vitamin A poisoning in animals causes remarkable bone lesions with predominant bone resorption (Clark 1971, Gallina et al 1971, Matrajt-Denys et al 1971, Barnicot & Datta 1972). Bone abnormalities with increased resorption also occur in human vitamin A poisoning and hypercalcaemia has been described (Caffey 1951, Wieland et al 1971, Katz & Tzagournis 1972).

Rare Causes of Hypercalcaemia

Hypercalcaemia caused by increased intestinal absorption of calcium (idiopathic hyperabsorption hypercalcaemia) has been described by Hornum et al (1968). This may be the same disease as idiopathic hypercalciuria (p. 113) but why hypercalcaemia develops is not clear. Chronic beryllium poisoning is often included in lists of causes of hypercalcaemia. Beryllium poisoning is now very seldom seen and even when it was more common, hypercalcaemia was a very infrequent complication (Tepper et al 1961).

Hypercalcaemia has been described with ill-planned intravenous therapy especially in hyperalimentation (Ulstrom & Brown 1972).

A temporary hypercalcaemia of obscure aetiology has been described at the onset of the diuretic phase of acute renal failure from muscle-damage (Grünfeld et al 1972, Wu et al 1972). Hypercalcaemia occurs in a few patients with acromegaly but this is probably an instance of multiple endocrine neoplasia. Hyperthyroidism and adrenal insufficiency as causes of hypercalcaemia are considered in chapter 17.

Chapter 7: Renal Stones

Renal stones are important as a presenting feature of hyperpara-thyroidism and other hypercalcaemias, but these are by no means the only causes of stone formation in the upper urinary tract. This chapter considers our present knowledge of urolithiasis and outlines the further investigation and management of stone-formers. Renal stones have been the subject of four recent symposia (Smith 1968, Hodgkinson & Nordin 1969, Finlayson et al 1972, Delatte 1973) and several useful reviews (Yendt 1970b, Prien 1971, King 1971, Lavan et al 1971, Smith 1972).

Stone formation in the upper urinary tract must be distinguished from stone formation in the bladder. These bladder stones were once common in Europe and provided the livelihood of itinerant lithotomists in the middle ages. Soon after the beginning of the twentieth century, bladder stone became almost unknown in Northern Europe and North America, but it remains a common disorder, especially in boys, in developing countries. In one hospital in Thailand, for instance, 1113 bladder stones were removed from boys aged less than nine years of age in 1960, 1961 and 1962. In the same period one third of all boys admitted were admitted for stone. Although changes in nutrition must in some way have contributed to the disappearance of bladder stones in Northern Europe, the precise factors underlying these remarkable historical and geographical differences are unknown (Andersen 1969, Prien 1971). Stone formation in the upper urinary tract is the subject of the rest of this chapter. This is a disease which was almost unrecog-nised before 1900 and which is now one of the most common reasons for admission to surgical wards. The increase in incidence is probably real and not just the consequence of improvements in diagnosis (Andersen 1969).

CHEMICAL COMPOSITION OF STONES

The main chemical varieties of stones from the upper urinary tract are stones containing calcium, phosphate, oxalate, uric acid and cystine but other substances also contribute rarely to stone formation (table 7.1). It is seen that most stones contain a mixture of substances. Calcium

TABLE 7.1. Results of the analysis of 10,000 urinary stones (Herring 1962). These stones were sent for analysis to a private laboratory and 99% of the sample came from the United States. No examples of silica stones were seen in this series.

Component	Number of stones with the substance as	
	Sole component (100%)	Principal component (50–99%)
Calcium oxalate dihydrate (Weddellite)	547	3,547
Calcium oxalate monohydrate (Whewellite)	690	2,446
Carbonate apatite	20	424
Hydroxyapatite	9	219
$Mg(NH_4)PO_4 . 6H_2O$ (Struvite)	12	900
$CaHPO_4 . 2H_2O$ (Brushite)	17	114
Other phosphates of Ca, Mg & NH_4	4	11
Uric acid	350	390
Urates of Na, Ca, Mg & NH_4	4	11
Haematin	3	23
Fibrin	2	53
Mucin	1	2
Steatin	3	1
Cystine	65	23
Xanthine	1	—
Indigo	—	1
Sulphonamides	1	1

oxalate stones often contain both hydrates, and hydroxyapatite is another common constituent. Another group of stones are the mixed phosphate stones whose principal constituent is magnesium ammonium phosphate. This is seldom found in the pure state but is usually associated with the apatites. Apatites, sometimes reported simply as calcium phosphates after chemical analysis, are seldom the principal component of stones but are often found as minor constituents. Uric acid stones are frequently pure or nearly pure: in Herring's series 857 stones contained some uric acid and of these 593 contained 90% or more uric acid. The main materials associated with uric acid stones were hydroxyapatite and calcium oxalate. Most of the cystine stones contained only cystine; a minority contained small amounts of apatite in addition. Haematin and fibrin were seldom found as major constituents of stones, but not uncommon as minor constituents.

A few alleged stones are artefacts: either part of a Munchausen syndrome (Herring 1962, Sutor & O'Flynn 1973) or part of a practical joke. Sir William Osler, who did have renal stones, is said to have sent a pebble to the laboratory for analysis (Yendt 1970b).

Chemical analysis of stones
The chemical analysis of stones makes a small, but definite, contribution to the diagnosis of the patient with recurrent renal stones. In some cases, notably patients with cystine or uric acid stones, information on the stone composition is most valuable. Various methods are used for stone analysis notably micro-chemical techniques (Westbury & Omenogor 1970, Hodgkinson 1971), optical crystallography (Prien & Prien 1973, Szabó 1973, Gaca et al 1973, Elliot 1973), x-ray diffraction (Sutor et al 1971), thermogravimetric analysis (Schneider & Heide 1971) and infra-red spectroscopy (Frye & Chan 1972, Grieve & Zarembski 1973, Delatte et al 1973). Despite this variety of methods, stone analysis is done badly in many hospital laboratories and there is a strong case for performing this work in centres with a special interest in the problem.

THE CAUSES OF RENAL STONES

There are many factors which contribute to stone formation (table 7.2). Even so, among patients who pass calcium containing stones no cause for the stone formation can be found in more than half. Urine is frequently supersaturated with respect to calcium oxalate and calcium phosphate. The tissue fluid of the renal medulla, especially at the tips of the papillae, contains calcium at a very high concentration (Cooke 1973). What is remarkable therefore is that renal calcification and stones do not occur more often than they do.

TABLE 7.2. Contributory factors to urinary stone formation.

Increased crystalloid concentration

Dehydration
Hypercalciuria (table 7.3)
Hyperoxaluria
Excess uric aciduria
Cystinuria

Low urine pH (uric acid stones)

High urine pH (mixed phosphate stones)

Renal tubular defects

Deficiency of a crystallisation inhibitor

Pyrophosphate
Magnesium
Citrate
Other factors

Urinary tract abnormalities

Urinary infection
Congenital abnormalities
Medullary sponge kidney
Polycystic kidneys

Deficiency of crystallisation inhibitors

Normal urine will delay the setting of cement; urine from most stone-formers will not (Howard 1961). Crystallisation inhibitors present in normal urine include magnesium, citrate and pyrophosphate (Sutton & Watson 1969, Dent & Sutor 1971). It is not clear how important these are in preventing stone formation; pyrophosphate, for instance, cannot be responsible for the whole inhibitory power of urine and in any case is present equally in stone formers and controls (Russell 1973b, Smith & McCall 1973). There is now evidence that normal urine contains a substance, whose nature is still unknown, which prevents the growth of calcium oxalate crystals. This substance is absent from the urine of recurrent stone formers (Dent & Sutor 1971, Robertson & Peacock 1972).

The inhibitors, or their absence, may well be the most important factor in stone-formation, but next in importance is likely to be the concentration of calcium, phosphate and oxalate ions. Normal urine is frequently supersaturated with respect to these ions but the degree of supersaturation is often greater in stone-formers (Marshall et al 1972). The most common metabolic abnormality among stone-formers is hypercalciuria.

Hypercalciuria
It is difficult to define the upper limit of the normal range for urinary calcium excretion (p. 48). However an increased urinary excretion of calcium is found at some time in between 30% and 40% of patients who form calcium containing stones. A few of these (between 1·3% and 16·8% of stone patients in different series, Lavan et al 1971) have hyperparathyroidism and a few others have hypercalciuria of other causes (table 7.3), notably immobilisation and chronic vitamin D excess (Taylor 1972). In most patients with hypercalciuria no cause can be found and this 'idiopathic hypercalciuria' has been very widely studied.

TABLE 7.3. Causes of hypercalciuria.

Hypercalcaemia of any cause (table 4.1)
Normocalcaemic patients with:
   Vitamin D excess
   Immobilisation and space-flight
   Sarcoidosis
   Malignant disease
   Hyperthyroidism*
Cushing's syndrome
Idiopathic hypercalciuria
Spironolactone therapy†

---

* Renal stones are uncommon in hyperthyroidism (Walker 1971).

† Probably an artefact caused by the calcium content of the tablets themselves (Prati et al 1972).

It is not clear whether patients with idiopathic hypercalciuria should be regarded as a different population from other stone-formers (Robertson & Morgan 1972), but there may be some practical value in treating these patients separately. Idiopathic hypercalciuria is more common in men than women and in many patients the cause appears to be an excessive intestinal absorption of calcium (Lavan et al 1971, Pak et al 1972a, Rose & Harrison 1973). The serum calcium is normal but some patients have a serum phosphorus at the lower end of the normal range; this has suggested that normocalcaemic hyperparathyroidism may be a cause of 'idiopathic hypercalciuria' (Yendt & Gagné 1968, Adams et al 1970b, Liberman & de Vries 1971, Shieber et al 1971a Coe et al 1971). In these series some of the patients should have been excluded because they had serum calcium levels which, by strict criteria, were abnormal. Other patients had normal serum calcium levels but parathyroid glands which were abnormal by electron-microscopy. Partial parathyroidectomy in those patients apparently reduced greatly the rate of stone formation. A few patients have had abnormally high serum PTH levels. Thus, hyperparathyroidism may be the cause of idiopathic hypercalciuria in some cases, but seems unlikely to be the whole explanation of this disorder.

Hyperoxaluria

The urinary excretion of oxalate is normally 1–4 mmol/day. Dietary factors influence oxalate excretion: the ingestion of purines (sardines, fish-roe, etc) increases oxalate excretion (Zarembski & Hodgkinson 1969). Unless in exceptional quantities, oxalate-rich food such as tea, rhubarb or spinach does not greatly influence urinary oxalate excretion because some oxalate is destroyed in the gut and some lost in the faeces. Oxalate excretion is increased and oxalate stones are formed in some patients with ileal disease and after intestinal shunt operations for the treatment of obesity (Dowling et al 1971, Dickstein & Frame 1973, Smith & Hoffman 1973, Williams et al 1973). The failure of bile salt reabsorption apparently leads to the bacterial breakdown of glycine-conjugated bile salts. The glycine is reabsorbed and converted to glyoxylate and ultimately oxalate. Lastly oxalate excretion is increased about tenfold in primary hyperoxaluria, a rare inherited metabolic disorder characterised by calcium oxalate stones and oxalate deposits in many tissues (Cochran et al 1968, Watts 1973).

Causes of uric acid stones

Uric acid stones form about 5% of all urinary stones in western countries. An increased urinary excretion of uric acid is found in some patients and causes include gout, myeloproliferative disorders with a secondary increase in purine turnover, and rare inborn errors of purine metabolism (Seegmiller 1973). Hyperuricaemia is not a prerequisite for uric acid stone formation. Indeed 80% of patients with uric acid stones have normal blood and urine levels of uric acid (Frank et al 1970) and it seems clear that the pH of the urine is more important than uric acid concentration in stone formation. Uric acid stones only form in an acid urine (Rapoport et al 1967).

Hyperuricaemia also predisposes to the production of calcium stones (Coe & Raisen 1973).

Cystinuria

Cystinuria accounts for between 2% and 3% of stones from the upper urinary tract. It is a recessively inherited disorder characterised by defects in the intestinal and renal transport of the basic amino acids, ornithine, arginine, lysine and cystine. Excessive quantities of all four amino-acids leak into the urine but cystine is very insoluble and stones are liable to form. A full account of this disorder and its treatment is outside the scope of this text but useful reviews include those by Crawhall and Watts (1968) and Stephens and Watts (1971).

Xanthinuria

Xanthine stones occur in xanthinuria, a very rare metabolic disorder caused by deficiency of the enzyme xanthine oxidase (Seegmiller 1968). Xanthine stones might also be expected to result from the treatment of gout with allopurinol, a xanthine oxidase inhibitor; this has been described but does not seem to be common (Greene et al 1969).

Causes of silica stones

Silica stones are common in cattle in the great plains of North America and among sheep and cattle in Australia. Polymers of silicic acid precipitate out in alkaline urine with a high protein content (Bailey 1972). Silica stones have been described in man but are very rare; they occur in patients who have taken large quantities of magnesium trisilicate for long periods (Joekes et al 1973).

Dehydration

Urinary stones of any type are more likely to occur in patients with a concentrated urine. In the Royal Navy for instance the incidence of stones is higher in personnel serving in the Mediterranean or in tropical areas than in Britain (Blacklock 1969). The incidence is also greater among cooks and engineers who work in a hot environment. Northern Europeans visiting areas with hot climates should be advised to increase their fluid intake deliberately. In Israel, for example, the incidence of urinary stones is low among Arabs and indigenous Israelis but high among recent immigrants from Europe.

Dehydration may underlie the increased incidence of urinary calculi which has been reported in ulcerative colitis (Bennett & Hughes 1972).

Urinary tract abnormalities, infection and stasis

Urinary infection is found in 12%–27% of stone formers in different series and is significantly more common than in controls (Jennis et al 1970). The link between infection and stone formation is not clear; one likely factor is the precipitation of magnesium ammonium phosphate in infections with urea-splitting organisms. Pyelography in some cases reveals renal abnormalities such as hydronephrosis, calyceal cysts, duplex kidney and horseshoe kidney. Medullary sponge kidney has been particularly associated with renal stone formation; some of these patients have hypercalciuria but most do not.

Stasis is likely to be important in stone-formation: recumbency leads to stasis in the upper calyces which, with the increased urinary calcium and the greater likelihood of urinary infection, contributes to stone formation (Smith & Robertson 1969). People in sedentary occupations have an increased incidence of stone formation. Seamen and Royal Marines have a lower incidence of renal stones than clerical staff in the Royal Navy (Blacklock 1969). In Czechoslovakia farmers have a much lower incidence of renal stones than civil servants (Mates 1969).

Nephrotoxic factors

The excessive use of analgesics affects the kidney in several ways but one result is an increased incidence of renal stones (Blackman et al 1967).

Calcium-containing renal stones have been described in addicts to Worcestershire sauce and among Indians in Fiji where it is known as the curry kidney. The Indian diet includes many spices which are also found in Worcestershire sauce but the nature of the toxic substances is not known (Murphy 1967, Holmes 1971).

Alcaptonuria
A high incidence of urinary calculi, composed principally of calcium oxalates and phosphates, has been noted in alcaptonuria (Křížek 1971). The reason is not known.

Vitamin A deficiency?
Rats and dogs on vitamin A deficient diets may develop renal stones. This seems to have no relevance to stone-formation in man as several surveys have failed to show any relationship between vitamin A deficiency and stone formation (Elliot 1954, McGeown & Bull 1957, Ramalingaswami & Aurora 1961). Although doubt was first thrown on the possible relationship between vitamin A deficiency and renal stones in man in 1935, vitamin A deficiency is still mentioned as a cause of stones in several currently available textbooks.

INVESTIGATION OF THE STONE-FORMER

In the patient with pain suggestive of renal colic, evidence in favour of a stone will be provided by microscopic haematuria, suggestive opacities on abdominal radiographs or by an abnormal pyelogram. No stone may be visible if it is too small (especially if radiolucent), if the stone was passed spontaneously, or if the pain had another cause such as pyelonephritis, depression or drug-addiction. Posen and Jerome (1971) remark that the larger the pile of films of negative intravenous and retrograde pyelograms a patient has, the lower is the probability that the symptoms are due to stones.

Once stone formation has been established and especially if it is recurrent, a search should be made for any underlying metabolic disorder. Estimations of serum calcium, uric acid and urea, and of urinary calcium excretion are worthwhile as is examination of freshly passed urine for crystals and cellular deposits. Many clinics do a screening test for excess urinary cystine on all stone-formers (Kelly et al 1972). Examination of a stone may be helpful particularly if it shows cystine or uric acid. While there is a tendency for hypercalciuria to be associated with caicium oxalate stones and urinary infection to be associated with mixed phosphate stones, the exact identification of the components of these calcium-containing stones is of limited value in practice. Even if a stone is not available the radiographic appearances of a stone in the kidney or ureter can be helpful. Calcium-containing stones are radio-opaque but some phosphate stones with a high proportion of magnesium ammonium phosphate have a low radio-density as have cystine stones and silica stones. Uric acid and xanthine stones are radiolucent.

In the majority of patients who form stones, no metabolic abnormality is found on investigation.

MANAGEMENT

The management of the patient with recurrent renal calculi consists of general measures and measures directed at any underlying metabolic disorder. In addition some patients may need surgical treatment for a particular stone.

Surgical intervention
Surgery is indicated for ureteric obstruction, or for partial obstruction when the stone has a size or shape which makes its spontaneous passage unlikely. Persistent or recurrent infection is another indication for surgery particularly when the stone is increasing in size during observation. Pain is more difficult to assess as an indication for surgery. The patient with recurrent bouts of typical pain associated with an identified ureteric stone usually benefits from surgery. In other cases, and particularly when the stone is in the renal pelvis, surgery often fails to relieve the pain (Taguchi 1970, Posen & Jerome 1971).

General measures
The patient with recurrent stones should increase his fluid intake. He needs not only a general exhortation to drink but specific advice, which will keep the urine dilute at night when ordinarily it is most concentrated. Thus he should be advised to drink before retiring and to drink again when he gets up to pass urine.

Treatment of any underlying disorder

Urinary infections should be treated. In some patients with renal calculi infections can be very persistent and difficult to eradicate, even after surgical removal of the stone and correction of any anatomical abnormality. However, promising results have been reported with a procedure in which surgical removal of stones is followed by pro-longed irrigation with buffered acid solutions to eliminate residual fragments of stones which may harbour bacteria (Nemoy & Stamey 1971). Acidification of the urine is of some value in patients with recurrent phosphate-containing stones but they benefit from treatment with phosphate binding antacids which greatly reduce the urinary excretion of phosphorus (Lavengood & Marshall 1972). Patients on this therapy should be checked regularly for hypophosphataemia.

Hyperparathyroidism This should be treated surgically; if possible the neck should be explored before any attack is made on the stone itself (p. 107).

Idiopathic stone formers and 'idiopathic hypercalciuria' Idiopathic hypercalciruia has been treated in a number of different ways, but in many patients a low dietary calcium and a high fluid intake suffices to reduce stone formation (Dent & Watson 1965). Other measures which are effective in reducing the urinary calcium include thiazides (Yendt et al 1970) and oral phosphate which also reduces urinary oxalate (Elliot et al 1970, Thomas 1971, Smith et al 1973c). Neither of these operate by reducing intestinal calcium absorption and the value of phosphate is partially offset by the increase in the urinary phosphate concentration (Pak & Ohata 1973). Cellulose phosphate reduces urinary calcium excretion by reducing its intestinal absorption (Parfitt et al 1964, Pak 1973); it causes only a minor rise in phosphate excretion.

Another group of drugs, the crystallisation inhibitors, are being investigated in the management of idiopathic calcium-containing stones as well as those associated with hypercalciuria. Both magnesium supplements (Melnick et al 1971) and the diphosphonates have been tried. Magnesium given as oral magnesium oxide, appeared to be effective in reducing the incidence of stones in one clinical trial in Virginia, an area with a high incidence of renal stones and a deficiency of magnesium in the soil. Diphosphonates (Fleisch 1973, Pak & Ohata 1973) are analogues of pyrophosphate but have a $-P-C-P-$ core instead of $-P-O-P-$. They are stable and can be given by mouth. In clinical use they inhibit crystal growth in urine *in vitro* but there are as yet no clinical trials of diphosphonates in urolithiasis.

Clinical trials in patients with idiopathic recurrent stone-formation are likely to be difficult because it is a condition with wide spontaneous variation in severity. At present there is insufficient evidence to know whether any of the measures described in this section have advantages over a regime consisting simply of a high fluid intake with or without a low calcium diet.

Uric acid stones These should be treated by making the urine alkaline. There have been objections that this treatment might precipitate the formation of calcium-containing stones but this has not been observed in practice. Allopurinol in a dose of 300–400 mg/day is also effective and is the treatment of choice for gout complicated by uric acid lithiasis. It is also the appropriate treatment for patients with hyperuricaemia and calcium stones (Coe & Raisen 1973)

PROGNOSIS

After passing a single stone a patient has an 80% chance of having no further episodes. It is debatable how extensively it is worth investigating such a patient. In a few patients with recurrent stones progressive renal damage may result from persistent pyelonephritis, and especially pyonephrosis. A very small number of patients die of gram-negative septicaemia. The great majority of patients with recurrent stones continue to have a normal renal function for many years.

Chapter 8: Hypocalcaemia: Causes and Clinical Features

Hypocalcaemia has many causes (table 8.1) but osteomalacia and uraemic osteodystrophy are the most common. The disorders listed are discussed individually in this chapter or elsewhere in the book (chapters 9–13). Neonatal hypocalcaemia is considered separately at the end of this chapter.

TABLE 8.1. Causes of hypocalcaemia outside the neonatal period.

Common

Uraemic osteodystrophy
Osteomalacia and rickets (table 10.1)

Uncommon

Hypoparathyroidism (post-surgical and idiopathic)
Pseudohypoparathyroidism
Acute pancreatitis
Magnesium depletion
Renal tubular disorders e.g. Fanconi syndrome

Very uncommon

Starvation
Malignant disease especially leukaemia
Citrated blood transfusion in neonates and in liver failure
Excessive ingestion of phosphate laxatives
White phosphorus burns
Colchicine overdose
Acute fluoride intoxication
Frusemide therapy
Therapy with viomycin, mithramycin or similar drugs
Malignant hyperpyrexia
Medullary carcinoma of thyroid (a minority of cases)

DIFFERENTIAL DIAGNOSIS

In the patient presenting with tetany or found to have hypocalcaemia the cause is seldom difficult to determine. There may be other features of uraemia, a history of intestinal or thyroid surgery or physical signs of osteomalacia or rickets. The drug history can be particularly relevant: anticonvulsants, phosphate laxatives, colchicine and frusemide (furosemide) can all cause hypocalcaemia.

The simpler chemical investigations appropriate to hypocalcaemia are indicated in table 8.2. Assay of parathyroid hormone (PTH)

TABLE 8.2. Clinical chemistry of hypocalcaemic disorders.

	serum phosphorus	serum alkaline phosphatase	urine calcium
Uraemic osteodystrophy	↑ ↑	↑ or Normal	↓
Osteomalacia and rickets (nutritional and due to intestinal disorders)	↓ or Normal	↑	↓
Hypoparathyroidism and pseudohypoparathyroidism	↑	Normal	↓
Acute pancreatitis	Normal	Normal	↓ or Normal
Fanconi syndrome	↓	↑ or Normal	↑
Hypoalbuminaemia	Normal	Normal*	Normal

* Unless increased as a result of liver disease.

in serum may become a valuable investigation in the future; at present none of the available methods distinguish completely between low values and normal values for PTH, but detectable PTH in serum from a hypocalcaemic patient makes hypoparathyroidism unlikely. Radiological studies in obscure hypocalcaemia should include a search for Looser's zones and for calcification of the basal ganglia. If the diagnosis is still not clear a bone biopsy should be done; bone histology distinguishes osteomalacia from hypoparathyroidism. The tests for distinguishing hypoparathyroidism from pseudohypoparathyroidism are described in the next chapter.

CLINICAL FEATURES

The most striking result of hypocalcaemia is tetany (p. 33) with carpo-pedal spasm or, in infants, laryngeal spasm (laryngismus stridulus). Some patients especially infants present with convulsions. Patients with hypocalcaemia have sensory abnormalities more often than tetany. These consist of paraesthesiae ('pins and needles') in the hands and feet, and less often, around the mouth. Abdominal pain is another feature of hypocalcaemia; the mechanism is obscure.

Cardiac changes, including bradycardia and hypotension, are sometimes noted in hypocalcaemia and are reversed when calcium is administered. The electro cardiogram shows prolongation of the QT interval especially the ST component (Boen et al 1962, Chaimovitz et al 1972). Hypocalcaemia potentiates and prolongs the action of curare in general anaesthesia (McKie 1969). Some infants with hypocalcaemia have congestive heart failure for which no other cause can be found (Troughton & Singh 1972).

Mental changes are described in hypocalcaemia of any cause. The most common is anxiety or depression. Chronic hypocalcaemia, especially in hypoparathyroidism, may be associated with progressive intellectual loss. The electroencephalogram in severe hypocalcaemia shows both spikes and bursts of high voltage slow waves. This association may be specific for hypocalcaemia (Swash & Rowan 1972). The abnormal EEG is not corrected as soon as the hypocalcaemia is treated but only after an interval. Some patients with hypocalcaemia severe enough to cause tetany have a normal EEG (Fourman et al 1963).

Other clinical features of chronic hypocalcaemia include skin changes (Reinberg & Sidi 1959) and cataract. White flecks in the nails are popularly thought to be associated with 'calcium deficiency' but I know of no evidence to support this view.

CAUSES

Uraemic osteodystrophy, osteomalacia and rickets, hypoparathyroidism and pseudohypoparathyroidism, and renal tubular disorders are considered in the next four chapters. This section is concerned with other disorders which cause hypocalcaemia.

A low total serum calcium is found in patients with a low serum albumin, because of a reduction in the serum protein-bound calcium fraction. Spuriously low serum calcium results have been noted after storage of plasma or serum from some uraemic patients on maintenance haemodialysis; the mechanism of this change is unknown (Coburn et al 1969a).

Starvation
Most medical students imagine that a low dietary calcium is an important cause of hypocalcaemia. However normal people adapt to low calcium diets by increasing the proportion of the dietary calcium which is absorbed (p. 9). There may be minor changes in the serum calcium but a normal calcium balance is soon re-established. One exception to this rule is in total starvation when adaptation fails and hypocalcaemia may ensue (Fromm et al 1970, Walker 1972a, Kumar et al 1972).

Acute pancreatitis
Hypocalcaemia has long been recognised as a complication of acute pancreatitis and the extent of the fall in serum calcium is some guide to the severity and thus the prognosis of the pancreatitis. Tetany has been described in severe cases (Cortese & Glenn 1968, D'Souza & Floch 1973).

Until recently it was thought that the hypocalcaemia was caused by precipitation of calcium with fatty acids released by enzymatic fat hydrolysis (Storck & Björntorp 1971). It is now appreciated that this mechanism is inadequate to explain the changes found and it is thought that glucagon released by the damaged pancreas causes hypocalcaemia (Shieber 1970). Glucagon causes hypocalcaemia by stimulating calcitonin release from the thyroid and perhaps also by other means (Birge & Avioli 1969, Hattner et al 1970, Scandellari et al 1972). In dogs the hypocalcaemia of pancreatitis is prevented by thyroidectomy (Shieber et al 1971b).

Magnesium depletion
Minor degrees of magnesium deficiency are common (table 8.3). Severe magnesium depletion may be a cause of hypocalcaemia. This is uncommon but occurs particularly in patients with severe intestinal

losses and in primary magnesium malabsorption, a rare disease of boys who present in the first year of life with convulsions or tetany (Vainsel et al 1970, Nordio et al 1971).

Magnesium is the principal divalent cation of cells and is important in the function of enzyme systems in all tissues (Fourman 1967, Wacker & Parisi 1968, Heaton 1973). Patients with magnesium deficiency often have other deficiencies as well; the main symptoms which can be attributed to the magnesium deficiency are muscular weakness, mood changes, especially restlessness and agressiveness,

TABLE 8.3. Causes of magnesium deficiency.

Intestinal loss*

   Severe and prolonged diarrhoea especially after intestinal resection
   Malabsorption
   Primary magnesium malabsorption

Renal loss*

   Diuretic therapy
   Renal tubular acidosis
   Diabetic ketosis
   Recovery from acute renal tulular necrosis
   Aldosterone excess
   Hyperparathyroidism with bone disease
   Alcoholism

---

   * Hypomagnesaemia also occurs rarely in hypoparathyroidism; defects both in intestinal absorption and in renal magnesium conservation are involved.

involuntary movements of an athetoid or Parkinsonian type, and epileptic convulsions. Tetany does occur in magnesium depletion but it is not clear whether it ever occurs in the absence of a simultaneous hypocalcaemia (Zimmet 1968).

Patients with magnesium deficiency have a low plasma magnesium and urine magnesium excretion, a negative potassium balance and often a fall in the serum calcium. The pathogenesis of the hypocalcaemia is controversial: one view is that in magnesium deficiency there is target organ unresponsiveness to parathyroid hormone (Heaton & Fourman 1965, Estep et al 1969, MacManus et al 1971, Nordio et al 1971, Connor et al 1972). This conclusion has been

challenged by Suh et al (1971) who found that puppies with hypocalcaemia due to magnesium deficiency responded to parathyroid
extract as well as control animals. Furthermore Suh et al (1973)
found that a child with hypomagnesaemia responded normally to
parathyroid extract and, when hypomagnesaemic, the serum levels
of parathyroid hormone became unmeasurably low. Both high and
low values have been found in other patients with hypocalcaemia
due to magnesium depletion (Connor et al 1972, Anast et al 1972).
This controversy cannot yet be resolved but whatever the mechanism
may be, it is clear that the hypocalcaemia of severe magnesium depletion is corrected by the administration of magnesium alone (Heaton
& Fourman 1965, Estep et al 1969). Oral therapy with magnesium as
magnesium hydroxide B.P. or as magnesium glycerophosphate in a
dose of 60–120 mEq/day or intravenous therapy with very slow
infusions of magnesium sulphate have been used; both are effective.

Magnesium administration

The intricacy of the relationship between calcium and magnesium
metabolism in man is illustrated by the occasional reports of acute
hypocalcaemia with tetany after intravenous therapy with magnesium
sulphate in eclampsia (Monif & Savory 1972). Possible mechanisms
include parathyroid suppression by the hypermagnesaemia (p. 15)
or the stimulation of calcitonin release (Nielsen & Jørgensen 1972).

Excessive phosphate ingestion

Phosphate-containing laxatives are widely used in North America
and there are case reports of severe hypocalcaemia resulting from
their use (Goldfinger 1969, McConnell 1971, Levitt et al 1973).
McConnell's case was fatal. A 48-year old housewife took '*Phospho-
Soda*', a mixture of sodium phosphates, daily in huge doses for
'chronic constipation'. An episode of severe constipation, pain and
distention led to the consumption of further large amounts of the
laxative and two days later she was admitted to hospital in semi-coma
where she died a few hours later. Her serum calcium was 1·2 mmol/l
(4·8 mg/100 ml), and serum inorganic phosphorus 15 mmol/l
(47 mg/100 ml). At autopsy there was faecal impaction, and massive
dilation and ulceration of the colon.

A similar mechanism may underlie the sudden deaths which occur
after white phosphorus burns (Bowden et al 1971).

Citrate administration in blood transfusion

Citrate infusion might be expected to cause a fall in serum ionised calcium but the citrate of ACD blood used in transfusion is normally metabolised by the liver sufficiently rapidly that little change in ionised calcium is seen (Hinkle & Cooperman 1971). However tetany, convulsions and death have been reported with the use of ACD blood in exchange-transfusions in neonates (Friedman et al 1972) and similar problems have been described with rapid blood transfusion in patients with liver disease (Ludbrook & Wynn 1958). I have seen hypotension and the electrocardiographic changes of hypocalcaemia in an adult having an exchange-transfusion in hepatic failure. In both situations intravenous calcium gluconate prevents or corrects the disorder.

Malignant disease

Hypocalcaemia is sometimes observed in patients with malignant disorders especially acute leukaemia in childhood. No single explanation can be given for this abnormality but in some cases the anti-tumour therapy may be responsible. In leukaemia hypocalcaemia appears to be an ominous sign (Jaffe et al 1972, Souillet et al 1973).

Other causes of hypocalcaemia

Hypocalcaemia has been noted in a patient who poisoned herself with colchicine. Colchicine in large doses appears to inhibit bone resorption (Heath et al 1972b). Hypocalcaemia is occasionally noted after therapy with frusemide (Toft & Roin 1971), with mithramycin (p. 75) or with viomycin (Vanasin et al 1972) and in acute fluoride poisoning (Waldbott 1963). Hypocalcaemia and hyperphosphataemia occur in malignant hyperpyrexia (Pollock & Watson 1971).

HYPOCALCAEMIA IN NEONATES

Hypocalcaemia is the most frequently identified disorder causing convulsions in the neonatal period (Keen 1969). There are many causes (Mizrahi et al 1968) but in the most common syndrome ('classic' neonatal tetany) the symptoms begin on or soon after the fourth day of life. It is particularly a disorder of bottle-fed babies and the use of cows' milk seems to be the main contributing factor (Barltrop & Oppé 1970). Cows' milk, even after dilution, has a high phosphorus content and a low calcium/phosphorus ratio compared with human milk (table 8.4). In these babies hypocalcaemia is associated with hyperphosphataemia. Unlike calcium, most of the phosphate in the diet is absorbed in the intestine and this excessive phosphate load is given to the child at a time when the capacity of the kidneys for phosphate excretion may be limited (Pierson & Crawford 1972). Some infants have hypomagnesaemia as well as hypocalcaemia; the significance of this is uncertain as the serum magnesium rises with calcium supplements alone (Chiswick 1971).

TABLE 8.4. Composition of breast milk and of a typical artificial milk, Ostermilk 1, which is produced by dilution of cows' milk with water and lactose (data of Barltrop & Oppé 1970). Similar values for the Ca/P ratio apply to other brands of milk for infant feeding (Shaw et al 1973).

Constituent	Breast milk (per 100 ml)	Ostermilk 1 (per 100 g)
Fat (g)	5·1	2·8
Carbohydrate (g)	6·7	8·3
Protein (g)	1·2	2·7
Calcium (mg)	29·0	93·9
Phosphorus (mg)	14·0	74·2
Ca/P ratio	2·1	1·3

Maternal factors may also contribute to neonatal hypocalcaemia: Watney et al (1971) noted that it was more common in the infants of Asian immigrants to Britain especially in winter. They suggested that marginal vitamin D deficiency in the mothers contributed to the hypocalcaemia. Hypocalcaemia is also more common in the infants of diabetic mothers (Tsang et al 1972); the mechanism is not clear but hypersecretion of glucagon could be a factor. Hypocalcaemia in the first 48 hours of life occurs in some premature infants delivered by Caesarian section; the cause is not known. Rare causes of hypocalcaemia in neonates include hypoparathyroidism and maternal hyperparathyroidism (pp. 108, 160).

Treatment of neonatal hypocalcaemia is that of the underlying condition as far as possible; most cases respond to calcium supplements or better still reduction of the phosphate content of the feeds. A few infants who do not respond to these measures require vitamin D. In most infants the hypocalcaemia is temporary and even the infants with convulsions seem to have no permanent mental damage (Knuckey et al 1971).

Chapter 9: Hypoparathyroidism

Hypoparathyroidism is an uncommon disorder which has several distinct causes (table 9.1). Pseudohypoparathyroidism is also discussed in this chapter because the chemical changes are similar.

TABLE 9.1. Causes of hypoparathyroidism.

---

1. Defect in parathyroid hormone secretion

Surgical damage to parathyroid glands or their blood supply in neck surgery.
Parathyroid damage by ^{131}I in treatment of hyperthyroidism.
'Idiopathic hypoparathyroidism', including
  Auto-immune hypoparathyroidism
  Congenital and familial hypoparathyroidism.
Haemochromatosis with iron deposits in parathyroids.
Metastatic neoplasm in parathyroid glands.

2. Defect in tissue response to parathyroid hormone

Pseudohypoparathyroidism.

CAUSES

Hypoparathyroidism after thyroid surgery

The incidence of hypoparathyroidism after thyroid surgery varies between 1 % and 6 % in different series; probably as a result of differences in surgical technique. In Australia for example Parfitt (1971) demonstrated a relationship between the incidence of hypoparathyroidism and the surgeon's experience of the operation. In partial thyroidectomy it seems likely that damage to the blood supply of the parathyroid glands is more often the cause of hypoparathyroidism than the removal of the glands. It is particularly important that the inferior thyroid artery should be preserved if possible. After partial thyroidectomy transient hypocalcaemia occurs more often than permanent hypoparathyroidism; while some of these patients may represent cases of temporary hypoparathyroidism, in others the hypocalcaemia could be the result of an increased bone avidity for calcium (Michie et al 1971).

Hypoparathyroidism is more common after total than after partial thyroidectomy; Thompson and Harness (1970) found permanent hypoparathyroidism in 5·4% of 184 cases. Hypoparathyroidism is even more common after the extensive neck surgery which is appropriate for carcinomas of the larynx and upper oesophagus (Sisson & Vander Aarde 1971). Hypoparathyroidism also occurs after parathyroidectomy.

Partial hypoparathyroidism In 1936 Kramer suggested that partial parathyroid insufficiency might be the explanation for the mental symptoms of some post-thyroidectomy patients with a normal serum calcium. This concept was extended by Fourman and his colleagues who showed that some normocalcaemic patients after thyroidectomy had an abnormal response to calcium depriviation with oral sodium phytate or intravenous sodium ethylene diamine tetra-acetate (EDTA). These patients had indefinite symptoms of lassitude and depression which apparently improved with oral calcium supplements. While Parfitt (1969a, 1972a) has confirmed that there are patients with abnormal responses to EDTA infusion after thyroidectomy, it is still not clear whether this represents a disorder of the parathyroids or whether it calls for treatment. Stowers et al (1967) conducted a double blind controlled trial of calcium therapy in a small group of patients with abnormal EDTA tests; they were unable to demonstrate any subjective or objective change in the patients.

Hypoparathyroidism after ^{131}I therapy

A few cases of hypoparathyroidism have been reported after the treatment of hyperthyroidism with [131]I (Orme & Conolly 1971). It has been inferred that the radio-iodine was the cause of the hypoparathyroidism although this may not be the explanation in every case.

Abnormal EDTA tests were reported in 10% of patients after ^{131}I therapy (Adams & Chalmers 1965). That this may not indicate a high incidence of 'partial hypoparathyroidism' is suggested by Goldsmith et al (1968b) who showed that a group of such patients were in fact hypothyroid and that the EDTA tests became normal when this was treated.

Idiopathic hypoparathyroidism

Hypoparathyroidism without a past history of neck surgery is rare and probably includes several different disorders.

Auto-immune hypoparathyroidism Some patients probably have an auto-immune disease for parathyroid antibodies were found in 38% of 74 patients with unexplained hypoparathyroidism by Blizzard et al (1966). The histology of the parathyroids in many cases is also suggestive of an auto-immune process: there is lymphocytic infiltration and atrophy (Irvine 1971). Parathyroid antibodies are also found in many patients with auto-immune Addison's disease and there is a clear association between auto-immune Addison's disease, idiopathic hypoparathyroidism, pernicious anaemia, moniliasis and occasionally hypothyroidism. These disorders occur together in families and the hypoparathyroidism is generally detected first in childhood or adolescence. This 'juvenile polyendocrine deficiency syndrome' appears to have an autosomal recessive mode of inheritance (Irvine & Barnes 1972).

Some patients with idiopathic hypoparathyroidism have a cell-mediated hypersensitivity against the parathyroids (Moulias et al 1971). It is not yet clear whether this is a different disease.

Familial hypoparathyroidism The juvenile polyendocrine deficiency syndrome has already been mentioned. Other families have been described with isolated hypoparathyroidism inherited in an autosomal dominant, autosomal recessive or sex-linked recessive manner (Barr et al 1971).

Iron storage diseases

Hypoparathyroidism has been described both in haemochromatosis (Vachon et al 1970) and haemosiderosis after repeated blood transfusions (Sherman et al 1970). The two reported cases of haemochromatosis also had diabetes mellitus, adrenal insufficiency and hypogonadism. The parathyroid pathology is not available for these cases, but in previous studies it has been noted that the parathyroid glands are 'invariably' infiltrated with iron in haemochromatosis.

Metastatic neoplasm

The parathyroid glands are sometimes the site of secondary malignant disease especially in carcinoma of the breast, leukaemia and melanoma. Hypoparathyroidism caused in this way appears to be uncommon but two cases have been described (Horwitz et al 1972).

CLINICAL FEATURES AND PATHOLOGY

The main clinical features of hypocalcaemia (anxiety, depression, paraesthesiae and tetany) were discussed in the previous chapter. Patients with hypoparathyroidism may have any of these symptoms or no symptoms at all. Some patients appear to adapt to hypocalcaemia with the passage of time. Other patients get worse during menstruation or pregnancy, or during an intercurrent illness.

Neurological and psychiatric disorders

Apart from tetany, the main neurological disorders associated with hypoparathyroidism are epilepsy, parkinsonism, chorea and dementia. The mechanism of these disorders is unknown but calcification within the brain is a feature of hypoparathyroidism and some patients have an increased cerebrospinal fluid pressure with papilloedema.

Epilepsy In one recent series epilepsy occurred in 12 out of 42 patients with hypoparathyroidism; it was particularly common in idiopathic hypoparathyroidism (Fonseca & Calverley 1967). All varieties of epilepsy occur: grand mal, petit mal and focal attacks. Few of the patients with epilepsy have tetany perhaps because this was abolished by the anticonvulsant therapy (Schaaf & Payne 1966). The epilepsy is usually abolished by treatment of the hypocalcaemia.

Parkinsonism and chorea The extrapyramidal disorders associated with hypoparathyroidism have been reviewed by Muenter and Whisnant (1968). Tremor, athetosis, rigidity, ataxia and oculogyric crises are found as well as chorea and rarely kinesio-genic choreo-athetosis (Tabaee-Zadeh et al 1972). Most patients have radiological evidence of calcification in the basal ganglia and these disorders are more common in idiopathic than in surgical hypoparathyroidism. These symptoms improve with correction of the serum calcium (Hossain 1970).

Mental changes and dementia In common with other hypocalcaemic disorders hypoparathyroidism causes mental changes such as anxiety and depression. A few patients have more dramatic symptoms including attacks of terror, hallucinations or delusional psychosis. These are relieved by treatment (Hossain 1970). Progressive intellectual impairment is another disturbing consequence of prolonged hypoparathyroidism. Treatment prevents further deterioration and restores some, but not always all, of the lost intellectual capacity. Permanent intellectual damage is found in children with untreated congenital or neonatal hypoparathyroidism (see below).

Papilloedema This is often found in hypoparathyroidism. In some cases it is associated with a rise in the pressure of the cerebrospinal fluid, but the reason for this is not known. A combination of epilepsy and papilloedema has more than once led to a provisional diagnosis of brain tumour (Drury et al 1971).

Brain pathology Calcification of the basal ganglia is a common feature of idiopathic hypoparathyroidism but is very uncommon in surgical hypoparathyroidism (Frame 1965).

The skin and nails
Moniliasis is a feature of some cases of idiopathic hypoparathyroidism, notably those with the juvenile polyendocrine deficiency syndrome. The candida infection, which may preceed the overt presentation of hypoparathyroidism appears to be a disorder of the cell-mediated response to candida albicans (Block et al 1971). The moniliasis can be difficult to treat and may persist even when the hypocalcaemia is treated.

Loss of hair, eczema and psoriasis occur in all forms of hypoparathyroidism and improve rapidly when the hypocalcaemia is treated. Brittleness of the nails is another common feature of hypoparathyroidism. This improves with treatment but moniliasis of the nails may also need attention.

The eyes
Cataracts occur in prolonged hypocalcaemia of any cause and were found in 24 out of 50 patients with idiopathic hypoparathyroidism (Bronsky et al 1958). It is not known why the cataracts develop but the calcium content of the lens appears to be normal. In a few patients gradual resolution of some lenticular opacities has been described after treatment of the hypocalcaemia (Drury et al 1971).

Intestine
Malabsorption is more common among patients with hypoparathyroidism than would be expected by chance and a few patients present with diarrhoea, or anaemia due to vitamin B_{12} deficiency. The malabsorption improves when the hypocalcaemia is treated with vitamin D (Clarkson et al 1960, Gay & Grimes 1972).

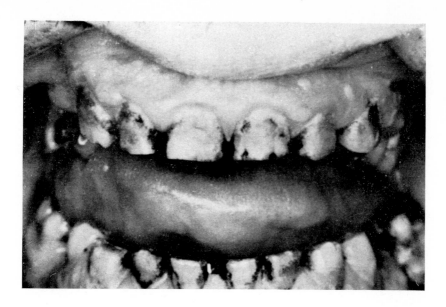

FIGURE 9.1. Teeth in a 42-year-old man with idiopathic hypoparathyroidism. There is hypoplasia of the enamel, abraded teeth and gross caries. (Courtesy of John A. Frensilli, D.D.S. and the American Dental Association).

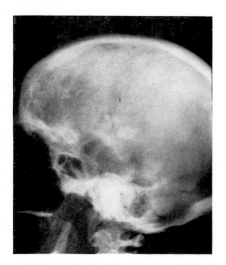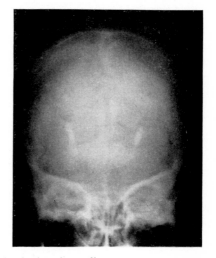

FIGURE 9.2. Calcification in the basal ganglia.

Teeth

In idiopathic hypoparathyroidism the teeth often show hypoplasia of the enamel (fig. 9.1) and blunting of the root apices. Some cases also have delayed dental development (Frensilli et al 1971).

Bone

There are no bone symptoms associated with hypoparathyroidism but the occasional association of hypoparathyroidism with spondylitis may be more than coincidence (Jimenea et al 1971). The histological appearances of the bone are generally normal in hypoparathyroidism although a few patients have an excess of osteoid (Woods 1972). Histochemical changes in the epiphyseal cartilage and bone matrix have been observed in parathyroidectomised rats (Bernick 1971).

RADIOLOGY

The radiological appearances of the bones are generally normal in hypoparathyroidism although there are a few reports of patients especially children with areas of sclerosis (Gibberd 1965). The most valuable radiological feature of idiopathic hypoparathyroidism is calcification in the basal ganglia (Frame 1965). This is illustrated in figure 9.2. Similar appearances are observed in pseudohypoparathyroidism, toxoplasmosis and in 'idiopathic familial calcification of the basal ganglia'.

CLINICAL CHEMISTRY

Blood chemistry

The serum calcium is always low in idiopathic hypoparathyroidism; no values greater than 1·8 mmol/l (7·5 mg/100 ml) were found in 60 cases collected by Parfitt (1972a). In surgical hypoparathyroidism the range of serum calcium depends on whether cases of 'partial hypoparathyroidism' are included; if they are, serum calcium values range between 1·1 mmol/l (4·5 mg/100 ml) and 2·5 mmol/l (10 mg/100 ml).

The serum inorganic phosphorus is almost always abnormal in idiopathic hypoparathyroidism but is frequently within the normal range in patients with milder degrees of surgical hypoparathyroidism (Parfitt 1972a). The plasma magnesium is low in some patients with idiopathic hypoparathyroidism (Jones & Fourman 1966, Niklasson 1970) and treatment may be difficult before magnesium depletion is corrected. Many patients with hypoparathyroidism have a mild metabolic alkalosis (Barzel 1969, 1971). Impaired glucose tolerance is found in some (Cushard 1971).

Urine chemistry

The daily calcium excretion is very low in hypoparathyroidism; this is the consequence only of the very low ionised calcium level in the serum as tubular calcium reabsorption is in fact diminished in hypoparathyroidism (Peacock et al 1969). Tubular phosphate reabsorption (measured by TmP/GFR) is increased in hypoparathyroidism (Bijvoet 1969).

Special tests

The EDTA infusion test for identifying patients with 'partial hypoparathyroidism' has been described by Parfitt (1969a). The nature of the disorder identified by this test and its need for treatment are both controversial, so that the place of the test cannot yet be defined. In any case the test is unpleasant for the patient and contra-indicated in any patients with hypocalcaemia.

Tests for effect of parathyroid hormone These tests are used to distinguish between hypoparathyroidism and pseudohypoparathyroidism. The tests are only needed in patients with no history of neck surgery and no family history or physical signs of pseudohypoparathyroidism. In all the varieties of this investigation, parathyroid extract (PTE) is administered and the test is of no value if the potency of the PTE is not confirmed in a normal person. A number of different measurements have been made to assess the response to PTE (Purnell 1971). These include phosphate excretion, as in the original Ellsworth-Howard test, serum calcium and urinary cyclic AMP. In normal subjects phosphate excretion increases three-fold or more after PTE while even greater proportional increases are found in patients with hypoparathyroidism. In pseudohypoparathyroidism the urinary phosphate seldom rises more than two-fold, but there is some overlap with the normal range. The most valuable index of response to PTE is provided by urinary cyclic AMP. With this measurement there is a clear distinction between patients with pseudohypoparathyroidism and all other disorders (table 9.2). Moreover several disorders (basal cell naevus syndrome, Gardner's syndrome and idiopathic familial calcification of the basal ganglia), once thought to involve resistance to parathyroid hormone, are also seen to have normal responses (Aurbach et al 1970). When the PTE test is needed the measurement of cyclic AMP provides the most satisfactory method of assessment but is not widely available.

TABLE 9.2. Urinary excretion of cyclic adenosine 3',5'-monophosphate (cyclic AMP) after infusion of parathyroid hormone (data of Chase et al 1969). Results are for a three hour period on a control day and the day of the infusion.

| Subjects | Cyclic AMP (μmoles in 3 hour period) | |
	Control day	Infusion day
Normal	0·62	3·90
Pseudohypoparathyroidism	0·47	0·63
Idiopathic hypoparathyroidism	0·38	4·43
Pseudopseudohypoparathyroidism	0·86	2·98
Surgical hypoparathyroidism	0·42	3·78

TREATMENT

The principal agents used for the control of hypocalcaemia in hypoparathyroidism are calcium, vitamin D and dihydrotachysterol. Parathyroid extract (PTE) has been tried in the past: it is of doubtful value because it must be given by injection and because the patient becomes resistant to its action within a few weeks. Intramuscular injection is painful and intravenous injection is not without risk of protein shock. The resistance to PTE, no doubt caused by antibody formation to the protein constituents of the extract, means that PTE has no place in the long-term management of hypoparathyroidism at present. Some authors feel that PTE may be useful in the early stages of acute hypoparathyroidism (Sisson & Vander Aarde 1971).

Acute hypoparathyroidism

In patients with symptoms of hypocalcaemia after thyroid surgery calcium should be given as a very slow intravenous injection of 10% calcium gluconate (containing 100 mg calcium gluconate or 9 mg calcium in 1 ml). The initial dose should not be greater than 10 ml although it may be followed by 20 ml to 30 ml calcium gluconate solution added to an intravenous infusion. Particular caution is needed in patients who are on digitalis. The treatment may be repeated appropriately according to the patient's symptoms or serum calcium results. As soon as possible oral calcium supplements should be started. In patients who are difficult to control there may be a place for PTE but after one or two weeks vitamin D or dihydrotachysterol should be started. However most patients with acute tetany after neck surgery do not go on to permanent hypoparathyroidism and the calcium therapy can be reduced gradually and stopped.

Chronic hypoparathyroidism

In some milder cases of surgical hypoparathyroidism oral calcium supplements may be adequate to control symptoms. In most cases of surgical hypoparathyroidism and all cases of idiopathic hypopara-thyroidism oral therapy with vitamin D or dihydrotachysterol is needed. The amounts of vitamin D used are grossly in excess of the physiological requirement; typical doses for the control of hypopara-thyroidism are in the range 1·25–5 mg (50,000–200,000 units) daily and a few patients require even more.

In these doses vitamin D raises the serum calcium mostly by an action on intestinal calcium absorption whereas dihydrotachysterol operates principally by promoting calcium release from bone (Mautalen 1970, Hunt & Morgan 1970, Kaye et al 1971). For these reasons vitamin D (usually D_2) is probably the treatment of choice, although it has the disadvantage of being rather slow in action and slowly eliminated after an episode of poisoning. In the future meta-bolites or analogues of vitamin D may become available for treatment (De Luca 1972).

The initial dose of vitamin D should be 1·25 mg daily by mouth and the amount should be increased by increments of 1·25 mg at intervals of not less than two weeks. When the serum calcium is approaching the normal range the dose should be adjusted monthly. The serum calcium should always be used for the control of therapy;

the Sulkowitch test on urine should be abandoned. While vitamin D is being given it is reasonable to give oral calcium supplements of 1–2 grams per day. Some authors use much larger calcium supplements but there is no good evidence of their value. Other authors recommend a low phosphorus diet or aluminium hydroxide in addition but there is little evidence that these measures contribute enough to justify the effort. Occasionally patients are resistant to the action of vitamin D in the doses described (Pak et al 1970). Some of these respond to much larger doses of vitamin D: one current personal patient requires 12·5 mg (500,000 units) vitamin D_2 daily to be symptom-free with a low-normal serum calcium. Some patients respond more readily to a different sterol such as cholecalciferol or dihydrotachysterol and others are resistant to the whole range of sterols. The reason for this resistance is not known although some patients have steatorrhoea and others are magnesium depleted and improve when this is corrected (Rösler & Rabinowitz 1973). Other patients respond to 25-hydroxycholecalciferol. A few patients have an intermittent resistance to vitamin D and so run a great risk of vitamin D poisoning.

A maintenance dose of vitamin D should be that which abolishes symptoms and brings the serum calcium into the lower end of the normal range. Even when this dose is reached the patients should be followed up indefinitely. Major changes in the sensitivity to vitamin D are found in some patients and intoxication has been reported on doses of vitamin D as low as 0·5 mg daily (Ireland et al 1968). An increase in sensitivity to vitamin D is often unexplained but recognised causes include thiazide therapy (Parfitt 1972b), pregnancy (Wright et al 1969) and vitamin D poisoning (Leeson & Fourman 1966a). In addition some patients with surgical hypoparathyroidism appear to recover their parathyroid function after a few months and attempts should be made in these patients to reduce the vitamin D dose as far as possible. The management of vitamin D poisoning is discussed on page 119. After an episode of poisoning vitamin D should be restarted with great caution.

There have been many attempts to treat hypoparathyroidism with parathyroid gland transplants. Until recently these have all been unsuccessful but in 1973 Groth et al reported survival of a homologous parathyroid gland implant in a patient on immuno-suppressive drugs for a renal transplant.

HYPOPARATHYROIDISM IN PREGNANCY

The symptoms of hypoparathyroidism may be made worse by pregnancy (Fourman et al 1963) but it is doubtful whether pregnancy ever causes hypocalcaemia in patients with 'partial hypoparathyroidism'. Treatment with vitamin D should continue in pregnancy and the dose carefully adjusted with particular attention during the immediate post-partum period when there is a danger of hypercalcaemia (Wright et al 1969). Although congenital hyperparathyroidism in the infant is a dangerous complication of untreated hypoparathyroidism, infants of normocalcaemic mothers are usually normal (Landing & Kamoshita 1970, Goodenday & Gordan 1971). Goldberg (1972) suggested that breast feeding should be discouraged because the milk contains 25-hydroxycholecalciferol.

Mothers with idiopathic hypoparathyroidism may have infants with congenital hypoparathyroidism (Gorodischer et al 1970, Barr et al 1971).

HYPOPARATHYROIDISM IN NEONATES

Congenital hypoparathyroidism is very rare; some cases are familial and others sporadic (Barr et al 1971, Orme 1971). One type is the III/IV pharyngeal pouch syndrome (Di George syndrome) in which there is hypoplasia of the thymus and parathyroids and impaired cellular immunity (Kretchmer et al 1968, Freedom et al 1972). Parathyroid gland aplasia has also been described in association with a ring chromosome 18 (Olambiwonnu et al 1972). Neonatal hypoparathyroidism resulting from maternal hyperparathyroidism has already been described (p. 108).

Congenital hypoparathyroidism usually presents with convulsions in early neonatal life and has to be distinguished from other, more common, disorders causing hypocalcaemia at this age (p. 147). Other patients, presumed to have had hypoparathyroidism since early childhood, present later with mental retardation or epilepsy. At one time it was suggested that hypoparathyroidism was an important cause of sudden unexpected death in infants. More recent studies have lent no support to this view (Valdés-Depena & Weinstein 1971).

In suspected neonatal hypoparathyroidism a parathyroid hormone

(PTH) test is needed to distinguish the disorder from pseudohypo-parathyroidism. However, a phosphaturic response to PTH is not consistently found at this age, and observation of the serum calcium and inorganic phosphorus concentrations is more reliable (Gorodischer et al 1970).

Treatment of neonatal hypoparathyroidism with vitamin D needs careful control and it is easy to cause hypercalcaemia. In one case a regime of weekly vitamin D administration was effective. Patients with good control of the plasma calcium develop with normal milestones and intelligence (Gorodischer et al 1970, Barr et al 1971).

PSEUDOHYPOPARATHYROIDISM

This inherited disorder was first described in 1942 by Albright and his colleagues who reported three patients with the chemical changes of hypoparathyroidism but no response to parathyroid extract. A variety of alternative names has been proposed such as Albright's hereditary osteodystrophy but Albright's original name, pseudo-hypoparathyroidism (PHP) has been generally accepted.

Pathogenesis

Albright concluded that the disorder was caused by a failure of the renal tubules to respond to parathyroid hormone. Many other views have been put forward to explain the disorder (Fourman & Royer 1968, Suh et al 1970), but Albright's suggestion has been substantially confirmed in recent years, from studies of cyclic AMP excretion. It is now clear that the basal excretion of cyclic AMP is low in PHP, but even more striking is the failure of urinary cyclic AMP to rise after the administration of parathyroid extract (table 9.2, Greenberg et al 1972). Thus PHP is a disorder at least of the renal cyclic AMP response to PTH. There is also evidence of an impairment of the response to PTH by the bone (McDonald 1972).

The exact nature of the defect in the response to PTH is not yet clear; there is no deficiency of adenyl cyclase in the kidney (Marcus et al 1971). The response mechanism to cyclic AMP also appears to be intact because patients with PHP respond to dibutyryl cyclic AMP (Bell et al 1972). Other hormones have actions mediated by cyclic AMP; at least in the case of glucagon there is no defect in the cyclic AMP response in PHP (Chase et al 1969).

Inheritance

In most families the inheritance of the disorder is consistant with an autosomal dominant pattern (Weinberg & Stone 1971). Some families include patients with the same physical signs but without hypocalcaemia ('pseudopseudohypoparathyroidism', see below). There appears to be an association of both disorders with Turner's syndrome but the significance of this is not known. In addition there is one case report of the coincidence of Turner's syndrome and idiopathic hypoparathyroidism (Gardner 1970, Tuvemo & Gustavson 1972).

Clinical features

The patients usually present in early childhood with convulsions, tetany, stridor or mental retardation. On examination they may have some of the physical features of hypoparathyroidism such as brittle nails, moniliasis and cataracts. In addition they have evidence of remarkable skeletal abnormalities which are not present at birth but probably result from early closure of certain epiphyses. Thus the patients are generally short with reduction particularly of the lower segment. They have a round face and, most characteristic of all, short metacarpal or metatarsal bones. These abnormalities affect particularly the fourth and fifth metacarpals although the phalanges

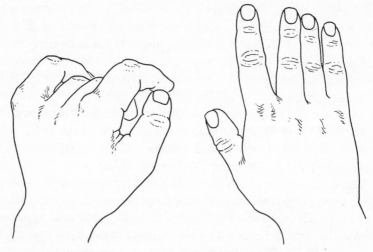

FIGURE 9.3. Hands of a 36-year-old patient with pseudopseudo-hypoparathyroidism. There is marked shortening of the third and fourth metacarpals.

and other metacarpals are also short in some cases. These changes lead to the unusual appearance of the hands which may be demonstrated particularly clearly by noting a dimple in the place of a knuckle when the patient makes a fist (fig. 9.3).

Other changes seen in some patients are ectopic bone formation especially in the skin (Barranco 1971, Eyre & Reed 1971, Brook & Valman 1971), and deformities due to chronic tetany. One 12-year old girl had adopted a 'sitting Buddha' position because of her tetany (Epstein et al 1971).

Radiology
The principal radiological abnormalities are in the skeleton, with the short metacarpals, metatarsals or phalanges. The teeth sometimes show enamel defects, hypoplasia or failure to erupt (Glynne et al 1972). X-rays may show calcification in the skin and other soft tissues and calcification of the basal ganglia is also common. A few patients have radiological evidence of osteitis fibrosa (Cohen & Vince 1969).

Clinical chemistry
The chemical changes in the blood are similar to those of hypoparathyroidism, with hypocalcaemia and hyperphosphataemia (Parfitt 1972a). The high serum phosphate is found in all patients including some with serum calcium levels at the lower end of the normal range. Serum immunoreactive parathyroid hormone levels are increased in PHP and are suppressed normally by induced hypercalcaemia (Chase et al 1969).

The tests of parathyroid hormone responsiveness have already been described. It is important to recognise that in PHP a small rise in urinary phosphorus is often seen after PTE administration, and that there is some overlap in this test between normal subjects and patients with PHP.

Treatment
Patients are treated in the same way as those with hypoparathyroidism with pharmacological doses of vitamin D. This not only relieves the tetany and epilepsy but also greatly improves the intellectual performance. There are few studies of the effect of treatment on growth but one boy grew normally from the twelfth to the sixteenth year on a regime consisting of vitamin D, calcium and aluminium hydroxide (Alterman & Leiber 1965).

Disorders related to pseudohypoparathyroidism

These disorders have a remarkable variety of names. Although Bronsky (1970) has attempted to create a rational classification, the older names are still widely used.

Pseudopseudohypoparathyroidism This name was applied by Albright et al (1952) to a 29-year-old woman with the skeletal anomalies of PHP but no chemical abnormality. While idiopathic brachydactyly might be a better name, pseudopseudohypopara-thyroidism (PPHP) is widely used (for example in *Index Medicus*) and is valuable in that it indicates the relationship of this disorder to PHP. Several families are described with both PHP and PPHP (Frech & McAlister 1970, Weinberg & Stone 1971, Brook & Valman 1971). It is said that PHP can turn into PPHP as the patient gets older (Fourman & Royer 1968).

Patients with PPHP have the same skeletal anomalies, ectopic calcification and mental retardation as patients with PHP (Jewelewicz & Nachtigall 1971). The plasma chemistry is normal but in one study the urinary excretion of cyclic AMP was significantly greater than normal (table 9.2).

Hypohyperparathyroidism This name was used by Costello and Dent (1963) to describe a girl of normal intelligence with bone pains and difficulty in walking. She had hypocalcaemia, hyperphosphatae-mia and the radiological changes in the bones of osteitis fibrosa. The symptoms and all the abnormalities improved with vitamin D therapy in a dose of (0·5–1·0 mg/day). While it is possible that this patient had an unusual form of rickets with secondary hyperpara-thyroidism, the hyperphosphataemia makes this unlikely and similar cases have been reported subsequently. In two cases reported by Frame et al (1972) there was evidence of a defect in the renal tubular response to parathyroid hormone. Although these patients do not have the physical signs of PHP it seems likely that this is a disorder with a similar pathogenesis.

A combination of PHP with radiological osteitis fibrosa has also been reported (Cohen & Vince 1969). Secondary hyperparathyroidism is a well recognised feature of PHP and there is probably no need for a special name for PHP with radiologically evident secondary hyperparathyroidism.

Chapter 10: Osteomalacia and Rickets

Osteomalacia in adults and rickets in children are the bone disorders caused by vitamin D deficiency. This can result from nutritional lack or from failure to absorb the vitamin. A similar syndrome results from defects of the metabolism of vitamin D as in anticonvulsant therapy, renal failure (chapter 11) and perhaps in some patients with liver disease. As these disorders have in common with nutritional vitamin D deficiency the defective production of 1,25-dihydroxy-cholecalciferol, it is reasonable to use the terms osteomalacia and rickets for all of them.

These names have also been applied to a number of disorders which resemble osteomalacia and rickets in some radiological and histological aspects but for which there is even today no evidence of defective metabolism of vitamin D. These include the bone defects associated with acidosis or renal tubular disorders (chapter 12), and metaphyseal dysostosis, hypophosphatasia, 'axial osteomalacia' and fibrogenesis imperfecta ossium (chapter 17).

Historical aspects of osteomalacia and rickets are well reviewed by Fourman and Royer (1968), Dent (1970) and Loomis (1970). The many opinions concerning the origin of the word 'rickets' have been outlined by Hunter (1972).

CAUSES

The principal causes of osteomalacia and rickets are shown in table 10.1.

Nutritional vitamin D deficiency
It is not always appreciated that vitamin D deficiency only occurs in patients who have *both* a dietary lack of the vitamin *and* lack of exposure to adequate ultraviolet light. The effective range of ultraviolet light is between 250 and 305 nm and the penetration of these short waves is limited by atmospheric pollution and by the obliquity

of the rays and thus latitude, season and time of day. Atmospheric pollution caused by coal-burning was a major factor in the great prevalence of rickets in European cities in the nineteenth century. Severe rickets was particularly common in London where it became a problem even among the lions in the zoo. The combination of high latitude with a mild climate is a unique feature of Northern Europe and Loomis (1970) suggested that unpigmented skin was evolved to allow the greatest possible use of such ultraviolet light as is available. Winter sunshine is a very poor source of ultraviolet light so that rickets in infants is most common between January and April.

TABLE 10.1. Causes of osteomalacia and rickets.

Nutritional vitamin D deficiency

Rickets in premature infants
Infantile rickets
Adolescent or late rickets
Osteomalacia in pregnant women
Osteomalacia in elderly women

Disorders of the intestinal absorption of vitamin D

Malabsorption of any cause including coeliac disease, pancreatic
    disorders and biliary obstruction
Partial gastrectomy

Defects of vitamin D metabolism

Anticonvulsant therapy
Renal failure
Liver disease (?)
Vitamin D dependency
Strontium excess (not yet recognised in man)

Similar factors may have contributed to the characteristic skeletal abnormalities of Neanderthal man who lived from 70,000 BC to 35,000 BC. Even in the 19th century palaeontologists suggested that the deformities were those of old rickets and these suggestions have been supported recently by Ivanhoe (1970). It is particularly interesting that the abnormalities are less obvious in remains from southern parts of Europe and that Neanderthal man disappeared, and modern (Cro-Magnon) man appeared, at a time when fishing implements were first noted among the associated remains. For ancient man at high latitudes fish and to a smaller extent eggs would be the only sources of vitamin D.

Today nutritional vitamin D deficiency is found particularly in certain groups of patients.

Neonatal and congenital rickets Rickets has been described as a cause of hypocalcaemic convulsions in the neonatal period. It occurs in infants born of mothers who are themselves depleted of vitamin D and responds rapidly to small doses of vitamin D (Ford et al 1973). On occasion rickets has been identified in antenatal radiographs and confirmed after birth (Russell 1973c).

Rickets in premature infants Premature infants have a very small intake of milk which, even if normally fortified, means that they get very little vitamin D. There is no reason to believe that their requirements are any less than usual and the rickets which might be expected in these infants has recently been described (Keipert 1970, Robertson 1970, Lewin et al (1971).

Rickets in other infants and young children In North America and Northern Europe, improvements in housing, the reduction of atmospheric pollution and the fortification of food with vitamin D led to a substantial fall in the incidence of rickets. In Dundee for instance 20–40 new patients were admitted to hospital yearly with rickets in the 1920's but less than five each year in the 1940's (Stewart et al 1964). In the 1950's a new problem became evident. The incidence of infantile hypercalcaemia in Britain rose and there was strong evidence to incriminate vitamin D sensitivity or excess as a cause (p. 125). Changes in government regulations in 1957 reduced vitamin D intake and led to a fall in the incidence of hypercalcaemia in infants.

In the past decade, an increase in the incidence of childhood rickets has again been noted in large cities such as London and Glasgow (Ford et al 1972a, Holmes et al 1973). This is a disorder both of immigrant and 'white' families, particularly families living in severely over-crowded conditions in central areas of cities. One contributory factor was a failure of the mothers to take advantage of welfare foods and services. It seems unlikely that there is any national food-fortification level for vitamin D which will completely eliminate both vitamin D deficiency and hypercalcaemia from the population; as hypercalcaemia carries a danger to life our present policies are probably satisfactory provided careful attention is paid to the families most at risk.

It is interesting that the modern successor to the slums, the multi-storey tower, may also contribute to the development of rickets. In Rouen in 1962 rickets was described in children from multi-storey flats. They had spent most of their time in rooms on the north side of the block and, because of the effort needed, were seldom taken outside by their parents (Evreux 1962).

Childhood rickets remains a major problem outside Europe. Rickets is well recognised in India (Agrawal et al 1969, Manchanda and Lal 1972) and tropical Africa (Antia 1970, Kendall 1972). Although sunlight is abundant in these areas exposure may be inadequate because the children spend much of their time inside dark huts or because they stay in purdah with their mothers. Rickets is found in urban children throughout the world including such unlikely places for a sunlight-deficiency disease as Australia, Texas, South Africa and the Middle East (Lipson 1970, Mayne & McCredie 1972, Nichols et al 1970, Robertson 1969 & 1970). These cases occur in children from underprivileged families with poor housing and without the will or the means to attend welfare clinics. In Texas one factor was the high price of milk and the lack of refrigeration. In India rapid industrialisation is sadly creating living conditions in towns similar to those of nineteenth century England.

Late rickets in adolescents There is a peak in the incidence of rickets in adolescents; it may be that the growth spurt at this age calls for an increased vitamin D intake. In Britain late rickets is particularly a disease of immigrants and both boys and girls are affected (Clark et al 1972, Ford et al 1972a). As in younger children this is a disease of urban life in smoky cities; additional factors among immigrants include the skin pigmentation and the traditions by which the girls tend to be confined to the house. That Asian immigrants to Britain have, as a group, a poor supply of vitamin D is suggested by the study of Preece et al (1973) who showed that they had lower levels of 25-hydroxycholecalciferol in the serum than European controls. One further factor has recently been explored: the diet of Iranians, Indians and Pakistanis includes a large amount of phytic acid, and this reduces calcium absorption in the intestine. Whether this contributes to the bone disease in these patients remains controversial for it responds promptly to the administration of vitamin D (Ford et al 1972b, Holmes et al 1973, Reinhold et al 1973, Dent et al 1973).

Osteomalacia in younger women In Britain osteomalacia has been described in pregnant immigrants by Felton and Stone (1966) and by Clark et al (1972). The same factors probably contribute to the vitamin D deficiency in this group as in the adolescent immigrants and it is likely that there is an increased requirement for vitamin D at this time; one of Felton and Stone's patients probably had osteomalacia in two successive pregnancies with symptomatic improvement in between. Severe dietary deficiency of vitamin D from religious restrictions or food fads was the cause of osteomalacia in a further group of young women, both Asian and European (Dent & Smith 1969). Outside Europe osteomalacia is common among women whose work or traditions preclude adequate exposure to sunlight. Thus it is common in Iran among carpet-makers who work for long hours in a dark and dusty environment (Chapman 1971). Osteomalacia is recognised too among Bedouin women, who expose very little skin to sunlight when they do leave their black goat-skin tents (Groen et al 1965).

Osteomalacia in elderly women Vitamin D deficiency osteomalacia has been increasingly recognised in the past decade among elderly women both in Britain and France (Chalmers et al 1967, Rosin 1970, Berthaux et al 1970). Some of these patients had had gastric surgery but most had not and were clearly examples of nutritional osteomalacia. In most cases it is possible to obtain a clear history of a diet with a poor vitamin D content; some elderly women insist on eating butter, which they can ill afford, when they would be wiser to use margarine with its higher vitamin D content. In addition it is usually possible to obtain a history of lack of exposure to sunlight. One of the patients of Gough et al (1964) had not left her room for ten years and another seldom went outside her small dark cottage. Sometimes a vicious circle seems to operate; an arthritis or the early symptoms of osteomalacia makes the patient even less likely to venture outside so that the disorder progresses rapidly.

Osteomalacia and rickets in malabsorption syndromes
Any malabsorption syndrome can cause osteomalacia or rickets but the differential diagnosis of malabsorption is outside the scope of this book. Useful reviews include those by Dyer and Dawson (1968), Ament (1972), Creamer (1974) and Losowsky et al (1974).

There is no consistent relationship between the severity of the steatorrhoea, the defect in calcium absorption and the likelihood of osteomalacia. In pancreatic disease fat malabsorption may be severe but osteomalacia is relatively uncommon, whereas after partial gastrectomy osteomalacia often occurs without steatorrhoea. Many factors contribute to the defects of calcium metabolism in patients with malabsorption.

Vitamin D is absorbed in the dueodenum and the jejunum, and bile salts are needed (Hollander et al 1971, Heaton et al 1972). Thus osteomalacia is recognised in obstructive jaundice (Sherlock 1968) and after therapy with cholestyramine which sequesters bile salts and reduces their entero-hepatic circulation (Heaton et al 1972). Vitamin D malabsorption may result from the blind-loop syndrome; it is suggested that the bacteria in the blind-loop promote the deconjugation of bile salts into bile acids (Tabaqchali 1970, Rogé et al 1973). Vitamin D malabsorption probably occurs in pateints who develop osteomalacia with chronic laxative abuse (Frame et al 1971a) and in patients with mucosal defects as in coeliac disease. However vitamin D deficiency is not the only cause of the defective absorption of calcium in these cases. Calcium absorption is diminished in coeliac disease, after extensive intestinal resection and in Crohn's disease but seldom in pancreatic insufficiency (Sjöberg & Nilsson 1970). This is probably the reason for the failure of physiological doses of vitamin D to heal the bone in patients with malabsorption.

Coeliac disease Nassim et al (1959) made balance studies on patients with osteomalacia due to gluten-sensitive enteropathy. They found that vitamin D (orally or parenterally) had no effect on calcium absorption until gluten was excluded from the diet. The gluten-free diet by itself improved calcium absorption considerably. They concluded that in coeliac disease there was a 'resistance' to the action of vitamin D. On the other hand two of their patients responded to oral vitamin D in a dose of 1·25 mg daily with a rapid rise in the serum phosphorus. Rose (1967) showed that ultraviolet light (equivalent, he felt, to a physiological dose of vitamin D) caused a marked increase in phosphorus absorption in two patients with coeliac disease and osteomalacia. The change in calcium absorption was small in one and negligible in the other. Figure 10.1 shows a response to parenteral vitamin D in another patient with coeliac disease.

These results suggest that there is a true vitamin D deficiency in coeliac disease. Patients with this disorder are resistant to vitamin D only in that oral vitamin D is not well absorbed and parenteral vitamin D is ineffective in promoting calcium absorption while the intestinal lesion persists.

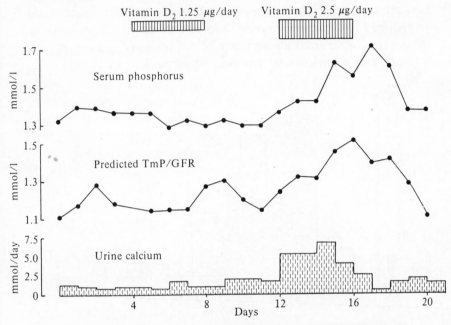

FIGURE 10.1. Acute effects of very small parenteral doses of vitamin D_2 in a 58-year-old woman with osteomalacia due to coeliac disease. With 2·5 µg vitamin D_2 there was a rise in the serum phosphorus which was associated with a rise in TmP/GFR. There was also an increase in the calcium excretion in the urine but no change in serum calcium or serum alkaline phosphatase (Unpublished study with Dr. D. B. Morgan).

Osteomalacia after partial gastrectomy

Incidence Partial gastrectomy became widely used in the management of peptic ulcer in the 1920's and osteomalacia was first reported as a sequel by Sarasin (1941) in Switzerland. Since then there have been at least 27 reports or series of patients with osteomalacia after gastrectomy and several attempts to define its incidence. Although biochemical abnormalities of the serum calcium or alkaline phosphatase occur in up to 15% of patients with a gastrectomy, osteomalacia can only be demonstrated in about 3% of the women and less than 1% of the men (Morgan et al 1965a, Higgins & Pridie 1966, Ambler et al 1970). Osteomalacia after gastrectomy provides a unique opportunity for examining the time course of vitamin D depletion. Figure 10.2 shows that there is an interval of five to fourteen years between the operation and the onset of symptoms. This period could be required for stores of vitamin D to be used up just as two or more years elapse after total gastrectomy before stores of vitamin B_{12} are depleted and megaloblastic anaemia develops (Cox et al 1963).

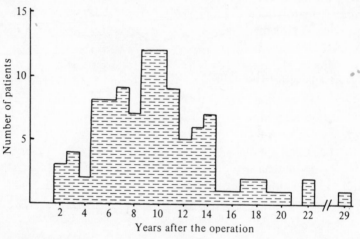

FIGURE 10.2. Interval between operation and onset of symptoms in 94 published cases and nine unpublished cases of osteomalacia after partial gastrectomy.

Osteomalacia appears to be uncommon after other operations for peptic ulcer. There have been four cases after gastroenterostomy (Nordin & Fraser 1956, Deuil et al 1963, Chalmers et al 1967) and one after vagotomy and pyloroplasty (Mitchell et al 1971). Most of these patients were elderly ladies however and it is difficult to be sure that the bone disease was a consequence of the gastric surgery.

Pathogenesis The pathogenesis of osteomalacia after gastrectomy is still not clear but it does respond to very small doses of vitamin D (2·5 µg daily by injection) (Morgan et al 1965b). Factors possibly contributing to the vitamin D deficiency include failure of intestinal absorption, dietary lack and lack of sunlight.

Malabsorption could be a factor. As many as half of the patients with a gastrectomy have steatorrhoea (Butler 1961, Clark 1963).

Possible mechanisms for this include precipitate gastric emptying, inadequate stimulation of the pancreas, inadequate mixing of pancreatic juice with food, or bacterial colonisation of the blind-loop in the Polya operation (Deller 1965, Wormsley 1972, Tomkin & Weir 1972). A few patients may develop malabsorption because of the unmasking of a previously asymptomatic gluten enteropathy (Hedberg et al 1966) or disaccharidase deficiency (Bank et al 1966). Whatever the mechanism of the malabsorption, the osteomalacia could result from it. However osteomalacia has been described in patients who do not have steatorrhoea (Thompson et al 1966, Morgan et al 1970). Furthermore Hillemand et al (1961) described a patient with steatorrhoea and osteomalacia nine years after a Polya gastrectomy. Conversion of the operation into a Billroth I type with re-establishment of the continuity of the stomach and duodenum cured the osteomalacia without affecting the steatorrhoea. Thus osteomalacia is not always related to fat-malabsorption. Vitamin D malabsorption however must be a factor in some cases. One of our patients had no steatorrhoea and a dietary intake of vitamin D in excess of 6 μg daily, yet her osteomalacia responded rapidly to parenteral treatment with vitamin D in a dose of 2·5 μg daily (Morgan et al 1970).

Another factor in a few patients may be dietary vitamin D lack. Some gastrectomy patients have a poor appetite and avoid particularly those foods, rich in vitamin D, which they were advised to eat before their operation as part of the peptic ulcer diet. Seven out of seventeen patients of Morgan et al (1970) took less than 2 μg vitamin D daily.

Osteomalacia and rickets in liver disorders
Bone disease is well recognised in patients with obstructive jaundice (Ask-Upmark 1939, Atkinson et al 1956) and consists of osteomalacia or osteoporosis or both. The osteomalacia responds well to small doses of vitamin D by injection (Sherlock 1968 & 1970, Dent 1970) and the disorder seems likely to be the result of vitamin D malabsorption. Rickets also occurs in neonates as a consequence of biliary obstruction or hepatitis (Bastis-Maounis et al 1973). While the likeliest explanation is vitamin D malabsorption, Yu et al (1971a) suggested that defective hepatic hydroxylation of vitamin D could be important. In adults with chronic hepatocellular jaundice osteomalacia is seldom seen perhaps because prolonged survival is uncommon (Paterson & Losowsky 1967).

Osteomalacia and rickets associated with anti-convulsant therapy.

Osteomalacia and rickets after prolonged treatment with anti-convulsant drugs has been reported since 1967 (Schmid 1967, Dent et al 1970, Genuth et al 1972, Borgstedt et al 1972).

Incidence There have been several attempts to determine the frequency with which this complication is found among patients on prolonged anticonvulsant therapy; most have consisted of studies of the incidence of a low serum calcium or a high serum alkaline phosphatase (ALP). Both in children (Hunter et al 1971, De Luca et al 1972) and in adults (Richens & Rowe 1970, Sotaniemi et al 1972, Hahn et al 1972a) abnormalities were found in between 20% and 40% of the patients. However, some of these studies failed to take account of the higher alkaline phosphatase values found in normal adolescents and the value of these surveys is further limited by the lack of confirmation that the patients with the biochemical abnormalities had osteomalacia. Some recent surveys have suggested that patients on prolonged anticonvulsant therapy have a reduced bone density compared with control subjects but only small numbers of patients have so far been studied (Linde et al 1971, Sotaniemi et al 1972, Christiansen et al 1973).

Pathogenesis Although there are deficiencies in many of the surveys discussed, some patients have undoubted osteomalacia or rickets after anticonvulsant therapy. How does this arise? One possibility is malabsorption of vitamin D. Some anticonvulsant drugs cause malabsorption (Reynolds et al 1965) and three of the four patients of Dent et al (1970) had some evidence of malabsorption. On the other hand Schaefer et al (1972) showed that patients with long-term anticonvulsant therapy appeared to absorb labelled vitamin D_3 normally. Another possibility, first suggested by Dent et al (1970), is that the anticonvulsant drugs induce the hepatic enzymes which degrade vitamin D to inactive products. There is now much evidence to support this view. Patients on anticonvulsant drugs have a low plasma concentration of 25-HCC and increased conversion of labelled vitamin D_3 to inactive polar metabolites (Stamp et al 1972, Hahn et al 1972a & b). A case of osteomalacia has been described after prolonged administration of glutethimide, another drug known to induce hepatic enzymes (Greenwood et al 1973).

In conclusion, it seems likely that enzyme-inducing drugs promote increased vitamin D catabolism. This in turn causes osteomalacia or rickets particularly in patients whose vitamin D intake is already marginal. On the basis of the present evidence it is reasonable to seek to prevent vitamin D deficiency in patients on anticonvulsant therapy by increasing the vitamin D intake to 100 μg weekly (Hahn et al 1972a).

Strontium poisoning

A disorder resembling rickets has been recognised for some time in livestock and experimental animals given excessive strontium. Omdahl and De Luca (1971) have now shown that these animals have defective calcium absorption which is improved by 1,25-DHCC but not by 25-HCC. They suggest that the strontium blocks the renal conversion of 25-HCC to 1,25-DHCC. A comparable disorder has not yet been described in man.

Itai-itai disease (? cadmium poisoning)

Soon after the 1939–1945 war a curious bone disease was recognised in the Toyama prefecture in Japan. This affected some 200 patients living near the Jintsu river which was at that time heavily polluted with cadmium, zinc and lead from a mine upstream. These patients had a syndrome resembling osteomalacia with severe bone pains and bone tenderness (hence 'itai-itai' approximately translated 'ouch!-ouch!'). Bone deformity was common and pseudofractures frequently seen. Investigation revealed evidence of severe intestinal damage as well as renal damage. There was a suggestion that the chronic cadmium poisoning was the cause of the disease because the patients had increased levels of cadmium in plasma and urine and because similar intestinal changes were reported in industrial workers poisoned with cadmium.

However this subject remains controversial and the nature of the bone disease is not clear. When investigated subsequently the patients often had evidence of renal tubular defects so that the bone disease could have resulted from phosphorus depletion. However, the serum phosphorus was not unduly low (0·7–0·8 mmol/l) and the urinary excretion of phosphorus was not raised. Furthermore many of the patients with renal tubular defects had previously received very large doses of vitamin D.

While malabsorption of vitamin D could be a factor in the disease, many Japanese authorities now feel that the disease represents nutritional vitamin D deficiency, for almost all the patients were elderly women with a poor diet and many had been confined to their homes (Tsuchiya 1969, Murata et al 1970, Lancet 1971, Takeuchi 1973).

Vitamin D dependency
This is an uncommon disorder which is also known as pseudo-vitamin D deficiency rickets. It is inherited in an autosomal recessive manner and is characterised by rickets, hypocalcaemia, hypophosphataemia and enamel hypoplasia in the teeth. Like vitamin D deficiency the disorder is characterised by impaired intestinal calcium absorption but unlike vitamin D deficiency it does not respond to physiological doses of vitamin D. It does respond completely however to doses of vitamin D of the order of 1 mg daily (although the enamel defects are permanent). These patients have a high serum parathyroid hormone level which becomes normal when the disease is treated. The disorder is now thought to be caused by a defect in the renal hydroxylation of 25-HCC to 1,25-DHCC; it responds only to large does of 25-HCC but improves rapidly when treated with small doses of 1,25-DHCC (Arnaud et al 1970b, Birtwell et al 1970, Mehls et al 1971, Jelonek et al 1971, Ozsoylu & Kaya 1971, Coburn et al 1974, Balsan & Garabedian 1974).

CLINICAL FEATURES

The clinical features of the disorder depend on the age of onset. It is therefore convenient to consider rickets and osteomalacia separately.

Rickets
In the first six months of life most infants with rickets present with tetany or convulsions; they may have only minor skeletal changes at this stage. After six months the child is as likely to present with bone pain or deformities as with tetany.

The classic skeletal disorders include enlargement of the bone ends especially in the wrists, ankles and knees (fig. 10.3). Changes in the costochondral junctions cause a 'rickety rosary'. Softening of the skull causes craniotabes in infants under six months and frontal boss-

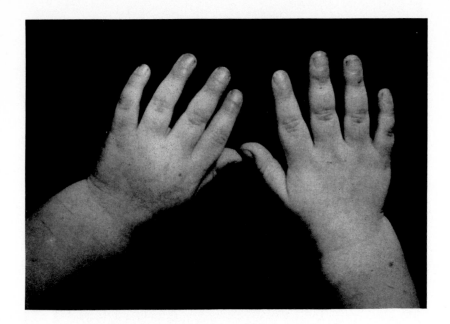

FIGURE 10.3. Enlarged wrists in a two-year-old child with nutritional rickets.

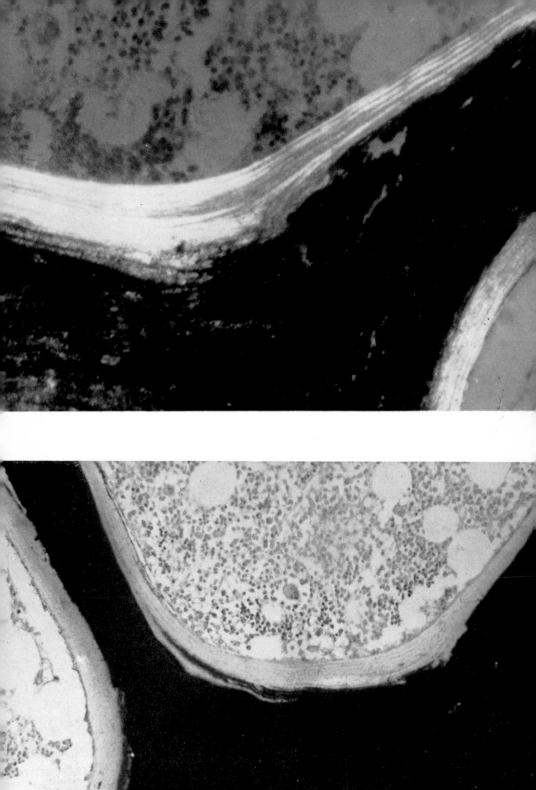

ing in older children. Softening of the ribs may predispose to chest infections and lead to the appearance of Harrison's sulcus, a groove at the points of attachment of the diaphragm. Softening leads to deformities in the long bones, for example knock-knees or bow-legs, while changes in the pelvis may cause serious difficulty in pregnancy in later life. Most of the bony abnormalities improve with vitamin D but some, such as the frontal bossing or bow-legs, persist into adult life as stigmata of former rickets.

In late rickets of adolescence most patients present with bone pain or tetany. Muscular hypotonia or weakness causing a waddling gait, is a prominent feature of some patients of any age.

Osteomalacia

The main symptoms of osteomalacia are bone pains and muscular weakness. The diagnosis is often delayed because the patients are thought to have rheumatoid arthritis, 'fibrositis' or 'lumbo-sacral strain', or simply regarded as neurotic. Jordan (1972) told the story of a 50 year-old school-teacher who came to him because she had run out of analgesic tablets. She complained of severe pains in the ribs and one foot. Fibrositis had been diagnosed but the pains were made worse by the vigorous physiotherapy which had been prescribed. On enquiry he found that she had had a partial gastrectomy four years earlier; she had widespread bone tenderness and radiographs revealed five pathological fractures. One of our own patients was regarded as neurotic for five years before his severe post-gastrectomy osteo-malacia was diagnosed.

Bone pains are a symptom of the majority of patients with osteo-

---

Facing page top
FIGURE 10.4. Histological appearance of bone from a 68-year-old woman with osteomalacia after gastrectomy. All bone surfaces are covered by osteoid, and an irregular zone of calcification extends into the thickness of one of the layers of osteoid. Magnification × 200. Von Kossa and neutral red staining of undecalcified double-embedded section. From Woods (1972) by permission.

Facing page bottom
FIGURE 10.5. Same patient as figure 10.4. Undecalcified section, with Von Kossa stain, with polarised light to show birefringent laminae. Magnification × 480. (Courtesy of Dr. C. G. Woods).

malacia. Many patients also have muscular weakness (p. 31) so that symptoms often include pain and disability in walking, in rising from a chair or in going up or down stairs. Some patients have a remarkable waddling or 'penguin' gait (Chalmers et al 1967, Morgan et al 1970). Clinical examination in most patients shows bone tenderness, elicited by springing the thorax or pelvis or by pressing on the shins. In some the bone tenderness is so severe that it is painful to turn over in bed. One elderly patient of mine could not walk and complained bitterly of the pain caused when the wheelchair jolted on the uneven floor.

Osteomalacia presents with fractures in a minority of patients. Greenstick fractures in adults appear to be unique to osteomalacia; subtrochanteric fractures of the femur occur particularly in osteomalacia as well as in Paget's disease, osteogenesis imperfecta and osteopetrosis (Chalmers et al 1967, Chalmers 1970).

A few adults with osteomalacia present with tetany. In my experience this is more common in osteomalacia due to coeliac disease than in nutritional or post-gastrectomy osteomalacia. One recent patient presented with tetany and no other symptoms at the age of 27 and was found to have osteomalacia and coeliac disease.

PATHOLOGY

Bone

The characteristic feature of both rickets and osteomalacia is a failure of new bone to calcify. This leads to the appearance of excessive quantities of uncalcified bone matrix, known as osteoid. It is not always appreciated that some osteoid is present in normal bone and that excess osteoid is found in some diseases other than osteomalacia (p. 60). However in osteomalacia the amount of osteoid greatly exceeds that found in normal subjects (table 10.2). Typical undecalcified bone sections from a patient with osteomalacia is shown in figures 10.4 and 10.5. Decalcified sections of bone in osteomalacia frequently provide histological evidence of secondary hyperparathyroidism in the excess of osteoclasts and Howship's lacunae. Special staining methods show that osteoid of normal bone has a 'calcification front' which is greatly reduced in osteomalacia (Bordier & Tun Chot 1972). Bone biopsy has an important place in the diagnosis of osteomalacia provided that the pathologist is able to prepare undecalcified sections.

The abnormal features of the bone in rickets have been recognised for many years (Park 1939, Engfeldt & Hjertquist 1960). Apart from osteoid the most remarkable changes are seen in the epiphyses where the formation of bone from cartilage is greatly disturbed. Normally the cells of the cartilage proliferate to form columns and calcium is deposited on the cartilage. Blood vessels from the metaphysis invade the calcified cartilage; this is then resorbed and replaced by osteoid which calcifies to give the primary trabeculae of bone. In rickets there

TABLE 10.2. The amount of osteoid in normal bone (41 specimens) and in osteomalacic bone (27 specimens). (Data of Woods et al 1968).

Estimate of osteoid	Range (and mean) in	
	normal bone	osteomalacic bone
Number of bright lines in polarised light	0–3	3–12
Proportion of trabecular surface covered by osteoid (%)	0–45 (13·8)	70–100 (93·7)
Area of osteoid in the section in relation to the total area of bone (%)	0–5·0 (1·1)	8·2–61·5 (28·3)

are defects in the calcification of cartilage, the invasion by blood vessels is irregular and the calcified cartilage is not resorbed. The proliferation of cartilage cells continues so that the zone of poorly calcified cartilage, and the epiphysis as a whole, becomes wider. There is an excessive number of osteoblasts in the metaphysis and marrow aspiration in rickets may produce both osteoblasts and osteoclasts in addition to the haemopoietic cells (Barak 1970). In starvation or a severe illness which stops growth the characteristic appearances of rickets are less obvious although osteoid may still be found in the trabecular bone (Park 1954).

Parathyroid glands

Happily the opportunity to examine the parathyroid glands in active rickets or osteomalacia seldom occurs nowadays. In the older literature most patients were found to have hypertrophy of the glands (Kaplan 1942, Bartos & Henneman 1965). Secondary hyperparathyroidism can today be inferred from the bone histology or from measurements of serum PTH levels (see below).

RADIOLOGY

Rickets

The radiological abnormalities of rickets reflect the pathological changes already described; they are best seen at the ends of the long bones although changes in the costo-chondral junctions and the inferior angle of the scapula may be noted on a routine chest radiograph (Greenfield 1969, Weiss 1971). The epiphyses are widened and, instead of being separated from the metaphyseal bone by a smooth line, the separation is irregular, cupped and indistinct (figs. 10.6 & 10.7). The epiphyseal centres appear late and are often indistinct. The bone shafts appear poorly calcified and especially in the legs may become deformed. In severe cases deposits of bone under the periosteum are seen. Fractures, especially greenstick fractures, are common but Looser's zones are seldom seen.

The first radiological sign of healing is the appearance in two to three weeks of a dense line in the epiphyseal cartilage, separate from the metaphysis. This results from mineralisation of the recently formed cartilage. Further mineralisation then continues between this line and the metaphysis. A ring of calcification may be seen around each ossification centre; this later fuses with the rest of the centre. Healing of the epiphysis is completed in the next few months and some of the deformities also correct themselves. Residual changes include translucent defects in the bone, consisting of islands of trapped cartilage, and areas of thickening of the cortex on the concave side of persistently bowed bones.

Changes very similar to those of rickets are seen in renal tubular disorders (chapter 12) and in some children with hyperparathyroidism. The changes of metaphyseal dysostosis and hypophosphatasia have some resemblance to rickets but those of scurvy and phenylketonuria are usually easy to distinguish (Greenfield 1969, Feinberg & Fisch 1972, Macpherson et al 1972).

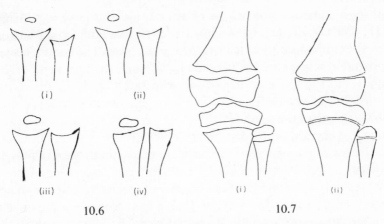

10.6   10.7

FIGURE 10.6. Rickets in an 18-month-old baby. Tracings from serial radiographs of the wrist (i) two months and (ii) one month before vitamin D. No change is seen. (iii) One month and (iv) two months after the start of vitamin D therapy, showing widening of the shafts of the radius and ulna, enlargement of the epiphyseal ossification centre and narrowing of the epiphyseal gap. From Fourman and Royer(1968) with permission.

FIGURE 10.7. Rickets in a 16-year-old Pakistani male. (i) Before vitamin D, (ii) Four months after a single dose of 1·5 mg vitamin D_2. From Fourman and Royer (1968) with permission.

Osteomalacia
As a group, patients with osteomalacia have thin bones. Morgan et al (1970) showed that seventeen patients with osteomalacia after gastrectomy had significantly thinner cortical bone than control subjects of the same age and sex who had had the same operation at the same time. However all but two of their patients were within a 95% range for the controls. Thus assessment of bone thinning contributes nothing to the diagnosis of the individual patient with suspected osteomalacia.

The hallmark of osteomalacia is the pseudofracture or Looser's zone (Looser 1920). This is sometimes known as Milkman's syndrome after an American who redescribed it some years after Looser. In France the pseudofracture has been called a Looser-Milkman-Debré zone. Pseudofractures consist of bands of decalcification two or three millimetres wide across or at one side of a bone (figs. 10.8–10.11). They resemble fractures but are sometimes symmetrical and on clinical examination there is little local tenderness. The common sites for pseudofractures are the ribs, the pubic rami, the upper end of the femora and the outer border of the scapulae. Fig. 10.12 shows the distribution of pseudofractures in thirty patients of Chalmers et al (1967). If present, pseudofractures are strong evidence for osteomalacia. They are not found in any other disorders although linear translucencies *through abnormal bone* are occasionally seen in fibrous dysplasia and in Paget's disease (fig. 15.3). Early fractures and stress fractures may resemble Looser's zones radiologically and are sometimes symmetrical; they may be found in osteogenesis imperfecta or after long-term steroid therapy (Camp & McCullough 1941, Chalmers 1968). Pseudofractures are not found in all patients with

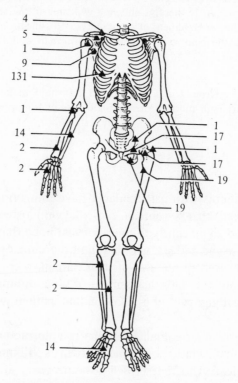

FIGURE 10.12. Positions of pseudofractures in 30 patients. Data of Chalmers et al (1967).

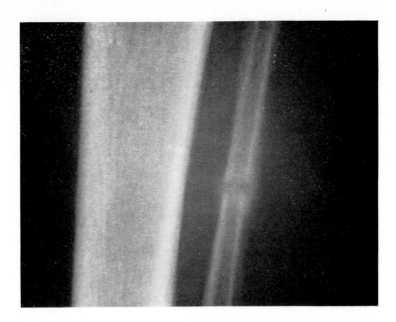

FIGURE 10.8. Pseudofracture in fibula. Man aged 52 with coeliac disease.

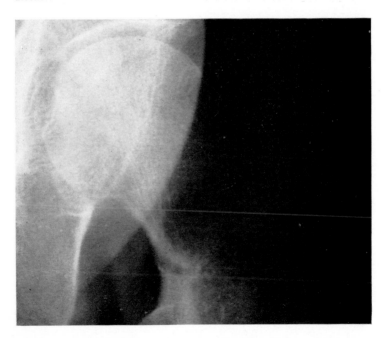

FIGURE 10.9. Pseudofracture in neck of femur. Osteomalacia in a 69-year-old woman who had had a total gastrectomy.

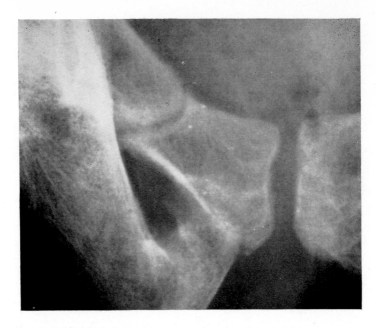

FIGURE 10.10. Pseudofracture in superior pubic ramus. Osteomalacia after partial gastrectomy in a man of 50.

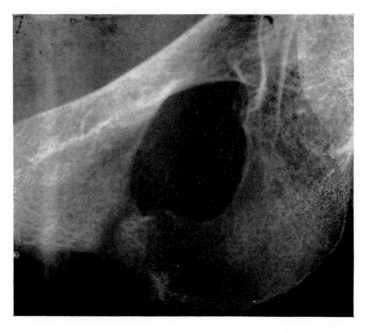

FIGURE 10.11. Pseudofracture in inferior pubic ramus in a woman of 55 with osteomalacia after gastrectomy.

osteomalacia. They were present in 30 of the 37 patients of Chalmers et al (1967) and 11 of the 23 patients of Morgan et al (1970). A failure to find pseudofractures (or any other abnormality) in no way rules out osteomalacia.

Less common radiological features of osteomalacia include fractures in the trabecular bone of the vertebrae which become bi-concave (the 'cod-fish vertebrae'). This appearance is not unique to osteomalacia; it is also found in osteoporosis and osteogenesis imperfecta. Other deformities, of the pelvis for example, are uncommon. Some patients have radiological evidence of secondary hyperparathyroidism notably subperiosteal erosions in the hands.

CLINICAL CHEMISTRY

Blood chemistry

Almost all patients with osteomalacia have a high serum alkaline phosphatase (ALP). Many have a low serum phosphorus and some also have a low serum calcium. A few patients with osteomalacia due to malabsorption have a normal serum ALP value; the same patients often have a very low serum calcium. Fig. 10.13 shows results found in

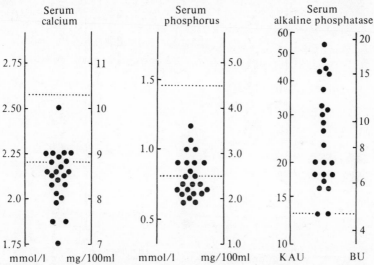

FIGURE 10.13. Serum calcium, phosphorus and alkaline phosphatase values in 23 patients with osteomalacia after gastrectomy (Morgan et al 1970). The approximate normal ranges are indicated by the dotted lines.

one large series of patients with post-gastrectomy osteomalacia. Similar results are found in nutritional osteomalacia. In children the biochemical diagnosis of osteomalacia is complicated by the lack of a satisfactory normal range for serum ALP, although very high serum ALP results are suggestive of osteomalacia. At this age radiology and the serum phosphorus are more valuable clues to the presence of rickets.

Ca × P product The product serum calcium × serum phosphorus has been widely regarded in the past as a useful diagnostic test for osteomalacia or rickets. This was particularly true when a low Ca × P product was thought to reflect an abnormality in the extra-cellular fluid important in the pathogenesis of the bone disorder. In practice the Ca × P product is of limited value even as an empirical test. Figure 10.14 shows the substantial overlap between patients with

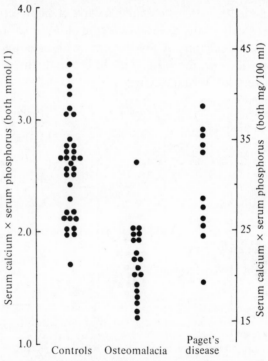

FIGURE 10.14. The product serum calcium × serum phosphorus in fasting patients with osteomalacia after gastrectomy and patients with Paget's disease of bone compared with control subjects with a gastrectomy but without bone disease.

osteomalacia and control subjects in one series. A similar overlap was noted by Chalmers et al (1967) and I do not feel that the Ca × P product provides any information not obtained from the original serum values themselves.

Plasma 25-hydroxycholecalciferol Methods have recently been devised for the estimation of 25-HCC in the plasma. These show low values in patients with vitamin D deficiency and high values in patients receiving treatment with vitamin D (Bayard et al 1972, Preece et al 1973).

Urinary chemistry and clearances
The urinary excretion of calcium is usually low in osteomalacia and rickets. Of 18 patients reported by Morgan et al (1970), 17 excreted less than 2 mmol daily while nine excreted less than 1 mmol daily. Hydroxyproline excretion in the urine is high in some patients but in

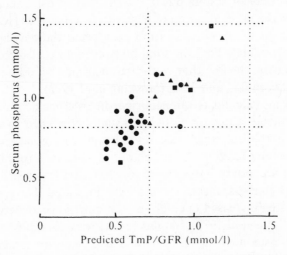

FIGURE 10.15. Relationship between predicted TmP/GFR and fasting serum phosphorus in 36 patients with osteomalacia. ■: Nutritional osteomalacia; ●: osteomalacia after gastrectomy; ▲: osteomalacia due to malabsorption.

our experience it is not abnormal as often as serum alkaline phosphatase and provides no additional information (Morgan et al 1970).

Patients with osteomalacia frequently have an impaired renal tubular reabsorption of phosphate (as measured by TmP/GFR) and amino-acids (Snapper & Kahn 1960, Fraser et al 1967, Dent & Stamp 1970). In a personal series of patients with osteomalacia (fig. 10.15) it was clear that predicted TmP/GFR was abnormal rather more often than the serum phosphorus. It should be recognised that amino-aciduria and phosphaturia in a patient with rickets or osteomalacia can be the result of vitamin D deficiency or malabsorption. This syndrome should not be taken as evidence of a primary renal tubular disorder without further investigation (MacCuish et al 1970).

Pathogenesis of the chemical abnormalities

A defect in calcium absorption and a negative calcium balance is a characteristic feature of osteomalacia and rickets even in patients without intestinal disease (Prakash & Ahuja 1971). At the same time there is a defect in the mineralisation of bone. Kinetic studies have yielded a variety of results but it is clear that in osteomalacia there is a delay in the mineralisation of new osteoid (Harris & Heaney 1969 or 1970). Even when mineralisation does occur the new bone has a low mineral content. That the total body calcium is also reduced can be inferred from the fact that, with treatment, the total body calcium rises by between 3% and 30% (Hosking et al 1972).

The serum calcium is often normal in osteomalacia despite the defect in calcium absorption. This is usually attributed to secondary hyperparathyroidism which releases calcium from bone and reduces urinary calcium excretion. Although not all patients have histological evidence of secondary hyperparathyroidism and fewer still have the radiological changes, recent reports have indicated that serum PTH levels are often increased in children with nutritional rickets (Arnaud et al 1972, Joffe et al 1972). Similar results were found in adults with nutritional osteomalacia or osteomalacia due to malabsorption (Bordier et al 1973b), so that it is likely that secondary hyperparathyroidism is a common accompaniment of rickets and osteomalacia.

The low serum phosphorus is closely related to the reduced tubular phosphate reabsorption. This in turn could be caused by the hyperparathyroidism (Fraser et al 1967) but the possibility that the vitamin D deficiency contributes directly to this defect has not been excluded (Morgan et al 1965b). The amino-aciduria could also be the result of the secondary hyperparathyroidism (Fraser et al 1967).

Special investigations in osteomalacia

The calcium infusion test Nordin and Fraser (1956) reported that patients with osteomalacia retain more of an infused dose of calcium than normal people. A high retention of the calcium has been regarded by many authors as diagnostic of osteomalacia. While subsequent work has confirmed the high calcium retention of osteomalacia, high retentions are also found in many patients without osteomalacia (Lever et al 1967). It is doubtful whether this test has any part to play in the diagnosis of osteomalacia.

TREATMENT

In vitamin D deficiency the response to vitamin D can be regarded as having two stages (Parfitt & Frame 1972). In the first stage, taking perhaps one day, the concentration of vitamin D metabolites builds up in their sites of action. In the second stage, covering a period of months or years, normal bone structure is restored by what must be a complex repair process, the parathyroid glands involute and stores of vitamin D are repleted. Giving excessive doses of vitamin D does not expedite the healing of the bone; it merely exposes the patient to the danger of vitamin D poisoning.

Preparations of vitamin D It is not always appreciated that the accuracy of the vitamin D content of many preparations is poor and that the shelf-life is limited. In view of this, reports that some groups of patients require unusually large doses of vitamin D for healing should be treated with caution. In particular vitamin D deteriorates when exposed to light and when mixed with other vitamins or with calcium (Parfitt & Frame 1972).

Nutritional rickets

Vitamin D in a dose of 100 μg (4,000 iu) daily should be given by mouth in the first instance. In almost all cases the serum phosphorus (and serum calcium if low) begins to rise within a week and radiological evidence of improvement is seen within eight weeks. When healing is well advanced the dose of vitamin D should be reduced to 10 μg daily. An alternative method is to give a single intramuscular injection of 10 mg (400,000 units). In patients with vitamin D deficiency this dose does not cause intoxication and the method is particularly useful for patients whose parents are unlikely to follow instructions carefully. Usually no further treatment is needed but an effort should still be made to follow up the child.

A few patients are said to require slightly larger doses of vitamin D than those described. This was particularly noted in late rickets in immigrants from North India and Pakistan. The patients could have failed to take their tablets, but it is possible that the phytate content of their diet contributed to the disorder of calcium metabolism. While some studies suggested a possible place for the elimination of chapattis from the diet, these patients also respond satisfactorily to vitamin D (Ford et al 1972b, Holmes et al 1973, Dent et al 1973). Very large doses of vitamin D are needed in 'vitamin D dependent rickets' which was discussed earlier.

Patients with tetany, convulsions or stridor need intravenous calcium supplements. Fraser (1971) advises the use of 10% calcium gluconate solution diluted five-fold with 5% glucose in water. The dose should be 2 ml of the diluted solution per kg per hour (3·75 mg calcium per kg per hour). The dose should be adjusted with reference to serum calcium values; results around the lower end of the normal range are quite satisfactory provided that the tetany has been relieved. The calcium infusion may need to be continued for as long as five days. The addition of heparin (1000 units per litre of diluted calcium solution) is valuable for preventing blockage of the infusion catheter.

In addition to vitamin D all patients should have an adequate calcium intake to allow for the repletion of the skeletal calcium content. A liberal supply of milk is the best method but Fraser (1971) suggests oral calcium supplements of 0·5 to 1·0 g daily as well for the first four weeks.

The deformities of the long bones in rickets improve with vitamin D and orthopaedic intervention is very seldom needed.

Nutritional osteomalacia in adults
This responds well to vitamin D orally in doses similar to those in infants but it is often simpler to use single large doses of vitamin D by injection. This is a reasonable course particularly for immigrants and for the elderly whose life may already be complicated enough with medicines which must be taken regularly. My policy with these patients is to give a single intramuscular dose of 1 mg (40,000 units)

when the chemical investigations have been completed and a bone biopsy has been done. This dose begins the healing of the osteomalacia and if osteomalacia is not present there is no danger of overdose. As soon as the histological diagnosis has been confirmed I advise an additional intramuscular dose of 10 mg (400,000 units). The patient is followed up regularly thereafter; in most cases healing progresses steadily and no further vitamin D is needed. A persistently raised serum alkaline phosphatase is not an indication for further vitamin D in a patient whose symptoms and other chemical tests are satisfactory. A high serum alkaline phosphatase may be found for as long as three years after treatment is begun (see below).

Patients should have oral calcium supplements of say 1 gram daily for six months to a year while the bone is healing.

Osteomalacia after gastrectomy
This is treated in the same way as nutritional osteomalacia but vitamin D should be given parenterally in all patients. Most patients respond well to a single intramuscular dose of 10 mg vitamin D_2.

Osteomalacia or rickets in coeliac disease
The bone changes of coeliac disease do not heal with the usual doses of vitamin D even by injection. With larger doses, 1 mg vitamin D daily or more by mouth or 0·25 mg daily by injection, partial healing of the bone takes place and tetany and bone pain are relieved. However the disorder responds well to a gluten-free diet and the bones heal eventually with this alone. It is reasonable to use vitamin D for two or three months in patients who have tetany or bone pains. As the gluten-free diet begins to be effective the sensitivity to vitamin D increases rapidly so that careful follow up is needed to avoid vitamin D poisoning in these cases.

Whether or not vitamin D is used, oral calcium supplements of 1–2 grams daily should be given for three to six months.

Osteomalacia or rickets with anticonvulsant therapy
Physiological doses of vitamin D have not been tried in this disorder but it does respond briskly to moderate doses (100 μg daily by mouth or parenterally) even if the anticonvulsant therapy continues (Dent et al 1970).

Features of the response to treatment with vitamin D

Both in children and in adults the first chemical sign of response to vitamin D is usually a rise in the serum phosphorus seen within one week. It is associated with an increase in renal tubular phosphate reabsorption (Morgan et al 1965b, Rosin 1970, Dent & Stamp 1970). The serum alkaline phosphatase (ALP) falls gradually to normal in most patients but in some with severe bone disease the fall is preceded by a substantial rise (fig. 10.16). In the extreme case shown, a woman

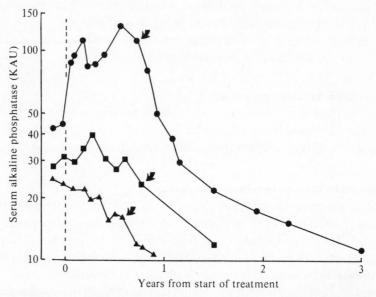

FIGURE 10.16. Changes in the serum alkaline phosphatase with vitamin D therapy in three patients with osteomalacia after partial gastrectomy. In this study the patients were treated initially with vitamin D_2 25 μg IM weekly. At the point indicated by the arrow this was discontinued and the patient was given a single intramuscular dose of 10 mg vitamin D_2. No further vitamin D was given.

aged 50, three years elapsed before the serum ALP became normal but her severe symptoms had been relieved within a month of starting treatment with vitamin D. A similar early rise in serum ALP has been reported among children with rickets (Bodansky & Jaffe 1934). It probably represented a temporary increase in bone cell activity while the osteomalacia was healing, for a rise in urinary hydroxyproline was

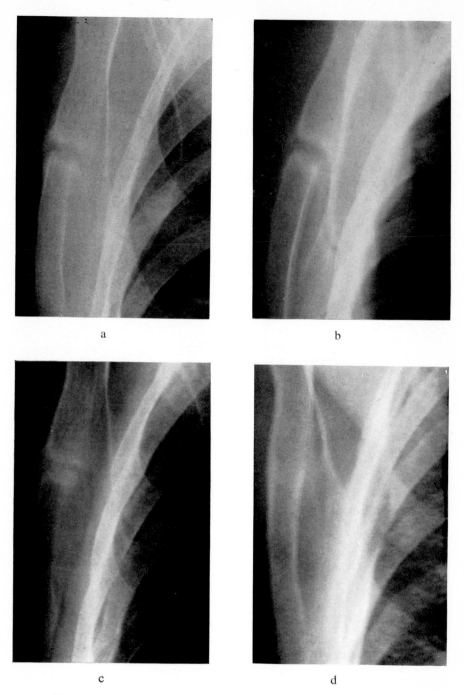

FIGURE 10.17. Changes in a pseudofracture in the right scapula in a 50-year-old woman with osteomalacia after gastrectomy; a: before treatment; b: after 1½ months treatment with vitamin D; c: after 4 months treatment; d: after 16 months treatment.

noted both in our patient and in another patient with osteomalacia treated with ultraviolet light (Nordin & Smith 1964).

The effects of treatment on the radiological appearances in rickets have already been described. On average 3–4 months is needed for healing in infants with 100 μg/day (Shelling & Hopper 1936). In adults the pseudofractures, if any, show changes within two months of the start of treatment. At first they are more prominent as their edges become more dense. They disappear althogether within six to eight months (fig. 10.17).

There is seldom any need to obtain histological evidence of response to treatment. When repeat biopsies are done, the earliest change is a marked increase within a week of the proportion of osteoid having a calcification front (Bordier et al 1969). Later, there is a progressive reduction of the quantity of osteoid. Some patients also show evidence of increased bone cell activity with numerous osteoblasts and osteoclastic resorption of osteoid (Fischer et al 1970).

One of the most satisfactory aspects of making a diagnosis of osteomalacia is the improvement in the patient's symptoms with treament. The patients often feel less miserable within a week, with reduction of bone pain in two to three weeks and loss of bone tenderness by three months. The muscle weakness and disability improve dramatically. Children with rickets improve rapidly; even the deformities of the long bones improve so that there is seldom a need for orthopaedic intervention.

Chapter 11 : Uraemic Osteodystrophy

The bone disease associated with chronic renal failure consists of osteomalacia (rickets in children) osteitis fibrosa and osteosclerosis, but the relative severity of these three components varies from patient to patient. In some patients on regular dialysis there is also a progressive loss of bone (osteopenia).

A variety of names have been used for this disorder. Uraemic osteodystrophy is the most satisfactory. Renal rickets or renal dwarfism should not be used because the disorder consists of more than rickets and because these terms have also been used for the bone changes associated with renal tubular defects. Useful reviews of uraemic osteodystrophy include those by Katz et al (1969), de Wardener (1972) and Stanbury (1972).

PATHOPHYSIOLOGY

Many factors contribute to the disturbance of calcium metabolism in uraemia. These have been well reviewed by Wills (1971c) and recent studies on vitamin D metabolism have made it easier to explain the physiological disturbance. Figure 11.1 illustrates some of the mechanisms involved.

Defects in 1,25-dihydroxycholecalciferol synthesis
Many patients with uraemia have defective calcium absorption and the radiological and histological features of osteomalacia or rickets. However these defects respond only to large doses of vitamin D and so have been described as 'vitamin D resistant'. Recent advances in our understanding of vitamin D metabolism (chapter 1) have clarified the nature of this resistance. In uraemic or in anephric patients there is no defect in the conversion of cholecalciferol to 25-hydroxycholecalciferol (25-HCC). There is good evidence that such patients have a defect in the hydroxylation of 25-HCC to 1,25-

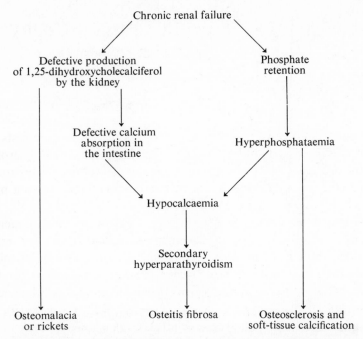

FIGURE 11.1. Probable mechanisms underlying the disturbances of calcium metabolism and the changes in the bones as a result of renal failure.

DHCC which takes place in the kidney (Mawer et al 1973). Furthermore Brickman et al (1972b) administered 1,25-DHCC in a dose of 2·7 μg daily for six to ten days to three patients with advanced renal failure. All three patients showed a rise in calcium absorption (fig. 11.2) and the patients who were not on long-term haemodialysis also showed changes in the serum calcium and phosphorus (fig. 11.3). This response to a very small dose of 1,25-DHCC makes it clear that defective production of the metabolite contributed to the disorder in these patients. Whether lack of this metabolite is also directly responsible for the defective mineralisation of bone is still uncertain (Bordier et al 1973a).

Phosphate retention

A high serum inorganic phosphorus is a common feature of uraemia. It is caused by the reduction in renal phosphorus excretion at a time when there is no defect in intestinal phosphorus absorption; the

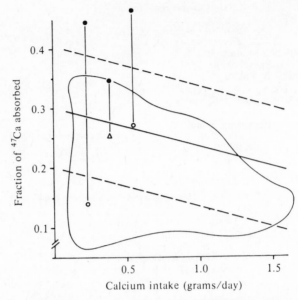

FIGURE 11.2. Effect of a small dose of 1,25-dihydroxycholecalciferol on the fraction of ^{47}Ca absorbed by patients with uraemia in relation to the previous dietary intake of calcium. The interrupted lines enclose the 95 per cent range in 50 normal subjects while the curved area encompasses the range of values obtained in 89 patients with advanced renal failure. Open circles (○) are values before treatment, closed circles (●) are values on treatment and the open triangle (△) a 'control' value for one patient obtained 26 days after the end of treatment. From Brickman et al (1972b) by permission.

phosphorus load may actually increase because secondary hyper-parathyroidism causes increased bone resorption (Krane 1970).

Hyperphosphataemia probably contributes to the hypocalcaemia of uraemic patients and it is suggested that as the plasma phosphorus rises salts of calcium and phosphate are precipitated in tissues (Bricker 1970). This cannot be the only cause of hypocalcaemia because many patients have hypocalcaemia with normal serum phosphorus concentrations (Cochran & Nordin 1971). The likelihood of calcium phosphate precipitation, often crudely related to the product serum calcium × serum phosphorus (Ca × P), increases as the serum phosphorus rises and is probably the main factor in the soft-tissue calcification and areas of bone sclerosis sometimes seen in renal failure.

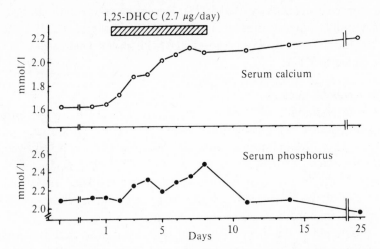

FIGURE 11.3. Changes in serum calcium and serum phosphorus in a 58-year-old man with chronic renal failure, who was given 1,25-dihydroxycholecalciferol for seven days. From Brickman et al (1972b) by permission.

Secondary hyperparathyroidism

Hypocalcaemia results from both the hyperphosphataemia (Slatopolsky et al 1972) and from the impaired intestinal absorption of calcium (Gregory & Messner 1969, Ogg 1969, Cochran & Nordin 1971, Hesch et al 1972). In turn hypocalcaemia causes secondary hyperparathyroidism and parathyroid hyperplasia has long been recognised as a feature of the pathology of chronic renal failure. More recently several studies have shown that the level of PTH in the serum is markedly increased in most patients with renal failure (Reiss et al 1969, Buckle 1970, O'Riordan et al 1970). Even a modest degree of renal failure, without hypocalcaemia, may be associated with an excess of PTH in the blood. In most cases calcium infusion causes a fall in the plasma PTH but there are some exceptions presumably in patients who have developed an autonomous hyperparathyroidism.

Resistance to the action of PTH The high plasma levels of PTH are associated with normal or low plasma calcium concentrations so the tissues may be said to be 'resistant' to the action of PTH. Similarly exogenous PTH causes a much smaller change in plasma calcium and phosphorus in patients with renal failure than in patients with hypoparathyroidism (Massry et al 1973). Recent work on the metabolism of vitamin D suggests that PTH influences the synthesis of 1,25-DHCC in the kidney and it may be a defect at this point which leads to the resistance to PTH.

Other possible factors

Acidosis Systemic acidosis is frequently found in renal failure and the factors responsible have been outlined by Muldowney et al (1972). In addition these authors suggest that the secondary hyperparathyroidism contributes to the acidosis. It is not known whether this acidosis in turn contributes to the bone disorder although an excess of osteoid is found in acidosis with other causes (Lennon 1969, Cochran & Nordin 1969).

Calcitonin It has been suggested that calcitonin secretion might contribute to the hypocalcaemia of renal failure or to the resistance to PTH. While assays for calcitonin are still very insensitive (p. 47), plasma calcitonin-like activity was normal in one group of patients with uraemic osteodystrophy (Chittal et al 1971).

Magnesium metabolism Hypermagnesaemia is often found in renal failure and acute hypermagnesaemia is known to inhibit the release of PTH in experimental animals. However there is as yet no evidence that hypermagnesaemia contributes to the bone disorder of uraemia (Kleeman et al 1970, Wills 1971c).

Effect of regular dialysis

The disorders of bone associated with uraemia are not relieved by dialysis, although with judicious dialysis the plasma level of calcium can become normal. There is no improvement in the intestinal calcium absorption (Messner et al 1969). Plasma levels of PTH remain elevated on dialysis (Genuth et al 1970, O'Riordan et al 1970, Goldsmith et al 1973) and some of the factors which contribute to the continuing hyperparathyroidism during dialysis can be identified. In some patients autonomous (tertiary) hyperparathyroidism must be a factor but other important factors include the calcium and magnesium content of the dialysis fluid (Fournier et al 1971a & b, Pletka et al 1971). Many factors could contribute to the progressive bone loss which is seen in some patients (p. 199) but the parathyroid overactivity is probably the most important for the loss is more severe when the dialysate calcium concentration is low (Bone et al 1972).

Women on regular dialysis bear children who have no apparent skeletal disease; it seems likely that the fetal kidney is able to produce 1,25-DHCC (Ritz et al 1973).

Effect of renal transplantation
In most patients successful renal transplantation leads to improvement in the intestinal absorption of calcium, a prompt fall in the serum PTH and a regression of the hyperparathyroid bone changes (Messner et al 1969, Hampers et al 1969, Johnson et al 1971b). In a few patients hypercalcaemia develops after transplantation (p. 202).

CLINICAL AND PATHOLOGICAL FEATURES

Despite the severe hypocalcaemia few patients with renal failure get tetany. The lack of tetany is usually ascribed to the simultaneous acidosis and this is reasonable because correction of the acidosis with intravenous sodium bicarbonate can precipitate tetany in uraemic patients.

BONE CHANGES

Pathology
The main histological changes in the bone are (a) those of rickets or osteomalacia, with an excess of osteoid, and (b) evidence of secondary hyperparathyroidism, notably excessive activity of osteoblasts and osteoclasts, and fibrous tissue deposition in the marrow. In some patients the osteomalacia is the dominant abnormality while in others it is the osteitis fibrosa. Ellis and Peart (1973) indicated that the osteitis fibrosa usually appeared early in the course of the renal disease while osteomalacia occured later. The secondary hyperparathyroid changes of renal failure differ from those of primary hyperparathyroidism in that bone resorption is seldom excessive and osteosclerosis with the patchy formation of woven bone is seen more often (Ingham et al 1973, Ellis & Peart 1973). Overall the total amount of bone in the skeleton does not greatly differ from that in normal people (Duursma et al 1972). Patients with chronic renal failure have these histological abnormalities in the bone much more frequently than they have radiological abnormalities or symp-

toms related to bone disease (Katz et al 1969, Kaye 1971, Ingham et al 1973).

Clinical features

Few patients with uraemia present with symptoms due to the bone disease. Occasionally children come with epiphyseal displacement or rachitic deformities and children are more likely than adults to get crippling deformities and bone pain. In adults bone pain and fractures are uncommon before dialysis.

Radiology

A great variety of radiological changes may be seen in the bones in uraemia; these reflect the pathological disorders already discussed.

Children The most common finding in children is a general loss of bone density with a thin cortex and indistinct trabeculae. Changes in the epiphyses resemble those of vitamin D deficiency rickets but the epiphyses are not cupped. Slipped epiphyses are more common than in vitamin D deficiency; they probably result from the hyperparathyroidism because they also occur in primary hyperparathyroidism and secondary hyperparathyroidism with other causes (Kirkwood et al 1972). Other consequences of hyperparathyroidism include subperiosteal resorption in the phalanges, metacarpals and other sites. In some areas the bone resorption is so severe that the radiological appearance has been compared with a 'rotting fence post'.

Bone growth is poor in children with uraemia and may be abnormal in character, with a thickening of the skull and an overgrowth of the mandible and maxilla (fig. 11.4). Some patients have an increased bone density in the base of the skull and in the vertebrae where it is best shown up by lateral radiographs. In some patients the whole of each vertebra is sclerotic; in others the increased density is confined to the upper and lower thirds of each bone and this appearance has been called the 'rugger-jersey spine'. Metastatic calcification is less common in children than in adolescents or adults.

Adults The radiological changes of hyperparathyroidism are found in 25% of the patients with histological abnormalities. Rather more patients show abnormalities if high resolution industrial film is used (Kaye 1971, Doyle 1972, Meema & Meema 1972). The bone resorption may be very severe including subperiosteal, subchondral and subtendineal resorption of any bone. The earliest changes are most easily detected in the hands, especially in the metacarpals and

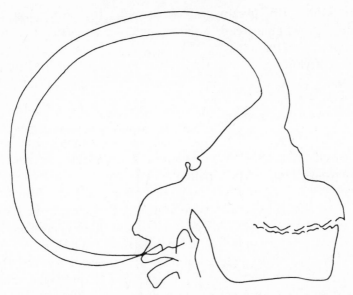

FIGURE 11.4. Uraemic osteodystrophy in a 17-year-old girl. Tracing from a skull x-ray to show the prognathism and the thickned calvarium. From Fourman and Royer (1968) by permission.

the proximal and distal phalanges. Parts of the distal phalanx may be completely resorbed causing shortening and 'pseudo-clubbing' of the fingers. The lamina dura usually disappears. The other bone changes of uraemic osteodystrophy include osteosclerosis, notably in the end plates of the vertebral bodies to give a 'rugger-jersey spine' as in children (Zimmerman 1962).

Results of dialysis
A progressive symptomatic bone disease has been recognised during regular haemodialysis especially in certain centres such as Newcastle-upon-Tyne (Siddiqui & Kerr 1971, Simpson et al 1973) and Los Angeles (Parfitt et al 1971 & 1972). These patients had bone pains and fractures and radiological evidence of progressive rarefaction. The cause of the disorder is uncertain; one factor may be a hitherto unidentified constituent in the tap-water used for making up the dialysis fluids.

In other dialysis centres this severe disease is less common but even among their patients there is persisting radiological and histological evidence of parathyroid overactivity. In addition the bone histology shows an increase in the amount of osteoid and a reduction in the amount of bone (Bishop et al 1972, Woods et al 1972). The bone changes of children on regular dialysis were outlined by Ritz et al (1973).

PARATHYROID GLANDS

In a series of patients with uraemic osteodystrophy, Katz et al (1969) found that 88% of those who came to autopsy had abnormal parathyroid glands. Most patients had chief-cell hyperplasia but the glands were rather larger than is usual in primary chief-cell hyperplasia and the cells were more uniform. A few patients had water-clear cell hyperplasia (p. 30). A full account of the pathology and ultra-structure of these glands has been given by Roth and Marshall (1969). The parathyroid glands of non-suppressible or tertiary hyperparathyroidism seldom show any additional morphological abnormality although adenomas are occasionally noted (Black et al 1970a, Grimelius et al 1972).

METASTATIC CALCIFICATION

Metastatic deposits of calcium are often found in uraemia. The principal sites are the arteries, cornea and conjunctiva, soft tissues particularly near joints, and rarely in the skin, lungs, stomach, heart and parathyroid glands (Parfitt 1969b, Caldwell et al 1971). Calcification is found in the kidney; while the location of this is often similar to that found in primary hyperparathyroidism, local factors in the renal disease also contribute ('dystrophic calcification'). Metastatic calcification is more severe and more extensive in patients whose product serum calcium × serum phosphorus is greater than 5·6 mmol/l × mmol/l (70 mg/100 ml × mg/100 ml).

Metastatic calcification occasionally causes clinical problems (Parfitt 1969b). Calcification around joints, notably in the shoulders, hands and elbows, sometimes causes distressing pain and limitation of movement. Calcification in arteries seldom causes ischaemia but occasional cases of ischaemic myopathy have been reported (Goodhue et al 1972). It may cause difficulties in the surgery of the arteries in inserting shunts or performing transplants. Calcification in the cornea (band keratopathy) is seen in a few patients with renal failure but calcification in the conjunctiva is more common and is probably the cause of the acute red eye sometimes found in renal failure (Berlyne 1968). Patients with uraemia often complain of pruritis and recent evidence has suggested that secondary hyperparathyroidism contributes to this; it is sometimes relieved by parathyroidectomy (Massry et al 1969).

There have been a few reports of patients with patchy necrosis and calcification of subcutaneous fat by a process which may be comparable to calciphylaxis (Anderson et al 1968, Rees & Coles 1969).

CLINICAL CHEMISTRY

Undialysed patients

There is some advantage in distinguishing between patients whose bone disease is predominantly osteomalacia and those who have predominantly osteitis fibrosa. There are significant differences in the plasma and urine chemistry between these two groups (Stanbury & Lumb 1966, Hioco et al 1972).

Serum calcium The total serum calcium is low in most patients with the osteomalacic form of the disease but rather higher, often within the normal range, in those with osteitis fibrosa. In the group as a whole the serum calcium is lower in the patients with the most severe renal impairment; there is a reduction in both protein-bound and ionised fractions of the serum calcium (Kleeman et al 1970, Weeke & Friis 1971).

Serum inorganic phosphorus The serum inorganic phosphorus is high in most patients whose creatinine clearance is less than 25 ml/min and may be very high; values up to 3 mmol/l are frequently seen and values as high as 6 mmol/l are reported. In general higher values are found in those patients who have marked osteitis fibrosa.

The calcium × phosphorus product Elsewhere in this book I have discouraged the calculation of the product serum calcium × serum phosphorus. It may however have some empirical value in the management of patients with renal failure. Very high Ca × P products, found in the patients with osteitis fibrosa, are associated with a greatly increased risk of metastatic calcification and values greater than 5·6 mmol/l × mmol/l (70 mg/100 ml × mg/100 ml) are an indication for the use of phosphate-binding antacids (de Wardener 1972).

Serum magnesium Most patients with renal failure have a mild to moderate elevation of the serum magnesium (Katz et al 1969, Kleeman et al 1970).

Serum alkaline phosphatase About one third of the patients in the series of Katz et al (1969) had high values for serum alkaline phosphatase. The highest values were found in the patients with marked osteitis fibrosa, but normal values did not exclude bone disease (Bishop & Smith 1971, Hioco et al 1972).

Serum acid phosphatase Katz et al (1969) drew attention to the high values of serum acid phosphatase in some patients with severe osteitis fibrosa. This was less frequently abnormal than alkaline phosphatase and the value did not exceed the upper limit of the normal range by a factor of more than two.

Plasma and urine hydroxyproline Although the urinary excretion of hydroxyproline is raised in some patients with the osteomalacic form of bone disease and many patients with osteitis fibrosa, this investigation is often impracticable in renal failure. The non-protein-bound fraction of the plasma hydroxyproline is increased particularly in patients with osteitis fibrosa and is probably a useful measure of bone resorption (Kaye 1971, Bishop & Smith 1971, Hioco et al 1972).

Patients on regular haemodialysis

In each dialysis the serum calcium rises and the serum phosphorus falls. The extent of the rise in serum calcium depends on the calcium content of the dialysis fluid and the factors which contribute to this acute rise are discussed by Tamm et al (1971). Over a long period of regular dialysis there is a slow rise in the pre-dialysis values for both phosphorus and calcium in most patients. At the same time serum alkaline phosphatase rises in a minority of patients but does not alter in the others (Katz et al 1969, Parfitt et al 1971).

There have been isolated case reports of patients who have developed severe hypercalcaemia while on regular dialysis. These are probably examples of autonomous hyperparathyroidism for they respond only to parathyroidectomy (Coburn et al 1969b, Grimelius et al 1972). Hypercalcaemia during regular haemodialysis has also been reported in patients treated with a calcium-containing ion exchange resin for hyperkalaemia (Sevitt & Wrong 1968, Papadimitriou et al 1968), and with oral calcium carbonate supplements (Ginsburg et al 1973).

Patients after renal transplantation

In the majority of patients who have successful renal transplantation the serum calcium and serum phosphorus rapidly return to normal. The serum PTH falls and the hyperparathyroid changes in the bones regress (p. 197). In a few patients hypercalcaemia develops after transplantation. In some of these patients it is temporary and represents perhaps the time needed for the involution of the hyperplastic parathyroids or the mobilisation of metastatic calcifications, In others the hypercalcaemia persists and calls for parathyroid surgery (Johnson et al 1971b, Hornum 1971, Grimelius et al 1972).

TREATMENT

The principles underlying the management of the disordered calcium metabolism of uraemic patients has been well reviewed by Kleeman et al (1970). The objective of therapy include (1) the maintenance of plasma concentrations of calcium and phosphorus as nearly normal as possible, (2) the correction and prevention of metastatic calcification, (3) the suppression of parathyroid overactivity and (4) the maintenance of a normal bone mass. In the light of the pathophysiology of uraemic bone disease (fig. 11.1) a rational approach to the disorder should include measures to reduce the phosphate retention and to mitigate the effects of the disordered vitamin D metabolism.

Correction of osteomalacia-like features

Some patients with uraemia have a clinical syndrome resembling osteomalacia and bone pains may become the dominant complaint. 1,25-dihydroxycholecalciferol promptly corrects the defect in intestinal absorption found in uraemia (Brickman et al 1972b) and this substance, or another vitamin D metabolite, should also prevent the osteomalacia or rickets. However, it is not yet available for routine use and a number of alternative methods have been advocated for controlling the osteomalacia-like aspects of the disease. These include vitamin D in large doses, dihydrotachysterol and oral calcium supplements.

Vitamin D Vitamin D in sufficiently large doses (more than 1·25 mg (50,000 units) daily is usually needed) improves calcium absorption, relieves the bone pain and heals the bones in patients with predominant osteomalacia (Fletcher et al 1963). The main worry about vitamin D is the possibility of vitamin D poisoning with the consequent dangers of metastatic calcification and further deterioration in renal function. Patients taking vitamin D should therefore be followed very closely; they should also receive aluminium hydroxide to lower the plasma phosphorus and reduce the chance of metastatic calcification developing (Mallick & Berlyne 1968).

Dihydrotachysterol In patients on regular dialysis modest doses of dihydrotachysterol (DHT) (0·25–0·375 mg/day) corrects the defect of calcium absorption and improves at least the osteitis fibrosa element of the bone disorder (Kaye & Sagar 1972). DHT may be effective because it is already hydroxylated at the position equivalent to carbon 1 of cholecalciferol. After hydroxylation in the liver at the 25 position DHT becomes an analogue of 1,25-dihydroxycholecalciferol (fig. 11.5). In support of this view Sagar et al (1972) reported a patient with hypoparathyroidism and renal failure who showed no response to 10 mg vitamin D_2 daily but was well controlled on 0·125 mg DHT daily.

Calcium supplements Liberal quantities of calcium carbonate (20–30 g/day) cause a greatly improved calcium absorption and also to a small extent binds phosphate in the gut and corrects a mild

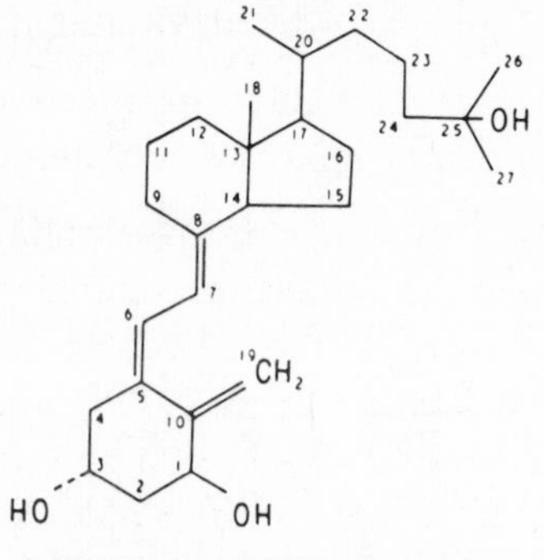

1,25 dihydroxycholecalciferol
(1,25-DHCC)

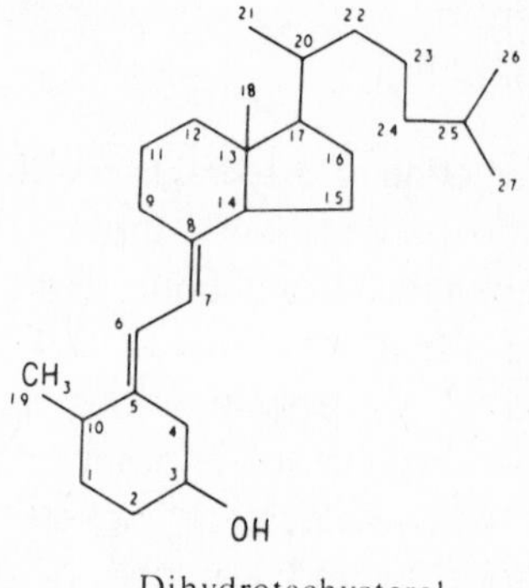

Dihydrotachysterol$_3$
(DHT$_3$)

FIGURE 11.5. Structural formulae of 1,25-dihydroxycholecalciferol and dihydrotachysterol$_3$ to show that the hydroxy-group attached at position 3 of DHT is equivalent to that at position 1 of 1,25-DHCC. The more usual form of DHT (DHT$_2$) differs from DHT$_3$ only in having a vitamin D_2-type side chain.

metabolic acidosis. According to de Wardener (1972) calcium supplements promote healing of the bones and relief of pain. As with
vitamin D therapy there is a danger of metastatic calcification especially in patients with marked hyperphosphataemia. The serum calcium
level should be followed carefully. In patients on regular haemodialysis calcium carbonate may cause hypercalcaemia (Ginsburg et al
1973).

Control of phosphate excess
Phosphate retention is a major cause of secondary hyperparathyroidism. Slatopolsky et al (1972) showed that if the phosphorus
intake of dogs was reduced at the same time as the renal function
was being reduced there was no evidence of parathyroid overactivity.
The same probably applies to man because in Israel, where dietary
intakes of phosphorus are generally lower than in Western Europe
and North America, uraemic bone disease is less common (Berlyne
et al 1973). In clinical practice phosphorus absorption can be reduced
by the administration of aluminium hydroxide or aluminium carbonate. These substances bind phosphate in the gut, cause a fall in the
serum phosphorus, a reduction in the serum PTH and an improvement both in the osteitis fibrosa and the metastatic calcification
(Pinggera & Popovtzer 1972, Clarkson et al 1972). The dose needed
is fairly large: 75–200 ml daily of the aluminium hydroxide Gel BP
or up to 24 grams of aluminium hydroxide in tablet form. Patients
may not be prepared to tolerate doses large enough to be effective
in reducing the plasma phosphorus. Proprietary mixtures containing
magnesium hydroxide in addition to aluminium hydroxide should
not be used because of the danger of hypermagnesaemia.

There are two possible side effects of aluminium hydroxide
therapy. Firstly overdose of aluminium hydroxide could lead to
phosphorus depletion and the superimposition of a phosphorus
deficiency bone disease (chapter 12). This can be avoided if the serum
phosphorus is checked regularly. Secondly some aluminium is
absorbed and deposited in the bone. However, there is so far no
evidence of any toxic results of aluminium absorption (Thurston
et al 1972).

Parathyroid surgery
In 1960 Stanbury and others first described the use of subtotal
parathyroidectomy for secondary hyperparathyroidism in uraemia.

Since that time several authors have explored the case for parathyroid surgery (Berens et al 1970, Hubay et al 1970, Fine et al 1970, Esselstyn & Popowniak 1971, Gordon et al 1972). Although in most patients secondary hyperparathyroidism is relieved by appropriate therapy with aluminium hydroxide, vitamin D, DHT or dialysis with an adequate calcium concentration, there remains a few patients who are very difficult to manage without parathyroidectomy. These include patients with continuing radiographic or clinical evidence of osteitis fibrosa, patients with severe or increasing soft-tissue calcification and patients with intractable pruritis. In addition parathyroidectomy is indicated in patients with 'tertiary' hyperparathyroidism, hypercalcaemia during regular dialysis or persistent hypercalcaemia after renal transplantation (Eilert et al 1971, Grimelius et al 1972).

Orthopaedic surgery
After successful renal transplantation patients may benefit from orthopaedic correction of deformities such as those resulting from slipped femoral epiphyses (Vanderhooft & Coleman 1972).

CHOICE OF METHODS OF TREATMENT
Almost all patients with an increase in the serum phosphorus should be given aluminium hydroxide. The dose should be carefully adjusted to bring the serum phosphorus into the upper part of the normal range but no lower. Liberal oral supplements of calcium carbonate should be given in most patients with persisting hypocalcaemia. Vitamin D should be given in patients with bone pain and radiological or histological evidence of rickets or osteomalacia provided that the serum phosphorus is not unduly high. It should be continued until the serum alkaline phosphatase is normal, but the patient should be seen regularly to check the serum calcium. In patients on regular haemodialysis the calcium concentration in the dialysis fluid may have an important bearing on the disturbance in calcium metabolism; a concentration of 1·3 mmol/l is thought to be associated with an increased incidence of osteitis fibrosa and 1·5 mmol/l is now more widely used. Higher calcium concentrations may increase the risk of metastatic calcification.

Patients with tertiary hyperparathyroidism and those with intractable secondary hyperparathyroidism should have a parathyroidectomy.

Chapter 12: Phosphorus Depletion and Acidosis

The bone disorders associated with phosphorus depletion and acidosis are considered together because they resemble each other in many respects and because phosphorus depletion and acidosis occur together in some renal tubular disorders. The bone abnormalities resemble osteomalacia or rickets in their histological and radiological features, but the underlying process differs in that there is no evidence of any defect in vitamin D metabolism. The nomenclature of these diseases is confused and inconsistent. For example if 'rickets' is applied to hypophosphataemic bone disease its use should logically be extended to include hypophosphatasia and metaphyseal dysostosis which also resemble rickets radiologically. If 'osteomalacia' is made to include the defects of chronic acidosis its use must logically be extended to include all other disorders characterised by excessive osteoid (table 3.4, p. 60). In my view this usage is likely to cause confusion and I suggest that the terms rickets and osteomalacia should be reserved for diseases with evidence of deficiency or defective metabolism of vitamin D (table 10.1, p. 166).

CAUSES OF PHOSPHORUS DEPLETION

Table 12.1 lists the principal causes of phosphorus depletion. Useful reviews of these disorders include those by Fourman and Royer (1968), Dent (1970) and Stickler et al (1970).

Familial hypophosphataemia
This disease has also been called primary hypophosphataemia, sex-linked phosphaturic rickets or hypophosphataemic vitamin D-resistant rickets. Familial hypophosphataemia is the most common of the disorders traditionally described as vitamin D resistant rickets. It is inherited in a sex-linked dominant manner; this unusual form of inheritance means that female patients pass the disease on to half of their sons and half of their daughters, while male patients pass the

207

TABLE 12.1. Causes of phosphorus depletion.

Inherited renal tubular disorders

Familial (sex-linked) hypophosphataemia ('phosphaturic rickets').
Cystinosis (De Toni-Debré-Fanconi syndrome).

Acquired renal tubular defects

Hereditary tyrosinaemia.
Wilson's disease (hepatolenticular degeneration).
Neurofibromatosis.
Mesenchymal tumours.

Prevention of intestinal phosphate absorption

Chronic excess of aluminium hydroxide antacids.

---

disease to all of their daughters and none of their sons. The dominance is incomplete: males tend to be more severely affected than females (Briard-Guillemot et al 1972).

Cystinosis

This disease of childhood was formerly called the Fanconi syndrome (or the De Toni-Debré-Fanconi syndrome). Since the term Fanconi syndrome has also been used to describe adults with acquired tubular defects it is probably best avoided. The disorder is inherited as an autosomal recessive and in Birmingham has an incidence of between 1 in 20,000 and 1 in 65,000 (Bickel & Harris 1952). It is characterised by the deposition of crystals of cystine in many tissues particularly the spleen, liver, kidneys and thyroid gland (Chan et al 1970). The main clinical consequences result from the renal changes which include characteristic abnormalities of the proximal tubules. These often have narrow segments with a flattened epithelium adjacent to the glomerulus (the 'swan-neck tubule'). The distal tubules also show abnormalities with flattening and atrophy of the epithelium and interstitial fibrosis sometimes leading to obstruction (Darmady & Stranack 1957, Teree et al 1970).

Reduced renal tubular reabsorption of phosphorus is a constant feature. In addition patients may have any of several other tubular defects such as defective reabsorption of glucose, amino-acids, potassium, calcium or water, or defects in urine acidification (Dent 1970). Cystine may be demonstrated in leucocytes, cultured fibroblasts and in biopsy specimens from the conjunctiva (Schulman et al 1970 a & b). Heterozygotes also have an increased cystine content in leucocytes and cultured fibroblasts (Kroll et al 1973). The natural history of the disease is characterised by the onset of uraemia in late childhood with death at about the age of 10.

A benign form of cystinosis has been described in adults who do not develop renal failure (Brubaker et al 1970).

Other inherited renal tubular defects
Besides familial hypophosphataemia and cystinosis it is likely that there are other inherited renal tubular defects. Some of these present only in adult life. For example Hunt et al (1966) described mixed renal tubular defects and osteomalacia with an autosomal dominant pattern of inheritance in one family.

Acquired renal tubular defects
Some of the diseases included in this section of table 12.1 are also inherited disorders. However the renal tubular defects are caused by post-natal metabolic defects as in tyrosinaemia and in Wilson's disease. If these are treated early renal tubular damage can be pre-. vented. Unexplained renal tubular disorders presenting in adult life are mostly sporadic (Dent & Stamp 1971).

Hereditary tyrosinaemia (tyrosinosis, tyrosyluria) This is a metabolic disorder of tyrosine metabolism and is inherited as an autosomal recessive; it is particularly common among French Canadians in some areas of Quebec. It is caused by deficiency of the enzyme responsible for the conversion of p-hydroxyphenylpyruvic acid (pHPPA) to homogentisic acid and results in accumulation of tyrosine, pHPPA and its metabolites. Untreated the patients develop symptoms in the first year of life and many die of liver failure. Those who survive have a chronic cirrhosis often going on to malignant hepatoma and renal tubular defects leading to hypophosphataemic bone changes. The disease, including the renal and bone defects, responds well to the restriction of dietary tyrosine and phenylalanine (Rosenberg & Scriver 1969, La Du & Gjessing 1972).

Wilson's disease Copper deposition in the renal tubules causes phosphorus depletion and bone disease in adults with untreated Wilson's disease (hepatolenticular degeneration) (Monro 1970, Aksoy et al 1972).

Neurofibromatosis About twenty cases of neurofibromatosis with an osteomalacia-like bone disease have been reported (Mittal et al 1971). The mechanism is not clear but as the patients almost always have hypophosphataemia, renal tubular phosphorus depletion has been suggested as the cause.

Mesenchymal tumours Nine cases of an osteomalacia-like syndrome have been reported in association with distinctive tumours probably of mesenchymal origin (Evans & Azzopardi 1972, Olefsky et al 1972). The tumours appeared to be benign and consisted of fibroblasts, giant cells and numerous blood vessels. The patients had phosphaturia and other evidence of tubular defects. The bone disease responds partially to large doses of vitamin D but, whether or not this is given, excision of the tumour cures the syndrome promptly.

Unexplained sporadic hypophosphataemia This is a disease of adults who present with bone pains and muscle weakness. There is no family history but there is often evidence of other tubular defects such as hyperglycinuria (Dent & Stamp 1971).

Other disorders with secondary tubular defects There are many other causes of defective phosphate reabsorption with or without other tubular abnormalities. These include hypercalcaemia (Lordon et al 1966), hypokalaemia (Vianna 1971) and myeloma (Costanza & Smoller 1963). In none of these conditions however has there been convincing reports of phosphorus depletion bone disease. Chronic poisoning with lead and other heavy metals is another recognised cause of renal tubular defects but the bone changes seen do not resemble those of phosphorus depletion.

Phosphate-binding antacids

Phosphorus depletion due to dietary deficiency is unknown but there have been occasional case reports of severe phosphorus depletion with bone changes and muscle weakness after prolonged treatment with large quantities of aluminium hydroxide (Bloom & Flinchum 1960, Lotz et al 1968, Boelens et al 1970).

PATHOPHYSIOLOGY

Familial hypophosphataemia is characterised by an impaired reabsorption of phosphorus by the renal tubules. Until recently there was controversy whether this was the result of secondary hyperparathyroidism or represented a primary defect in phosphorus transport.

It is now clear that, while most untreated patients have raised plasma levels of PTH, normal values of PTH are found when the serum calcium is raised by vitamin D therapy or calcium infusions (Arnaud et al 1971, Lewy et al 1972). Thus a disorder of the renal tubular reabsorption of phosphorus seems likely to be the primary defect (Glorieux & Scriver 1972). In addition these patients have impairment of the intestinal absorption of phosphorus.

The pathogenesis of the bone disease of phosphorus depletion is still not understood. Because of its resemblance to osteomalacia or rickets, there have been many attempts to find evidence of defects in the metabolism of vitamin D. There is no evidence of defects in the hepatic hydroxylation of cholecalciferol to 25-HCC either in familial hypophosphataemia in man or in phosphorus-depleted rats (Haddad et al 1972 & 1973). Patients with hypophosphataemia respond no better to 25-HCC than to vitamin D itself (Balsan & Garabedian 1972, Pak et al 1972c, Cohanim et al 1972). There is no evidence of defects in the further hydroxylation of 25-HCC to 1,25-DHCC, because the capacity of the intestine for calcium absorption appears to be normal in familial hypophosphataemia (Condon et al 1971b) and because the defect is not corrected by therapy with 1,25-DHCC (Glorieux et al 1974, Coburn et al 1974). The high faecal calcium seen in these patients could be a consequence of the disturbed phosphorus absorption. There are other respects in which phosphorus depletion differs from vitamin D deficiency: clinically these patients seldom get deformities of the pelvis; chemically many patients have a normal serum calcium; histologically there are differences in the orientation of the collagen fibres of compact bone (Engfeldt & Hjertquist 1960).

CLINICAL FEATURES

Children
Familial hypophosphataemia At birth children with this disorder have no abnormal physical signs and usually a normal serum phosphorus for their age. The serum phosphorus falls during the first year. Between the second and fifth year of life growth slows and the signs of the rickets-like bone disease become evident. These include bow-legs or knock-knees, enlarged epiphyses and skull changes such as a prominant forehead or occiput. Other deformities are found in the ribs or clavicles; a rachitic rosary was present in one quarter of the

patients of Stickler et al (1970). Defects in the pelvis or spine are uncommon.

The severity of the disease and the age at which it is recognised varies greatly between families and within families. Untreated the deformities gradually increase during childhood and adolescence but do not progress in adult life. Some patients are not recognised until adult life; they are usually small in stature, with some deformities, and occasionally they present with fractures or spinal cord compression (Highman et al 1970). Other clinical features of vitamin D deficiency are seldom seen. Bone pain not always present and tetany is not seen.

Cystinosis In cystinosis the disorder is usually recognised in the first two years of life and sometimes in the first few months. The bone disease is like that of familial hypophosphataemia but other symptoms due to water depletion or potassium depletion may dominate the clinical picture. Later these patients develop renal failure.

Adults
Adults with phosphorus depletion have a syndrome including bone pains, muscle weakness and sometimes loss of height due to vertebral fractures (Boelens et al 1970, Dent & Stamp 1971).

BONE CHANGES

Pathology
The bone in children with phosphorus depletion resembles that in vitamin D deficiency rickets. One difference has been noted: the cortical bone in phosphorus depletion shows a mineral deficit around the osteocyte lacunae and the canaliculi (Steendijk 1971). In cystinosis the bones may also show the changes of uraemic osteodystrophy. There are relatively few studies of the bone histology in phosphorus-depleted adults; in general the appearances resemble those of osteomalacia with a large excess of osteoid on all trabecular surfaces (Dent & Stamp 1971).

Radiology
The radiological changes of familial hypophosphataemia are occasionally seen in the first six months of life but more commonly they develop between six and eighteen months. The appearances cannot be

distinguished from those of vitamin D deficiency rickets. In adolescence or adult life the bones may show persisting deformity, fractures, pseudo-fractures and exostoses (Stickler et al 1970, Serre et al 1972).

CLINICAL CHEMISTRY

A low or very low serum phosphorus for the patient's age is a uniform feature of this group of disorders. When the cause of the phosphorus depletion is a tubular defect this can be demonstrated by the very low TmP/GFR; sometimes the excreted phosphorus appears to exceed the filtered phosphorus. The serum phosphorus becomes normal or high in patients who develop uraemia.

The serum calcium is normal in patients with familial hypophosphataemia and in most of the other disorders described here. It is low in some cases of cystinosis, either because of the tubular calcium losses or because of uraemia. Hypercalcaemia due to the development of tertiary hyperparathyroidism is rare; only two cases have been reported (Thomas & Fry 1970).

The serum alkaline phosphatase is sometimes very high in children with hypophosphataemia although in many the values are not outside the range found in normal children of the same age. A moderately raised serum alkaline phosphatase is also found in about half of the adults with phosphorus depletion but at no age is there any correlation between the alkaline phosphatase value and the severity of the bone disease.

Patients with cystinosis or acquired tubular defects have other chemical changes appropriate to the tubular lesions. Thus there may be a metabolic acidosis, hypokalaemia, renal glycosuria and aminoaciduria. In cystinosis the blood chemistry is later modified with the onset of uraemia.

TREATMENT

Familial hypophosphataemia
The treatment of familial hypophosphataemia has been the subject of considerable controversy. Until recently the mainstay of treatment had been vitamin D in large doses. Ths induces at least partial healing

of the bones but does not improve growth. The doses of vitamin D needed are close to the toxic range and hypercalcaemia from vitamin D poisoning has been reported frequently. This is a particularly undesirable complication in these patients as it causes renal damage (Moncrieff & Chance 1969, Stickler et al 1970 & 1971, Glorieux et al 1972).

The alternative approach to the management of familial hypophosphataemia has been the use of phosphate supplements. Phosphate by itself had been reported to induce healing of the bone in two patients (Nagant de Deuxchaines & Krane 1967). Some subsequent studies failed to confirm these results perhaps because doses of phosphate were inadequate and phosphate has until recently been used mainly as an adjunct to therapy with vitamin D. Oral phosphate supplements permit healing of the bone with much smaller doses of vitamin D and so reduce the risk of vitamin D poisoning. Recently treatment consisting of high doses of phosphorus together with relatively small doses of vitamin D to prevent hypocalcaemia has been used (McEnery et al 1972, Glorieux et al 1972); this appears to be the method of choice not least because it restores normal growth. Patients should be treated with oral vitamin D (dose range 0·25–1·0 mg daily) and phosphate (1–4 grams of phosphorus daily) and followed up very carefully. The dose of phosphate should be adjusted so that the serum phosphorus is not less than 1·0 mmol/l (3·0 mg/100 ml). The dose of vitamin D should be adjusted so that hypocalcaemia (and therefore secondary hyperparathyroidism) is avoided.

Other patients with phosphorus depletion
In general these patients should also be treated with phosphate supplements and moderate doses of vitamin D. In adults Dent and Stamp (1971) recommend oral calcium supplements for the first year while the bone disease is healing.

Patients with cystinosis may require potassium supplements and alkalis such as sodium citrate and the possible value of thiazide diuretics was explored by Callis et al (1970). In these patients the treatment will need modification when uraemia supervenes. Attempts to delay the progress of the disease with a diet low in cystine and methionine have given encouraging early results (Christensen et al 1970). Renal transplantation from a parent has been used in terminal uraemia with good results (Briggs et al 1972).

BONE DISEASE IN CHRONIC ACIDOSIS

Bone changes resembling those of rickets or osteomalacia have been described in patients with chronic acidosis. While there is little evidence that the acidosis of chronic renal failure contributes to uraemic osteodystrophy (p. 192) there are other patients in whom it does seem likely that chronic acidosis is the cause of the bone disease. This is particularly true of some renal tubular defects and of the acidosis which follows ureterosigmoidostomy.

Pathophysiology There are two views on the cause of the bone disease of chronic acidosis. One is that the acidosis has a direct effect on bone mineralisation, bone-salts being mobilised to act as buffers. The other view is that acidosis promotes phosphorus depletion. There is evidence that systemic acidosis reduces the tubular maximum for phosphorus reabsorption. Balance studies indicate that an improvement in phosphorus balance can be achieved by alkalis alone (Donohoe et al 1969).

Renal tubular acidosis
Acidosis occurs in a number of renal tubular disorders both as the principal abnormality and as a feature of patients with the general tubular defects, which have already been discussed. Chronic renal tubular acidosis is known as the Butler-Albright syndrome but is probably not a single disorder. Most cases occur sporadically but a few are inherited in an autosomal dominant manner (Richards & Wrong 1972). The patients have poor growth and short stature in adult life. Thirst and polyuria are common features and renal stones occur. Bone disease with symptoms is a feature of a minority of the patients; when it occurs it resembles rickets or osteomalacia.

Investigation provides evidence of a metabolic acidosis with a defect in urine acidification. Most patients have a low serum phosphorus and a high serum alkaline phosphatase. The serum calcium is usually normal. Some patients have hypokalaemia. The bone x-rays show a rickets-like disorder in children and pseudofractures in some adults. Most patients have nephro-calcinosis.

The patients respond quickly to correction of the acidosis with oral soium bicarbonate or Shohl's mixture (citric acid 140 g, sodium citrate 90 g, water to 1 litre). On this treatment the bone symptoms are quickly relieved, the bone disease heals completely and growth improves (Richards et al 1972). Vitamin D is probably not indicated; although it may expedite healing, the danger of increasing the nephrocalcinosis and provoking renal failure outweighs this possible advantage.

Lowe's syndrome

In 1952 Lowe et al described three unrelated boys with glaucoma, cataracts, mental retardation and defects in renal ammonia production. Two of them had acidosis and bone defects resembling those of rickets. These could be healed with alkali therapy alone. Further cases have been described subsequently (Holmes & Tucker 1972).

Ureterosigmoidostomy

A bone disease characterised by severe bone pains and resembling osteomalacia has been described in a number of patients with a metabolic acidosis after ureterocolic anastomosis. Although most patients have been treated at least initially with vitamin D it is not clear how necessary this is, since healing continues and further bone disease is prevented with oral alkalis alone (Donohoe et al 1969).

Chapter 13: Disorders of Calcitonin Secretion

The physiology of calcitonin was outlined in chapter 1 and as with other hormones one would expect to be able to identify syndromes resulting from deficiency or excess of calcitonin. There has been a disappointing search for such disorders. There is no convincing evidence of calcitonin deficiency syndromes even after thyroidectomy and the one disease known to cause calcitonin excess, medullary carcinoma of the thyroid, is seldom characterised by hypocalcaemia.

Possible causes of calcitonin deficiency

Hypercalcaemia sometimes occurs in hyperthyroidism and like other hypercalcaemias shows some response to calcitonin therapy. The factors which contribute to this hypercalcaemia are discussed in chapter 17 but calcitonin deficiency does not seem to be one of them. Calcitonin deficiency has been suggested as a possible cause of the difficulty in controlling the serum calcium after thyroidectomy (Hazard et al 1969). Again there has been no evidence to support this; it is unfortunate that methods are not yet available for the estimation of calcitonin in normal human plasma (p. 47). Paget's disease of bone (chapter 15) responds to treatment with calcitonin but there is no evidence yet that calcitonin deficiency plays a part in its pathogenesis.

Medullary carcinoma of thyroid

Medullary carcinomas of thyroid constitute about 7·5% of cases of thyroid carcinoma (Keynes & Till 1971) and are probably derived from the parafollicular cells (C-cells) of the thyroid (Williams 1966, Ljungberg 1972). An excess of calcitonin was first demonstrated in a tumour by Milhaud et al (1968); this has been confirmed on numerous occasions since then as has an excess of calcitonin in the peripheral blood of these patients (Deftos et al 1971).

Clinical features Medullary carcinoma is a slow growing tumour; in one series the average interval between first symptom and hospital attendance was 6·6 years (Williams et al 1966). Typically it presents with a goitre but some patients have metastases in lymph nodes, liver or bone at the time of presentation. Many patients die from the eventual spread of the tumour but survival is often prolonged (Keynes & Till 1971). Patients frequently have a number of symptoms not obviously related to the presence of metastases. These include diarrhoea, flushing attacks and skin pigmentation. Although the diarrhoea is often relieved by removal of the tumour it does not seem to be caused by the calcitonin excess. Prostaglandins may be responsible since they have been found in the blood draining the tumours, and sometimes, in the peripheral blood as well (Bernier et al 1969, Higgins & Braunwald 1972).

Medullary carcinoma may be familial and a particularly remarkable family with 11 affected members was reported by Melvin et al (1971). Many of the familial cases represent examples of multiple endocrine neoplasia type 2 (p. 95) and are associated with phaeochromocytomas, parathyroid adenomas and occasionally Cushing's syndrome. As these patients also have an increased incidence of neural tumours and neurofibromatosis it seems likely that this disorder represents a general defect in neuroectodermal tissues. This view is supported by the demonstration that a calcitonin-like substance can be extracted from the adrenal medulla of pigs (Kaplan et al 1970, Paloyan et al 1970, Keynes & Till 1971, Keiser et al 1973). The nature of the association between parathyroid adenomas and medullary carcinomas is not clear (Keynes & Till 1971, MacGillivray & Anderson 1971). Some patients may represent cases of tertiary hyperthyroidism as a result of hypocalcaemia. Equally it is conceivable that proliferation and neoplasia of the parafollicular cells could result from a long-standing hypercalcaemia (Ljungberg & Dymling 1972).

Radiology The radiological appearances of medullary carcinoma are characteristic (Pearson et al 1973). Most tumours are heavily but irregularly calcified and may be seen to be indenting the trachaea. Metastatic tumour in lymph-glands may also calcify so that chronic tuberculous lymphadenitis may be considered. Hepatic metastases may also calcify but those in the lung do not.

No abnormality has been described in bone radiographs.

Clinical chemistry Most patients with medullary carcinoma have a serum calcium within the normal range although a minority have hypocalcaemia (Keynes & Till 1971, Markovitz 1971). The most likely reason for the usual lack of hypocalcaemia is compensatory hyperparathyroidism. Although parathyroid hyperplasia was not noted in many of the early reports of medullary carcinoma, it does appear to be common and an increase in plasma levels of PTH has also been noted frequently (Melvin et al 1971). Both in experimental animals and patients with Paget's disease of bone evidence of secondary hyperparathyroidism has been found after prolonged administration of calcitonin (Sørensen et al 1972, Dubé et al 1972). The serum phosphorus is generally normal but sometimes low especially in the patients with hypocalcaemia. The serum alkaline phosphatase is usually normal unless there are hepatic metastases.

Plasma levels of calcitonin are high or very high but the secretion of calicitonin is not autonomous. It can be supressed by infusion of EDTA and increased by calcium infusion (Deftos et al 1971). Serum histaminase levels have recently been shown to be elevated in some patients with medullary carcinoma. This test is not as sensitive as serum calcitonin but it has a possible place in the detection of residual tumour after surgery (Keiser et al 1973).

Treatment The usual treatment of medullary carcinoma is total thyroidectomy and removal of the regional lymph nodes. This is particularly appropriate in familial cases where the tumour is frequently multicentric. Keynes and Till (1971) suggest that in non-familial cases with the disease confined to one lobe it may be reasonable to limit the surgery to the affected lobe. In such cases block dissection can be deferred until a recurrence occurs perhaps years later. In patients with inoperable carcinoma great relief of symptoms such as diarrhoea can be achieved by the removal of a major part of the tumour.

Both at presentation and during the follow-up period a search should be made for phaeochromocytoma and hyperparathyroidism. A family study may also be worthwhile as patients detected in this way are likely to be early cases (Melvin et al 1971).

Other disorders with possible calcitonin excess
An excessive production of calcitonin has been found or inferred in a few cases of benign parafollicular cell adenoma of the thyroid, carcinoid tumours, oat-cell carcinoma of bronchus and in cases of

phaeochromocytoma without recognised medullary carcinoma of thyroid (Milhaud et al 1972, Whitelaw & Cohen 1973).

The possibility that calcitonin excess causes osteopetrosis in man has been canvassed particularly because it appears to be the cause of osteopetrosis in the 'grey-lethal' strain of mice (Murphy 1972, Walker 1972b). However there is no evidence yet that the human disease is caused by calcitonin excess (Verdy et al 1971). At one time it was thought possible that calcitonin excess contributed to the hypocalcaemia of pseudohypoparathyroidism and a high concentration of calcitonin was found in the thyroid gland in some cases. However, thyroidectomy did not lead to any improvement in the condition and it is now clear that the increased calcitonin content of the gland results from the inhibition of calcitonin release (Anast & Conaway 1972).

Chapter 14: Bone Loss and Osteoporosis

Albright's classical definition of osteoporosis was 'too little bone, but what bone there is, is normal'. This basic definition still stands not least because it makes no assumptions about the cause of the condition. It is now clear that bone loss is a universal process with aging especially in females (Newton-John & Morgan 1970). This results in 'post-menopausal' or 'senile' or 'primary' osteoporosis but these are very unsatisfactory as diagnostic labels because they have been given different meanings by different authors. Some have limited the terms to patients with symptoms due to fractures; others have defined osteoporosis as a condition with a measured amount of bone which is less than an arbitrary limit. Such definitions have at least the merit of recognising that while patients with thin bones have an increased incidence of fractures, there are many patients with equally thin bones but no fractures. By no technique for assessment of bone density can a distinction be made between normal subjects and patients with fractures.

Secondary osteoporosis is the term which has been applied to patients with bone loss with a recognised cause. In the light of the above argument this bone loss is seen to be superimposed on that of normal aging and should therefore be regarded as accelerated bone loss. Osteopenia is a term which has been introduced recently to describe any condition with a diminished amount of calcified bone whether or not the bone appears normal. Table 14.1 is an attempt to provide a rational classification of these disorders.

ASSESSMENT OF BONE MASS

Subjective evaluation of bone radiographs

This practice is mentioned only to be dismissed. Although it is not difficult to distinguish by eye between the bones of young adults and those of the very elderly, this is too crude a method to be of any value in clinical practice. Lachman (1955) estimated that the loss of between 30% and 60% of the bone was needed before the unaided observer was likely to be confident about bone rarefaction. Furthermore quite minor differences in the radiological factors and in the amount of overlying soft-tissue may make major differences in the apparent density of the bones.

Slightly less crude is the assessment of the appearance of the trabecular bone in the upper end of the femur. With increasing bone rarefaction the major trabeculae became less obvious and this has been made the basis for a system of grading (Singh et al 1972). The authors found that this technique distinguished between patients without fractures and patients with vertebral fractures but this result was inevitable from the manner in which the patients in each group were selected. The same result would have been obtained with any other technique applied to the same patients, and it is doubtful whether this technique provides any information which cannot be obtained from more objective measurements.

TABLE 14.1. Causes of reduced calcified bone mass ('osteopenia').

A. With bones of apparently normal microscopic structure ('osteoporosis').

Bone loss associated with aging ('primary osteoporosis').
Accelerated bone loss ('secondary osteoporosis').
Glucocorticoid excess including steroid therapy.
Immobilisation and space-flight.
Vitamin C deficiency and iron overload.
Hypogonadism.
Alcoholism.
Malabsorption and after partial gastrectomy (other than with osteomalacia).
Liver disease.
Heparin therapy.
Idiopathic juvenile osteoporosis.

B. Usually with abnormal bones.

Hyperparathyroidism.
Hyperthyroidism.
Osteomalacia.
Uraemia with regular haemodialysis.

C. Inherited disorders.

Osteogenesis imperfecta.
Chromosome disorders (XO, XXXXY).

Methods of bone densitometry

The optical density of the image of a bone on an x-ray film is of little value by itself but if a standard, such as an aluminium step-wedge, is included the variations due to radiological factors and soft-tissue can be reduced. In general these techniques are more successful when applied to the peripheral skeleton than to the spine because of the smaller effect of soft-tissue. In the hand for instance the image of the soft-tissue can be eliminated by immersing the hand in water (Morgan et al 1967).

Another method uses two sources of widely different energies. The differences in the absorption of x-rays by bone and soft-tissue decreases at higher energies so that the use of two sources allows the contribution of bone and soft-tissue to be determined separately. Several methods have been devised on this principle and they provide the only worthwhile method for examining the vertebral bodies *in vivo* (Oeser & Krokowski 1963). The absorption of photons from gamma-emitting isotopes provides another technique for bone densitometry (Jelliffe & Strickland 1970, Atkinson et al 1970, Smith et al 1972b, Zimmerman et al 1973). Although elaborate equipment is needed for this purpose, an instrument is now available commercially. It is potentially the most reproducible method available for studies on the individual.

Cortical thickness and derived indices

Measurement of cortical thickness has been widely used for the assessment of the amount of bone. The metacarpals, particularly the right second metacarpal, have been used most extensively for this but other bones used include the femur, the radius, the humerus and the clavicle. The results of such measurements have been expressed in a number of different ways (fig. 14.1). Morgan et al (1967) showed that changes in the simplest measurement $(D - d)$ correlated very closely with the amount of bone measured by x-ray densitometry at the same site and fairly closely with that of the trabecular bone in the base of the proximal phalanx (fig. 14.2). Furthermore the incidence of bones with values of $D - d$ less than arbitrary limits correlates closely with the incidence of fracture (see below). Morgan et al also showed that dividing $D - d$ by D to get the 'metacarpal index' confused rather than clarified the results. Similar comparisons have not yet been made for the other indices but Dequeker (1970) showed that of four different

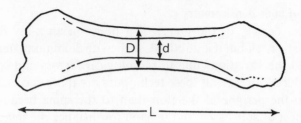

FIGURE 14.1. Indices related to measurements of the thickness of the metacarpal cortex.

$D - d$ (Morgan et al 1967)

$D^2 - d^2$ (Dequeker 1972)

$\dfrac{D - d}{D}$ i.e. 'metacarpal index' (Barnett & Nordin 1960)

$\left(\dfrac{D^2 - d^2}{D^2}\right) \times 100$ i.e. 'percent cortical area' (Garn et al 1971)

$\dfrac{D^2 - d^2}{DL}$ (Gryfe et al 1971)

indices $D - d$ was influenced least by variations in D within a group of subjects aged from 25 to 34 (table 14.2). It is likely therefore that all the procedures for 'correcting for body size' introduce greater errors than they eliminate and that $D - d$ is the most satisfactory of the simple indices proposed.

TABLE 14.2. Indices of amount of bone in 50 adults aged 25–34 years. Measurements at the mid-point of the second metacarpal for bones of different external diameters (Dequeker 1970). All measurements in millimetres.

D	$D-d$	$\dfrac{D-d}{D}$ %	D^2-d^2	$\dfrac{D^2-d^2}{D^2}$ %
7·0	4·8	68·5	44·2	90·1
8·0	4·9	61·3	54·4	85·0
9·0	5·0	55·6	65·0	80·2
10·0	5·1	51·0	76·0	76·0
Percent change between D = 7·0 and D = 10·0	+6·2	−25·8	+71·9	−15·6

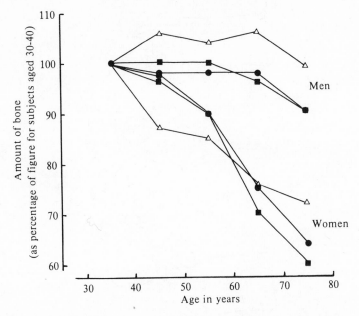

FIGURE 14.2. The amount of bone in normal men and women at different ages measured by three different techniques (Morgan et al 1967). In each case the results are expressed as a percentage of those found between the ages of 30 and 40. ●: thickness of metacarpal cortex; ■: optical density of image of metacarpal (aluminium equivalent); △: optical density of image of base of proximal phalanx (aluminium equivalent). The two measurements on the metacarpal agree very closely with each other. The measurements on the phalanx are subject to greater imprecision (there is less bone to measure) and the number of subjects was smaller. Despite these limitations the figure demonstrates that the changes in the trabecular bone at this site are very similar to those in the cortical bone of the metacarpal.

Evidence of structural failure

One of the hallmarks of bone loss is an increased liability to fracture. This is true particularly of fractures of the neck of the femur, the distal radius and the vertebrae (fig. 14.3). At different ages the incidence of fracture or spinal deformity correlates with the incidence of thin bones, whatever method is used for its assessment (Newton-John & Morgan 1970). On the other hand the presence or absence of fractures or deformed vertebrae is a very poor guide to the bone mass of the individual patient.

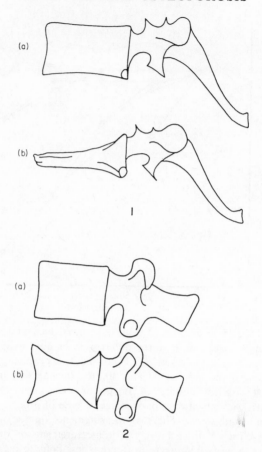

FIGURE 14.3. Deformity of 1) thoracic and 2) lumbar vertebrae associated with thin bones. (a) Normal, (b) after typical crush fractures. From Fourman and Royer (1968) by permission.

Histological assessment of bone loss

As with radiological methods, histological examination of the bone at different ages has led to the conclusion that aging is associated with progressive reduction in thickness of cortical bone and in the number and thickness of the trabeculae in cancellous bone (Ellis & Peart 1972, Nordin 1973). These conclusions are mainly based on autopsy material and although similar changes are seen in biopsy specimens, it is very doubtful whether assessment of the amount of bone in a biopsy sample ever provides any more information about the individual patient than can be obtained by radiology. Moreover Ellis and Peart (1972) showed that in histological sections from different parts of the iliac crest the proportion of bone could vary greatly. For these reasons bone biopsy has no place in the 'assessment' of osteoporosis.

Choice of methods for the assessment of bone loss

The recent advances in our understanding of the nature of osteo-porosis have all come from epidemiological studies on large numbers of patients with very simple methods notably measurement of cortical thickness (Newton-John & Morgan 1970). Such measurements correlate well with the incidence of fracture in large groups of patients and there is no evidence that measurements on the peripheral skeleton are in any way irrelevant to the changes in the axial skeleton. Indeed several authors have noted that structural failure in the vertebrae correlates better with the thickness of cortical bone in the limbs than with the density of trabecular bone in the spine or any other site (Meema & Meema 1963, Dequeker et al 1971a, Goldsmith et al 1971). There is no evidence that fractures of the femur represent a different disorder from that which causes fractures in the spine (Nilsson 1970).

Studies in the individual patient are much more difficult. All the methods have a wide normal range so that the extra precision of the complex methods of assessment is of no advantage. The simple methods are adequate but even here unless the amount of bone is severely diminished, as in juvenile osteoporosis (Exton-Smith et al 1969), the information is of little clinical value. There is no evidence that any useful purpose is served by screening for a 'preclinical osteoporosis'.

Methods are needed for the assessment of changes in bone mass with time, particularly in studies of medical measures which might be effective in modifying the rate of loss of bone. For such research projects the precision of photon absorptiometry is likely to make it the method of choice as changes can be measured with some con-fidence at relatively short intervals.

BONE LOSS ASSOCIATED WITH AGING

Fractures associated with thin bones are most common in elderly women. The present evidence is not that these women are in any way a different population from those without fractures but that all women and, to a smaller extent, all men lose bone with advancing age. Evidence of bone loss with age has been provided both by radiological and by histological techniques and in many populations both modern and ancient (Garn et al 1967, Newton-John & Morgan 1970, Van Gerven & Armelagos 1970, Dequeker et al 1971b, Ellis & Peart 1972).

When the numbers of subjects is sufficiently large it can be shown that the standard deviation does not increase as the aging continues (fig. 14.4). Thus all women over 40–50 and all men over 50–60 lose

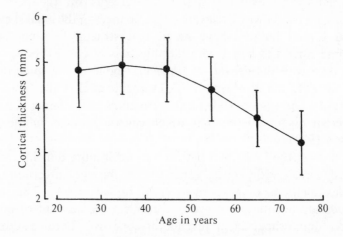

FIGURE 14.4. Thickness of the metacarpal cortex in 125 normal women of different ages. The vertical lines represent one standard deviation. Data of Morgan et al (1967).

bone. Once bone loss has started it is linear with age so that the patients who have the least bone at any age are probably those who had the least bone at maturity. One consequence of this linear loss of bone with age is that the proportion of patients with amounts of bone below arbitrary limits increases rapidly with increasing age (fig. 14.5). Newton-John and Morgan (1970) have shown that the frequency of thin bones at different ages defined in such a manner correlates well with the frequency of fractures in the femoral neck or radius (fig. 14.6). In an individual patient the occurrence of a

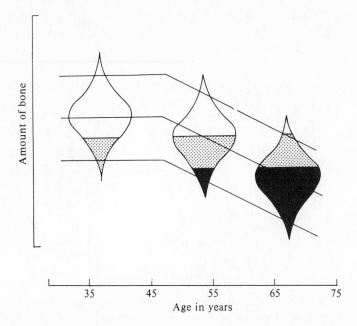

FIGURE 14.5. A model for the loss of bone with age. The dotted and black areas represent the proportion of the population at each age who have an amount of bone less than arbitrary figures corresponding to (mean − 1 standard deviation) and (mean − 2·5 standard deviations) respectively for women aged between 30 and 40. From Morgan and Newton-John 1969 with permission.

fracture is a random event to which factors other than the thinness of the bones contribute so that for each patient with a fracture there are many with equally thin bones but no fracture. However these studies indicate that the age-related bone loss is the principal factor in the increased liability to fracture experienced by elderly people. Whether this universal change should be regarded as a disease is a semantic argument outside the scope of this review.

The evidence for the concept of a universal loss of bone with age has been fully reviewed by Newton-John and Morgan (1970). The many studies which support this conclusion have been cross-section studies—that is studies of a population at one point in time. Much more telling information would be obtained with longitudinal studies; there are very few of these. Garn et al (1967) reported the changes in the metacarpal in 53 women and 34 men at average intervals of

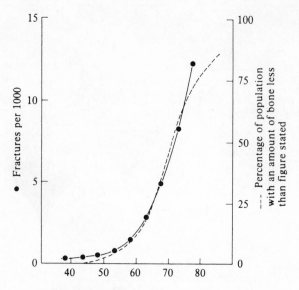

FIGURE 14.6. Frequency of fractures of the femur (●) in women at different ages, compared with the frequency of amounts of bone less than an arbitrary figure corresponding to 2·5 standard deviations below the mean for women aged between 30 and 40. From Newton-John and Morgan (1968) by permission.

23 years and 15 years respectively. Overall there was a loss of bone with age but the apparent rate of loss varied greatly from one individual to another; some even 'gained' bone. A limitation of this type of study is that, in the individual, the error of the difference between two measurements compounds the errors of each measurement. Similar results were obtained by Adams et al (1970a) who also found overall a loss of bone with age in 62 men and 55 women initially aged between 55 and 64 and studied again 11 years later. As with the study of Garn and colleagues there was a great variation between individuals in the rate of loss but the same technical limitations apply. It seems likely that even moderately accurate estimates of the rate of loss of bone in the individual will not be possible without densitometric techniques.

Pathogenesis of the bone loss
Many theories have been proposed to account for the loss of bone with age; some have been proposed and discarded more than once.

Even the nature of the change in the skeleton is not clear: kinetic studies have given a wide variety of results (Fourman & Royer 1968).

One suggestion has been that the bone loss is caused by marginally increased parathyroid activity; this view has not been supported by studies of serum parathyroid hormone levels measured with specific radioimmunoassays (Riggs et al 1973a). Another suggestion is that bone dissolution is a result of the necessity to buffer the fixed acid load which results from a meat-rich diet. In one study reported by Ellis et al (1972) some data to support this view was presented but the number of subjects was very small. Fluoride deficiency may be another contributory factor as crush fractures in the vertebrae appear to be more common in women from areas with a low fluoride content in the water supply (Berstein et al 1966). The possibility that calcium depletion contributes to osteoporosis has been repeatedly investigated (Riggs et al 1967, Hurxthal & Vose 1969). Although calcium deficiency causes osteoporosis in experimental animals it is very uncertain whether comparable situations often occur in man. Normal people adapt to a diet with as little as 200 mg calcium daily by increasing the proportion absorbed by the intestine (p.9), and epidemiological studies have provided very little evidence that a low calcium diet is a significant cause of bone loss (Garn et al 1967). Immobilisation and inactivity could contribute to the progressive bone loss with age particularly in western societies but some bone loss with age has been demonstrated in many populations. A primary change in the collagen of bone has been suggested as a cause of the

TABLE 14.3. Possible factors contributing to age-related bone loss.

Likely

Changes in oestrogens and/or androgens.
Inactivity.
Protein-rich diet.
Fluoride deficiency

Unlikely on present evidence

Parathyroid overactivity.
Calcium deficiency in diet.
Vitamin D deficiency.
Protein deficiency.

---

bone loss by Black et al (1970b) but further evidence of this is needed. Vitamin D deficiency is not uncommon among elderly women in some populations and it has been suggested (Bullamore et al 1970) that a widespread subclinical vitamin D deficiency causes defective calcium absorption and osteoporosis without osteomalacia. While vitamin D deficiency may contribute to the bone loss in a few patients it seems likely this could account for the bone loss which is a universal phenomenon. Perhaps the likeliest factor in age-related bone loss is hormonal changes particularly in oestrogens and androgens. The fact that the loss is more severe in women and starts near the time of the menopause supports this view, but the precise changes which are important are still unknown.

These conclusions are summarised in table 14.3

Clinical features
Symptoms in patients with thin bones are the result of fractures. The increased liability to fractures of the femur and of the forearm has already been described. Episodic back pain occurs in some patients. Each episode probably represents a crush fracture of a vertebra, and the pain typically lasts about a month. Other patients have little history of back-ache but are found to have loss of height and radio-logical evidence of crushed vertabrae. Few patients have marked bone tenderness over the spine and remarkably few develop neurological complications of spinal root compression. In some patients the scoliosis leads to deformity of the thoracic cage and impairment of the vital capacity.

Although there are some patients in whom the principal cause of symptoms is vertebral fractures, there is no evidence that 'Spinal osteoporosis' represents a different disease from that in patients who present in other ways (Morgan 1973).

Prevention and management
In the light of our knowledge that bone loss appears to be an inevitable companion of normal aging, there are three possible objectives: to restore the bone mass, to prevent continuing loss of bone and to provide relief for patients with symptoms.

Restoration of bone mass The identification of possible drugs for the restoration of bone mass has been greatly hampered by the lack of valid methods for assessing small changes in the amount of bone. There is evidence that some drugs notably phosphate, di-phosphonates, oestrogens and anabolic steroids can cause calcium retention but there is no evidence that the retained calcium goes into the bone (Riggs et al 1972a). Another indirect measure of bone turnover is provided by micro-radiography. Promising changes in the numbers of bone forming and resorbing surfaces have been noted with oestrogens and with a combination of fluoride, calcium and vitamin D (Riggs et al 1972a, Jowsey et al 1972) but there is still no evidence that these changes are sustained or lead to an increase in the amount of bone in the skeleton. Thus there is little evidence that there is any measure available at present which can restore the amount of bone. Even in disorders such as glucocorticoid excess where the cause of the bone loss is known the bone loss appears to be irrevers-ible and the same is true of immobilisation osteoporosis in rats (Rose 1967, Mattsson 1972).

Prevention of continuing bone loss There have been no controlled trials of any form of therapy for a long enough period to assess its effect on bone loss although Meema and Meema (1968) produced some evidence that oestrogen replacement therapy possibly reduced bone loss in post-menopausal women, and oestrogens have been shown to increase intestinal calcium absorption (Caniggia et al 1970). Immobilisation osteoporosis is a possible model for age-related bone loss and there have been several studies of various forms of treatment on the rate of loss of bone. In man phosphate supple-ments have no effect on the rate of loss of bone in immobilised adults (Hulley et al 1971). In experimental animals calcitonin administra-tion does not influence the rate of loss of bone but in one study diphosphonates were found to reduce bone loss from immobilised rat limbs (Singh & Jowsey 1970, Orimo et al 1971, Mühlbauer et al 1971). Diphosphonates are unlikely to be of practical value in human osteoporosis (Jowsey et al 1971) so that there is little evidence of any practical long-term measure which is likely to prevent or reduce bone loss with aging.

If bone loss is inevitable and irreversible the best way of ensuring immunity from unnecessary fractures in later life is to acquire a large mass of bone in childhood. However we do not even know what factors are important in this.

Management of the patient with symptoms It will be seen from the preceding discussion that there is insufficient evidence yet to justify the 'treatment' of symptomless patients found to have radiological evidence of thin bones. The information available at most suggests that oestrogen therapy merits further study but at present we have no way of knowing whether any reduction in the likelihood of fractures in later life outweighs the side effects of long term therapy.

The patients with symptoms due to fractures have been very extensively studied and subjected to a wide variety of treatments including calcium (both orally and parenterally), phosphorus, fluoride, vitamin D, diphosphonates, calcitonin, oestrogens, androgens and synthetic anabolic steroids, in addition to mixtures of these agents (Dent 1969, Melick & Baird 1970, Brown et al 1970, Riggs et al 1972a & 1973b, Ryckewaert et al 1972, Wallach 1972, Belchetz et al 1973). There is no reliable evidence that any of these treatments promote the relief of symptoms or reduce the incidence of further fractures. The strong pressure on the clinician to provide some form of treatment has endangered the design of experimental studies on the treatments of osteoporosis. Few trials have had controls let alone a double-blind protocol. Furthermore the symptoms of the condition are episodic and a spontaneous improvement is often attributed to the therapy which happened to be given at the time.

The clinician must therefore be aware of the unproved value of any active therapy he gives. His main responsibility is to exclude other possible causes for the patient's symptoms and to give general advice. Thus he should exclude particularly metastatic bone disease and osteomalacia as well as the other conditions listed in table 14.1. He should recognise that while the clinical chemistry of the serum is generally normal in osteoporosis, a high serum alkaline phosphatase occurs after a fracture. The patients should be given general advice to avoid falls and knocks and lifting heavy weights. At the same time they should avoid inactivity. After particular episodes of spinal collapse splinting or plaster casts are seldom needed and probably not desirable. A handout on the lines of that by Dent (1971) may be helpful, and a good general account of the place of rehabilitation in these patients has been provided by Tobin (1970).

ACCELERATED BONE LOSS

The disorders which cause accelerated bone loss or 'secondary osteoporosis' are listed in table 14.1. The bone changes associated with glucocorticoid excess are described in chapter 17.

IMMOBILISATION AND SPACE FLIGHT

It has long been recognised that bone loss is a consequence of immobilisation both in man and experimental animals (Griffith 1971, Hulley et al 1971, Hardt 1972, Mattsson 1972). In man prolonged immobilisation leads to a loss of 0·5% of the calcium stores each month, but the mechanisms underlying the bone loss are not yet known (Hulley et al 1971). In growing animals bone growth is impaired (Pennock et al 1972). At one time there was concern about the evidence of severe bone loss during prolonged space flight. These results came from radiological studies and the conclusions conflicted with those from metabolic balance studies. More recent studies both with photon absorptiometry and with neutron activation analysis have indicated that the loss of bone was no more than 0·05% of the total stores daily. In the more recent Apollo missions (10 and 11) the loss of calcium was very much less (Douglas 1970, British Medical Journal 1971).

It is not yet clear whether the restoration of activity restores the bone mass fully. Bones which normally bear weight such as the calcaneum show a detectable bone loss in a relatively short period of immobilisation and do recover fully at least in young men (Hulley et al 1971). Whether the same is true at all ages is not known; in adult rats disuse osteoporosis appears to be irreversible (Mattsson 1972). Many attempts have been made to find drugs which reduce the effect of immobilisation on the bone but with the possible exception of the diphosphonates these have not been successful (p. 232).

VITAMIN C DEFICIENCY AND IRON STORAGE DISEASES

Vitamin C has a role in the hydroxylation of proline to hydroxyproline and when it is deficient there is a disturbance of collagen formation and thus bone formation. Osteoporosis is a consequence of vitamin C deficiency in children and experimental animals, but there have been few instances yet of thin bones in adults as a result of vitamin C deficiency, perhaps because patients are unlikley to be allowed to have prolonged untreated deficiency. A probable example is provided by the incidence of osteoporosis in negro males in South Africa (Lynch et al 1970, Wapnick et al 1971). These patients have severe siderosis caused by the consumption of alcoholic beverages which are stored in iron containers. It is thought that the iron stores lead to vitamin C depletion by promoting its oxidation in patients who already have a relatively poor dietary intake. Bone changes similar to those in the patients could be induced in guinea pigs by iron injections and could largely be prevented by the administration of ascorbic acid.

In haemochromatosis bone loss would be expected for the same reason but the incidence of thin bones has varied between different series no doubt because of variations in the criteria for the identification of undue bone thinning. While the vitamin C depletion could again be a factor another possible factor could be hypogonadism due to iron deposits in the testes (British Medical Journal 1969).

Hypogonadism

Oestrogens act on bone to oppose the action of parathyroid hormone and to reduce bone resorption (Atkins et al 1972). The fact that bone loss in normal women starts near the time of the menopause and that oophorectomy in younger women may expedite bone loss has suggested that oestrogen deficiency is a factor in the bone loss (Meema et al 1965, Utian 1971, Aitken et al 1973). Whether hypogonadism is an important factor in idiopathic juvenile osteoporosis (see below) or in the osteoporosis of Turner's syndrome remains controversial.

Whether hypogonadism in males contributes to bone loss is uncertain but there have been a few suggestive cases (Dent 1971).

Liver Disease and Alcoholism

Osteomalacia due to liver disorders especially obstructive jaundice has been discussed earlier (p. 173). Undue bone loss may occur in patients who do not have osteomalacia and sometimes fractures are major symptoms. The cause is not known and more than one factor may be involved. Impaired intestinal absorption of calcium has been demonstrated in icteric patients with chronic parenchymatous liver disease and also in a few patients without jaundice (Whelton et al 1971). In some patients parenteral vitamin D therapy improves calcium absorption but it does not always prevent the progress of the bone loss.

Saville (1965) has noted thinner bones in young alcoholics at autopsy than in other subjects of similar ages. While hepatic cirrhosis is one possible cause of the bone loss in these patients another possibility is that magnesium depletion leads to stimulation of the parathyroid glands.

MALABSORPTION SYNDROMES

While malabsorption syndromes are well recognised causes of osteomalacia, bone loss without osteomalacia may also occur (Parfitt et al 1962). It is likely that this is caused by malabsorption of calcium in patients who still absorb sufficient vitamin D or who have adequate vitamin D stores. One example is the osteopenia of lactose intolerance in which there is evidence of impaired calcium absorption (Condon et al 1970, Güller et al 1973).

PARTIAL GASTRECTOMY

Osteomalacia after partial gastrectomy has been described earlier (p. 171). This complication affects a small proportion of the patients but it is now clear that as a group these patients have an accelerated loss of bone after the age of sixty in men and fifty in women (Morgan et al 1966, Fujita et al 1971).

HEPARIN THERAPY

Long-term therapy with heparin has been reported to cause serious loss of bone with spontaneous fractures (Griffith et al 1965). Several suggestions have been made about the pathogenesis of this complication; one is that heparin reduces the stability of lysosomes which release collagenase. Long term heparin therapy is now seldom used, but a similar mechanism may underly the bone loss which is sometimes seen in urticaria pigmentosa where there are increased numbers of mast cells (Ives & Thompson 1973).

LACTATION

While acute studies in small numbers of patients have suggested that bone may be lost during lactation (Atkinson & West 1970), epidemiological studies have not shown that multiparity and repeated periods of lactation lead to a reduced bone mass in the long term or an increase in the incidence of fractures (Walker 1972a).

IDIOPATHIC JUVENILE OSTEOPOROSIS

This is a rare disorder found both in boys and girls who, when aged between 8 and 15, suddenly develop bone pains, fractures with minimal trauma and usually loss of height (Dent 1969, Görgényi 1969, Lapatsanis et al 1971, Jowsey & Johnson 1972). Radiologically there is evidence of thin bones and of vertebral collapse. Serum levels of calcium, phosphorus and alkaline phosphatase are generally normal for the patient's age but the urinary excretion of calcium is sometimes increased. Untreated most patients recover in four or five years, although there may be persisting deformities. In long bones the bone laid down during the acute episode remains less dense than normal.

TABLE 14.4. Differences between idiopathic juvenile osteoporosis and osteogenesis imperfecta.

Idiopathic juvenile osteoporosis	Osteogenesis imperfecta
No family history.	Family history usually.
No blue sclerae.	Blue sclerae in most cases.
Normal teeth.	Abnormal teeth.
Onset at age 8–15; normal in early life.	First fractures in early childhood or even *in utero*.
Severe disease in adolescence.	Tendency to have fewer fractures in adolescence.
Most fractures in vertebrae.	Most fractures in long bones.
Characteristic x-rays with very thin new bone at the metaphysis. Vertebrae sharply outlined.	Typical x-rays (chapter 16).
Bone histology: normal appearances but diminished amount of bone.	Bone histology: cortex consists mainly or entirely of woven bone.

Diagnosis Idiopathic juvenile osteoporosis is uncommon and should not be diagnosed unless there is no suggestion of osteogenesis imperfecta and all other causes of thin bones in adolescence have been eliminated. Thus a search should be made for Cushing's syndrome, hypogonadism, hyperparathyroidism, malabsorption and osteomalacia. Osteogenesis imperfecta differs from idiopathic juvenile osteoporosis in several ways (table 14.4).

Treatment It is very difficult to evaluate the possible place of any form of therapy in this condition with its tendency for spontaneous improvement. The fact that it begins around the time of puberty suggests that changes in hormones have a part in the production of the disorder. However there is no clear advantage in the use of oestrogens or anabolic steroids (Dent 1969). Indeed these agents may be inadvisable in some patients because they could possibly cause premature fusion of the epiphyses. During the acute phase of the illness splints may be needed for fractures. Inactivity should be avoided as much as possible both to prevent a superimposed bone loss due to immobilisation and to prevent obesity which is frequently a problem in these patients.

TRANSIENT OSTEOPOROSIS

Transient osteoporosis or regional migratory osteoporosis are names given to a local bone loss usually in the upper femora but also sometimes in other sites. The patients present with bone pain, later develop rarefaction of the bone, but eventually heal completely. The cause is unknown but there may be an association with type IV hyperlipoproteinaemia (Hunder & Kelly 1971, Pinals & Jabbs 1972).

DISAPPEARING BONES

This remarkable condition is also known as phantom bones or massive osteolysis (Phillips et al 1972). In this disorder a part of the skeleton usually one or two bones in an arm or a leg is resorbed and replaced by fibrous or vascular tissue. There is no evidence of a metabolic disturbance and the cause is quite unknown although in most cases there is a history of a fracture or other injury

Chapter 15: Paget's Disease of Bone

The classical description of this disorder by Sir James Paget in 1871 remains an accurate account of the severe form of the disease as it is seen today. There are a few earlier case reports which almost certainly refer to the same disease, notably that of Dr. (later Sir) Samuel Wilks of Guy's Hospital, London in 1869 (Barry 1969). Paget called the disease osteitis deformans because he did not think that hypertrophy or new growth could have been the cause for enlargement of the bone, and concluded that it had an inflammatory basis. However osteitis deformans is not a satisfactory name because there is no evidence of an inflammatory element in its pathogenesis and because many patients are now recognised who have no deformity. The eponymous title, Paget's disease of bone, is more satisfactory. Useful reviews of this disorder include those by Barry (1969) and Woodhouse (1972).

Age and sex incidence Paget's disease is rare before the age of forty but thereafter occurs with increasing frequency with advancing age (table 15.1). Schmorl (1932) found Paget's disease in 3% of 4,614 unselected autopsies on patients aged over forty in Dresden, Germany and a similar proportion was noted by Collins (1956) in Yorkshire, England. In a radiological study Pygott (1957) found Paget's disease in the spine or pelvis in 3·5% of patients aged 45 or more. Since only these two parts of the skeleton were studied the true incidence must be higher, but the similarity between the autopsy and the radiological studies is striking. Collins estimated that Paget's disease had been diagnosed before death in no more than a third of his patients while less than 5% had been admitted to hospital because of the disease. This illustrates the limitations of any estimate of incidence which is based on the incidence of symptomatic or recognised cases. Occasional patients with Paget's disease are recognised before the age of forty. The two youngest patients recorded were aged 18 and 27 (Collins 1966). The term juvenile Paget's disease has been used to describe an unusual bone disease of childhood also known as hereditary hyperphosphatasia (Woodhouse et al 1972). There is no good evidence of the identity of this disorder with Paget's disease in adults and it is considered in the next chapter.

In most series males slightly outnumber females; a male : female ratio of about 4 : 3 is probably realistic (Collins 1966).

TABLE 15.1. Incidence of Paget's disease of the spine and pelvis at different ages. From a radiological study by Pygott (1957).

Age (years)	Incidence of Paget's disease (%)	
	Men	Women
35–44	0·4	0·3
45–54	0·4	0·5
55–64	2·9	1·4
65–74	7·4	3·6
75–84	7·0	2·9
more than 85	8·6	11·4

Racial and geographical incidence Paget's disease appears to be common in Europe, North America and Australia but few cases have been described in Indians, Africans and Chinese (Barry 1969, Bohrer 1970, Dastur & Kaji 1971). Lawrence (1970) found that the disease was almost as common among Negroes in Jamaica as in Europeans but found no cases among American Indians. There have been no large scale studies of age-matched groups from different races so that it is not yet clear whether these differences in incidence are real.

Familial incidence There have been many case reports of Paget's disease in several members of a family (Barry 1969). It has been described in siblings and in parents and children. One family had six cases in three generations. Although only a small proportion of cases can be explained in this way, the disease in these families appears to be inherited in an autosomal dominant manner.

AETIOLOGY

The aetiology of Paget's disease remains as obscure as it was when the disorder was first described. The many theories which have been advanced have been reviewed by Nagant de Deuxchaines and Krane (1964). There is no evidence that parathyroid hormone is necessary for the development of the disease (Genuth & Klein 1972).

BONE CHANGES

Pathology

Three phases can be distinguished in the bone disorder (Collins 1966). The first defect appears to be abnormal destruction of bone by excessive numbers of osteoclasts. This is best seen on the skull and at the advancing edge of the disease area in a partially affected bone. The osteolysis is followed by new formation of primitive, coarse-fibred bone and the development of a very vascular fibrous marrow. Third, waves of resorption and new bone formation ebb and flow to produce the features specific to established Paget's disease. Irregular un-oriented trabeculae contain blocks of bone with their lamellae oriented in many different ways (fig. 15.1) and separated by irregular cement lines (fig. 15.2). The bone at this final stage has been described as 'jerry-built'. At this time the marrow becomes less vascular and is re-occupied by haemopoietic tissue or fat cells.

The gross appearances of affected bones may be very striking with thickening, particularly in the skull, and deformity, particularly in long-bones such as the femora or tibiae. Many bones may be affected but the most common sites for Paget's disease are the spine, the pelvis and sacrum, the skull and the femora.

Clinical features

Most patients have no symptoms. Those who have complain of pain or deformity or present as a result of a fracture. The bone pain is most commonly localised in long bone such as the tibia, but other patients complain of back-ache or headache. The severity of the pain varies greatly and bears no relationship to the apparent extent of the disease as indicated by radiology. In one recent personal case the principal symptom was pain in the right tibia which was little affected, while the grossly abnormal left tibia was pain-free. The cause of the pain is not known, although in some cases it results from a secondary arthrosis. The onset or rapid worsening of pain may be a sign of the development of a sarcoma (see below).

On clinical examination the characteristic deformities may be

FIGURE 15.2. Paget's disease: a relatively quiescent area of bone without excessive cellular activity. The mosaic pattern of the cement lines is evident. Part of the intertrabecular tissue consists of fibrous tissue. Decalcified section stained with haematoxylin and eosin. Magnification × 50. From Woods (1972) by permission.

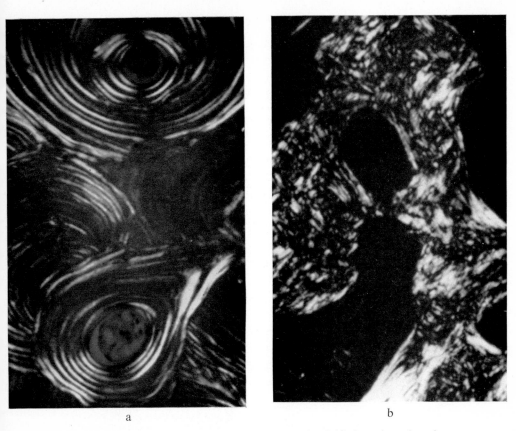

a   b

FIGURE 15.1. a: Normal compact bone, decalcified section viewed under polarised light. Magnification ×260. Note the orderly arrangement of birefringent lamellae around the Haversian canals. From Woods (1972) by permission. b: Bone from a patient with Paget's disease under polarised light to show the disorganised pattern of bone architecture. Courtesy of Dr. C. G. Woods.

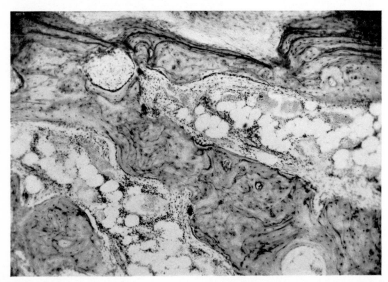

15·2

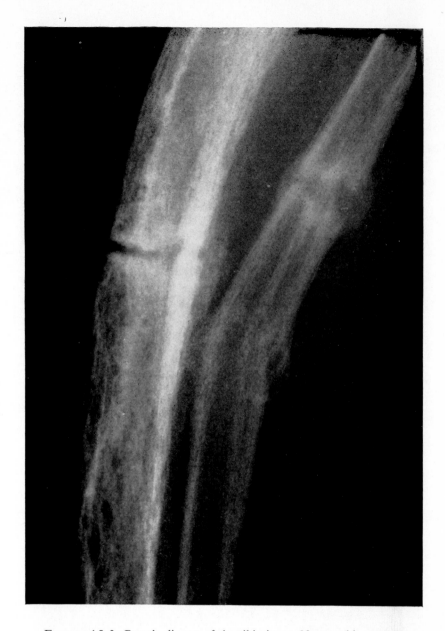

FIGURE 15.3. Paget's disease of the tibia in an 80-year-old woman. A band of decalcification in the affected bone resembles a pseudofracture. The fractures in the otherwise unaffected fibula probably result from the bowing of the tibia.

seen: notably anterior bowing of a femur, lateral bowing of a tibia or enlargement of the skull or of a clavicle. When the Paget's disease is extensive, the skin overlying an affected bone may be considerably warmer and a bruit is sometimes heard.

Radiology
Radiographs reveal abnormalities which correspond to the pathological changes already described. There is an early phase of osteolytic activity sometimes seen clearly in the skull as 'osteoporosis circumscripta' or at the V-shaped advancing edge of a lesion in a long bone (Ravault et al 1970). The second ('combined') phase, with evidence of both bone dissolution and sclerosis, corresponds to the active phase. In the third phase bone sclerosis predominates but the extent of the sclerotic change does not correspond with the activity of the disease as estimated in other ways. In this phase the skull and the cortex of long bones are greatly thickened while the trabecular pattern is coarse, disorganised and bears no relation to the stresses to which the bone is subject. Deformities are sometimes characteristic such as the 'shepherd's crook' appearance of the upper end of the femur. Good accounts of the radiographic appearances of Paget's disease have been given by Wilner & Sherman (1966), Barry (1969), Greenfield (1969) and Murray and Jacobson (1971).

In Paget's disease bands of decalcification resembling fractures are sometimes seen (fig. 15.3). These would be difficult to distinguish

TABLE 15.2. Anatomical distribution of lesions of Paget's disease in 46 patients at necropsy (Collins 1956).

	Number of cases
Lumbosacral vertebrae	35
Skull	30
Pelvic bones	22
Femur (one or both)	16
Tibia (one or both)	14
Clavicle (one or both)	5
Sternum	3
Fibula	2
Scapula, humorus, radius, phalanx, mandible, ribs and patella	1 each

from pseudofractures (p. 180) except that they occur through bone which is clearly abnormal.

Although most of the bones in the skeleton have been reported to be sites of Paget's disease, the bones most commonly affected are shown in table 15.2. Bones in which Paget's disease has been detected less often include scapula, patella, radius, ulna and calcaneus; it is even more rarely found in the fibula, mandible, the facial bones and the bones of the hand (Barry 1969, Uthman & al-Shawaff 1969, Grundy & Patten 1969).

Involvement of a single bone (monostotic Paget's disease) is found in between 10% and 40% of the patients in different series (Suchett-Kaye 1970). Even when widespread, Paget's disease does not become generalised and is not symmetrical. Although the disease spreads within a bone it does not cross a joint.

The radiographs of the bones in Paget's disease are often characteristic and there is no difficulty in making the diagnosis, particularly if the deformities are also seen. There may be a difficulty in patients with a mixture of lytic and sclerotic lesions in the pelvis where the appearances can resemble closely those of metastatic neoplasm. In such cases bone biopsy is valuable in diagnosis. Occasionally polyostotic fibrous dysplasia can be difficult to distinguish from Paget's disease but a thickened cortex in long bones is characteristic of the latter. The differential diagnosis of sclerotic lesions of bone is discussed on page 265.

Complications

Fractures Fractures occur both during the early phases of Paget's disease when bone rarefaction is taking place and in the established disease. They may result from minimal trauma. The long bones notably the femur and the tibia are the common sites of fractures. Less common are fractures in the pelvis or of the vertebrae. The fractures of long bones with sclerotic Paget's disease are characteristically transverse and, at least in the femur, are unusual in the parts of the bone involved (table 15.3).

Fractures in Paget's disease generally form callus and heal well. The management of femoral fractures may be difficult because severe bowing of the femur may make intramedullary fixation impossible without an additional osteotomy. The fractures of the shaft can be treated conservatively with immobilisation on a Thomas splint and most of these patients heal well in between six weeks and five months. Non-union is common with the fractures through the neck of the femur (Grundy 1970).

Neoplastic change Paget's original patient developed a sarcoma and four other early cases which he collected also died from malignancy. Two forms of malignancy are recognised: sarcomas and giant-cell tumours. The sarcomas arise in affected bone in parts of the skull where Paget's disease itself is common, but are particularly frequent in the humerus and skull and unusual in the spine. They may complicate monostotic Paget's disease. Histologically most resemble the osteosarcomas of younger patients but fibrosarcomas and chondrosarcomas have also been reported. In many cases the tumours are pleomorphic with different histological types in different areas (McKenna et al 1964, Barry 1969).

TABLE 15.3. Sites of fractures in the femur in Paget's disease of bone. Combined data of Barry (1969) and Grundy (1970) to include 153 fractures in 113 patients.

	Number of fractures
Femoral neck	19
Trochanteric region	13
Subtrochanteric	48
Uppermost third of shaft	23
Middle third of shaft	29
Lowest third of shaft	21
	153

The principal clinical features of sarcoma are severe pain and swelling; the onset of pain in a patient known to have Paget's disease should suggest the development of malignancy. The pain may precede the development of the radiological changes of sarcoma. In some cases the pain is intractable demanding ablative surgery, local radiotherapy or cordotomy; in other cases such as those with tumours in the skull, there is little pain. Radiological signs of sarcoma formation may include both osteolytic or sclerotic lesions but the lytic changes predominate. Unlike the osteosarcomas of youth there is no predilection for the ends of the long bones; any part of the bone may be affected. Sunray spicules of new bone formation are seldom seen and the early sign is usually medullarly bone destruction. This is followed by cortical destruction and the development of a soft-tissue mass. In many cases pathological fractures develop at the site of a sarcoma. Metastatic deposits may be found both in normal and abnormal bone and in the lungs.

The prognosis of sarcoma superimposed on Paget's disease is generally poor. While there have been isolated case reports in which prolonged survival has followed an appropriate amputation, most patients die within one year. Treatment is difficult. An amputation is worthwhile if there is no evidence of metastases and in other patients may be called for by intractable pain or fungation. Radiotherapy does not seem to influence prognosis but may be valuable for the relief of pain. In a single case, calcitonin did not appear to slow the progress of the disease (Barry 1969, Walton & Strong 1973).

Giant-cell tumours are much less common than sarcomas and both benign and malignant types are recognised (Brooke 1970). Many arise in the skull or facial bones and although benign tumours have a better prognosis than sarcomas, they may cause considerable problems by encroachment on vital tissues. Malignant giant-cell tumours have a prognosis similar to that of sarcomas.

EXTRAOSSEOUS COMPLICATIONS

Neurological complications
The main neurological complications of Paget's disease result from pressure of the abnormal bone on cranial or spinal nerves or the spinal cord, or from softening of the base of the skull leading to pressure of the odontoid process on the brain stem (Friedman et al 1971).

Deafness The most common cranial nerve defect is deafness resulting from pressure on a cochlear nerve or from rigidity of the footplate of the stapes. In a few patients with a conductive type of deafness stapedectomy has led to a useful improvement in hearing (Waltner 1965, Henkin et al 1972). There is a suggestion that Paget's disease was responsible for Beethoven's deafness (Naiken 1971).

Visual disorders Four out of 23 patients described by Paget had become blind and in some cases optic atrophy is due to obliteration of the optic foramen. Diplopia due to pressure on other nerves also occurs.

Platybasia This is the name given to the invagination of the base of the softened skull so that there is pressure on the brainstem from the odontoid process. A variety of neurological problems may result including ataxia, muscle weakness due to long-tract defects, and disturbances of the control of respiration. Distortion in the region of the foramen magnum and the aqueduct of Sylvius may lead to hydrocephalus and dementia. Surgery has been of value in some cases (Friedman et al 1971). Although a grossly thickened skull must encroach on brain tissue it is remarkable how few patients with Paget's disease in the skull have symptoms.

Spinal column defects Few patients with Paget's disease of the spine have symptoms, but both spinal cord compression due to enlargement of vertebrae and defects of spinal nerves due to pressure at the foramina have been described (Klenerman 1966, Direkze & Milnes 1970, Brown et al 1971, British Medical Journal 1973).

Cardiovascular complications
The increase in the blood flow in bones with active Paget's disease has long been recognised and very occasionally extensive Paget's disease can cause high-output cardiac failure. Recent evidence supports the view that the increase is due to a vast increase in the capillary bed in the bone rather than to any arterio-venous anastomoses (Rhodes et al 1972).

Dental changes
It has already been mentioned that the mandible is sometimes affected by Paget's disease and this can cause as much difficulty to wearers of dentures as the skull changes cause to wearers of hats. It is not widely recognised that the teeth themselves can be affected by Paget's disease (Lucas 1955, Cooke 1956). The roots of the teeth may show knob-like irregularities due to the excessive deposition of cementum and histologically the new cementum has a mosaic pattern not unlike that of affected bone. The lamina dura of affected jaws is missing. The dental changes of Paget's disease may cause difficulties with extractions.

CLINICAL CHEMISTRY

The main chemical changes in patients with Paget's disease reflect the great increase in both bone formation and bone resorption (Nagant de Deuxchaines & Krane 1964). Thus there may be enormous increases both in the serum alkaline phosphatase and in the urinary excretion of hydroxyproline.

Almost all patients have a marked increase in the serum alkaline phosphatase. In a few with very local disease the alkaline phosphatase is normal Most studies have indicated that the alkaline phosphatase is derived from bone (Woodard & Marcove 1969) but in one some evidence was presented that the hepatic isoenzyme was increased (Sussman 1970). Nevertheless the serum alkaline phosphatase value provides a good guide to the activity and extent of the disease and correlates with the urinary excretion of hydroxyproline (fig. 15.4).

The serum calcium and phosphorus levels are generally normal

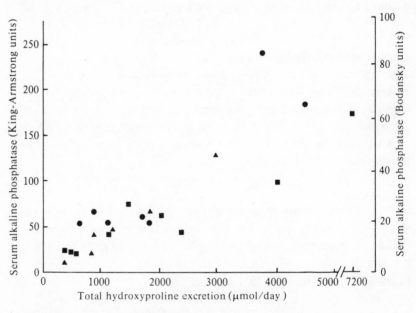

FIGURE 15.4. Relationship between the serum alkaline phosphatase values and the urinary excretion of hydroxyproline in 22 patients with Paget's disease. Data of Nagant de Deuxchaines and Krane (1964) (●), Woodhouse (1972) (▲) and Smith et al (1973a.) (■).

but the serum calcium may increase markedly when a patient with Paget's disease is immobilised (fig. 15.5). The serum acid phosphatase is occasionally increased; this may reflect the increased activity of osteoclasts (Woodhouse 1972). The urinary excretion of calcium is generally normal but high values are found during a period of predominant bone resorption and when a patient is immobilised. The urinary excretion of pseudouridine, which reflects the turnover of ribonucleic acid, is increased (Fennelly & Hogan 1972).

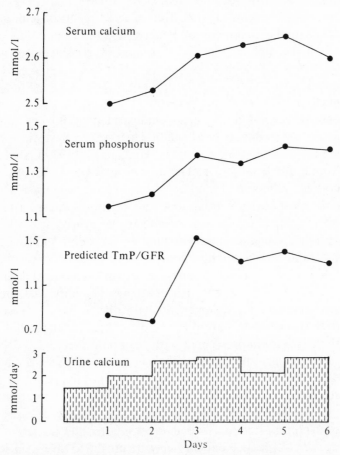

FIGURE 15.5. Effect of bedrest on a 62-year-old man with Paget's disease. There is a rise in the serum calcium and the urine calcium excretion. There is a fall in TmP/GFR which suggests that there is suppression of the activity of the parathyroid glands. Unpublished study with Dr. D. B. Morgan.

TREATMENT

Many forms of treatment have been advocated in the past for Paget's disease of bone including, phosphate supplements (Goldsmith 1972), calcium supplements and radiotherapy (Levison 1970). While all these have apparently been of benefit to some patients none has been consistently useful. Fluoride therapy has also been thought of value to some patients (Riggs & Jowsey 1972) but while it does reduce bone turnover it does not produce normal bone (Lukert et al 1972). The last ten years has seen the identification of three agents of undoubted effectiveness in the treatment of Paget's disease: calcitonin, mithramycin and the diphosphonates; these will be considered in more detail.

Calcitonin

A response to calcitonin was first demonstrated by Bijvoet and his colleagues in 1967 (Bijvoet et al 1968). Their results have since been confirmed by numerous other workers (Haddad et al 1970b, Shai et al 1971, Woodhouse et al 1971a, De Rose et al 1972, Goldfield et al 1972). Porcine, salmon and human calcitonin have been used; all are effective. In most patients, treatment with calcitonin causes a reduction in serum alkaline phosphatase and in the urinary excretion of hydroxyproline. Other results of treatment include an improvement in calcium balance, reduction in bone turnover and a decrease in the skin temperature over affected bones. Bone pain is frequently relieved but pain due to a secondary arthropathy is not improved, nor is there any consistent improvement in pain due to nerve root compression. In two patients with spinal cord compression in the thoracic region there was an improvement with calcitonin therapy.

The dose of calcitonin has usually been in the range 50–200 MRC units daily (20–80 μg salmon calcitonin) by intramuscular or subcutaneous injection. The ideal duration of a course of treatment is not yet known but patients with symptomatic Paget's disease have remained symptom-free for several months after the treatment has been stopped. In practice patients may be taught to give themselves the injections of calcitonin.

The injections are associated with some local pain and other side effects sometimes noted are flushing or nausea with the larger doses. The effectiveness of the treatment varies from patient to patient particularly with porcine and salmon calcitonin. Some patients improve and, as judged by serum alkaline phosphatase and urinary hydroxyproline measurements, remain well controlled. In some patients there is only a limited response, the 'plateau' effect. A few patients respond initially to treatment, but later the biochemical findings return to base-line values despite continuing treatment. The plateau effect and this failure of treatment is associated with the development of antibodies (De Rose et al 1972, Singer et al 1972 & 1974). Although the only calcitonin available commercially is the porcine form, human calcitonin is more potent weight for weight, and salmon calcitonin more potent still in their effects on the serum calcium in Paget's disease (Galante et al 1973). However, the effectiveness of therapy and the incidence of side effects are similar for the porcine and the salmon forms (Lesh et al 1974).

Mithramycin

Mithramycin is an antibiotic which operates by inhibiting RNA synthesis (Yarbro et al 1966). It has been used as an antitumour agent but is also effective in relatively small doses in reducing bone turnover. It has a place in the management of hypercalcaemia (p. 75) and is also effective in patients with Paget's disease of bone. A single course of treatment may produce a remission lasting one or two years. However, mithramycin must be administered by intravenous infusion and it has side effects, particularly a temporary liver cell damage (Condon et al 1971a, Aitken & Lindsay 1973, Ryan 1973).

The diphosphonates

The diphosphonates are a group of substances with a $-P-C-P-$ core and are thus analogues of pyrophosphate. Unlike pyrophosphate they are not broken down by phosphatases and they can be administered by mouth. No diphosphonate is yet available for routine clinical use but sodium etidronate (EHDP) has shown some promise in the management of Paget's disease of bone (Smith et al 1973a).

$$O=P - C - P=O$$

with OH, OH, OH above the three central atoms and ONa, CH_3, ONa below.

This substance blocks growth and dissolution of apatite crystals *in vitro* and reduces bone turnover in experimental animals. It is effective in reducing the serum alkaline phosphatase and the urinary excretion of hydroxyproline. In addition it relieves the bone pain in some patients. After a period of treatment the histological appearance of the bone is not normal; there is often an excessive quantity of osteoid. When treatment has been stopped the biochemical evidence of improvement continues for some months.

Indications for drug therapy

Paget's disease only calls for treatment when it is causing symptoms notably bone pain or neurological problems. It is difficult to know whether calcitonin or disodium etidronate (when it becomes available) should be regarded as the drug of choice. Calcitonin produces a prolonged remission of symptoms in some patients; however it is expensive, it must be given by injection and, until human calcitonin becomes available, it is limited by the development of resistance. Mithramycin may be of value in patients who have become resistant to calcitonin. Disodium etidronate also produces some prolonged remissions and has the great advantage that it can be given orally. Although normal bone is not produced it is not known whether this is a serious disadvantage. Further clinical trials are needed to resolve this question.

Chapter 16: Some Inherited Bone Disorders

There are a very large number of intrinsic bone disorders whose aetiology is quite unknown and whose nomenclature is confusing (although Maroteaux et al (1971) have attempted to give some uniformity to this). In this chapter I shall cover a few of the more common disorders which enter into the differential diagnosis of metabolic bone disease. The other disorders are reviewed by McKusick (1972) and Wynne-Davies (1973).

OSTEOGENESIS IMPERFECTA

This is a disease caused by defective collagen throughout the body; the main disability results from frequent fractures. An excellent review of historical and other aspects of the disease has been given by McKusick (1972). Two forms of osteogenesis imperfecta have been delineated: osteogenesis imperfecta congenita (OIC) where the disease becomes evident soon after birth or even before birth and osteogenesis imperfecta tarda (OIT) which presents later. Although not all cases fit into this classification it still provides a useful framework for discussing inheritance and prognosis. It is not clear whether there is a single disease with varying severity or whether there are several diseases with a similar phenotype. A wide variety of names have been used for this condition and as several still appear in the literature they have been listed in table 16.1.

Osteogenesis imperfecta has been described in all races and is not particularly uncommon. In Germany, Schröder (1964) estimated that OIC had a frequency of 2·6 per 100,000 live-births and still-births while for OIT the figure was 4·7 per 100,000 births. OIC is not a new disease; one case has been recognised in the skeleton of an infant from Egypt dating from about 1000 BC (Gray 1969).

TABLE 16.1. Some synonyms for osteogenesis imperfecta.

Fragilitas ossium
Mollities ossium
Eddowes' syndrome (fragile bones and blue sclerae)
van der Hoeve's syndrome (fragile bones, blue sclerae and deafness)
Osteopsathyrosis idiopathica

Osteogenesis imperfecta congenita

Vrolik's disease
Periosteal dysplasia of Porak and Durante (France)

Osteogenesis imperfecta tarda

Maladie de Lobstein (France)

Inheritance and genetic counselling

In almost all cases of OIT and in many cases of OIC there is clear evidence of an autosomal dominant mode of inheritance (McKusick 1972). However the severity of the disease varies greatly from patient to patient, and this variable penetrance sometimes makes inter-pretation of a family tree difficult. This is illustrated by one recent personal case, a severely affected woman of 37 whose father had an oddly shaped head and only four fractures during his lifetime. Careful study of a family may make a valuable contribution to the diagnosis of the patient presenting with unexplained fractures.

A patient with OIT who seeks advice on the possibility of trans-mitting the disease to offspring should be aware that the children have a 1 in 2 chance of being affected to some degree. The situation is much more difficult for siblings of patients. Because of the wide variation in the penetrance of the disorder an apparently unaffected sibling may be a carrier. However it is probably fair to state that a sibling who has no evidence of the disorder on clinical or radio-logical examination is very unlikely to be affected or to pass on the disease.

Some patients with OIC come from families with the dominantly inherited disorder; in such cases the parents will need to know that further children have a 1 in 2 chance of being affected. In other cases of OIC there is no evidence of abnormality in either parent. These cases could result from new mutations or could represent an autoso-mal recessive inheritance pattern. McKusick (1972) has reviewed the evidence for such an inheritance and it seems likely that autosomal recessive inheritance does occur but that it is rare. Many of the patients in sibships consistent with an autosomal recessive pattern have an atypical osteogenesis imperfecta without blue sclerae. New mutation seems to be a more frequent cause of OIC so that in the case of parents who are definitely normal and have one child affected by OIC the chance of having a further affected child is very small.

At present there is no way of detecting osteogenesis imperfecta *in utero* at a stage when termination could reasonably be considered.

Pathology and aetiology
Bone changes The cortex of long bones is usually thin and the trabeculae in cancellous bone are thin and sparse. There is a greater defect in periosteal bone deposition at the diaphyses than in bone formation at the epiphyses so that the bones themselves are slender though often of nearly normal length. Histological examination shows normal numbers of osteoblasts and osteoclasts and although the quantity of bone salts is greatly reduced, its chemical composition appears normal. However the composition of the bone matrix appears to be quite abnormal. Instead of osteoid there is a basophilic material containing reticulin fibres but not mature collagen. Although there have been reports of deficiency of glycosamino-glycans (Solheim 1969) most studies have concentrated on the collagen component of the matrix; it seems likely that there is a defect in the cross-linking of collagen molecules at least in some patients (Francis et al 1973).

Other tissues The structure of other collagen containing tissues has also been studied. There is a reduction in the collagen content of the skin (Stevenson et al 1970). The cornea and sclera have also been studied with the electron microscope. In two patients with OIT Eicholtz and Müller (1972) showed abnormalities in the fibroblasts with vacuolar changes in the endoplasmic reticulum. The collagen itself showed minor abnormalities in its cross-striations. In one patient with OIC Blümcke et al (1972) showed that the collagen was markedly abnormal with small fibres and very little cross-striation.

Pathophysiology Thus these patients have a generalised defect in collagen-containing tissues which is probably related to a defect in the maturation of collagen. The cause of this defect is quite unknown. One speculation is based on analogies between osteogenesis imperfecta and vitamin A excess in experimental animals

(Bovill 1972). Another suggestion is that there is a defect in energy metabolism like that of hyperthyroidism, since there is some evidence of a high metabolic rate in these patients (Cropp & Myers 1972).

Clinical features

It is helpful to divide cases into those whose symptoms begin around the time of birth and often have fractures before birth (osteogenesis imperfecta congenita, OIC) and those whose symptoms begin later (osteogenesis imperfecta tarda, OIT). There is however no clear dividing line between these.

Most of the patients with OIC have evidence of fractures before birth; some even have callus at birth indicating the age of the fractures. The diagnosis is sometimes made by antenatal radiography. In others it is suspected from the 'boggy' feel of the fetal skull on pelvic examination.

Some of these infants are stillborn and most of the others die within the first few weeks of life as a result of intracranial haemorrhage or respiratory difficulties. On examination there are deformed and often shortened limb bones with multiple fractures while the skull is usually large and soft on palpation (caput membranaceum). The differential diagnosis is from chondrodysplasia fetalis (achondroplasia) and from hypophosphatasia. Radiological examination serves to distinguish these and other conditions which cause dwarfism at birth (Bailey 1971). Blue sclerae are not always found in OIC. Many of the male infants have inguinal hernias (Laverty et al 1971, Tan & Tock 1971). Children who survive infancy often have less frequent fractures with increasing age but may have persisting deformity of the limb bones and very poor growth. This is due in part to the fractures and deformities and in part, it is thought, to microfractures at the epiphyseal plate. A few patients also have hypopituitarism (McKusick 1972).

In OIT the first fractures may occur soon after birth or be delayed for a year or more. During childhood there may be very many fractures: some children have more than one hundred. The fractures occur with at most minimal trauma; many parents insist that the fractures occur without trauma: 'I hear a crack and then she cries and falls down'. One French author has described these patients as 'les hommes de verre'. In another family the affected children were referred to as 'china dolls' (McKusick 1972). The fracture rate often

falls considerably at puberty; indeed there may be no further fractures although x-rays show no improvement in the bone density.

Deformities The characteristic deformities include those resulting
from fractures in the limb bones and the characteristic shapes of
the thorax and skull. There is frequently anterior bowing of the tibiae,
the back is rounded so that the thorax often has a 'beehive' shape.
Gross deformities of pectus excavatum and kypho-scolosis are not
uncommon. The skull is broad and flattened with temporal bulging
and an overhanging occiput. Many similies have been used for this
but one of the most apt is 'Tam-o'-Shanter skull' (fig. 16.1). One
result of this is that unrelated patients often have a striking resemblance to each other, and another is that old photographs can be
valuable for family studies.

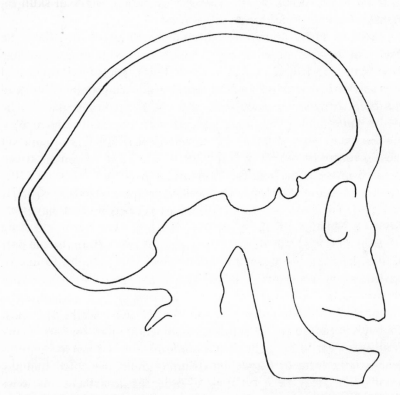

FIGURE 16.1. Osteogenesis imperfecta: tracing from a skull x-ray to
show the sloping cranium and overhanging occiput of the 'Tam-o'-
Shanter' skull. From Fourman and Royer 1968 with permission.

Eye signs One of the most useful physical signs of this disorder is the blue sclerae, resulting from the transparency of the sclerae. Although there are a few undoubted cases of OIT who lack this sign most do have sclerae whose colour varies from a vivid 'Wedgewood blue' to a dull slate-blue. Normal children may have slight blueness of the sclerae but in adults this sign is seldom seen in conditions other than osteogenesis imperfecta. It has been noted in iron-deficiency anaemia (by Sir William Osler), in rheumatoid disease, in the Ehlers-Danlos syndrome and in pseudoxanthoma elasticum (Agnoletto 1971, Pope 1971). Other eye signs of OIT include a relative whiteness around the cornea ('Saturn's ring'), a thin cornea with some danger of perforation, a circular corneal opacity known as embryotoxon or 'arcus juvenilis' and an increased danger of glaucoma (Bonnet et al 1969, McKusick 1972). The eyes are often rather prominent, perhaps because of deformity in the orbit.

Deafness This is a common complaint and usually begins in the third and fourth decades of life although cases with an earlier onset have been reported (Kosoy & Maddox 1971). The possible relationship between otosclerosis and the deafness of osteogenesis imperfecta has been extrensively discussed; while both conditions may occur in the same family and some patients with otosclerosis have blue sclerae, there does seem to be morphological differences between the disorders (Srivastava & Gupta 1969, Bretlau & Jorgensen 1969). In osteogenesis imperfecta the footplate of the stapes is enlarged and consists of soft friable bone. The hearing defect is conductive in type and often responds well to stapedectomy (Patterson & Stone 1970, Kosoy & Maddox 1971).

Dental changes The dental changes of OI result from the softness of the dentine; the teeth are often unusually yellow or may be opalescent in transmitted light. The root canals often becomes obliterated and although the enamel is normal in this condition it fractures readily because of the soft dentine underneath. The teeth gradually wear down, sometimes reaching the gum margin. Some families appear to have the dental abnormalities, known as dentinogenesis imperfecta or Capdepont teeth, without the other manifestations. This may be a different disorder because there are some histological differences in the teeth and because, unlike osteogenesis imperfecta it is almost completely limited to families with a European ancestry.

Other clinical features Many patients complain of excessive sweating. This is probably related to the high metabolic rate (Cropp & Myers 1972). Backache and leg pains are common; these may result from arthropathy at deformed joints or from nerve-root compression. Some patients have unusual laxity of the joints. One won prizes as a contortionist; he was able to put his feet into his trouser pockets (McKusick 1972). Neurological problems are uncommon but basilar invagination occasionally occurs and may cause various cerebellar or upper or lower motor neurone disorders (Evans 1971). Cardiovascular defects recognised in OIT include dilation and incompetence of the mitral and aortic valves (Wood et al 1973).

The patients generally have normal intelligence and even severely handicapped children are often remarkably well adjusted psychologically (Reite et al 1972).

Radiology

Ante-natal radiographs in OIC show extreme radiolucency of the fetal skeleton and fractures often with callus formation are common. At birth, the most striking finding is the large number of wormian bones in the skull. The long bones are usually slender with a thin cortex but OIC patients with a recessive inheritance often have broad bones with a cystic cortex. Frequent fractures lead to gross deformity. As in other types of osteopenia the vertebrae become biconcave due to the pressure of the nucleus pulposus (which may actually herniate into substance of the vertebra to give a Schmorl's node). The remarkable changes in the shape of the skull have already been mentioned.

Clinical chemistry

The plasma levels of calcium, phosphorus, alkaline phosphatase and acid phosphatase are generally normal although a high value for alkaline phosphatase may be found while fractures are healing. Abnormalities in collagen metabolism are indicated by the changes in plasma and urine hydroxyproline (Langness & Behnke 1970 or 1971). In the plasma there is an increase in the protein-bound but not the peptide or free hydroxyproline. In the urine there is an increased excretion of total hydroxyproline. Reports that there is an increased serum level of pyrophosphate (Hathaway et al 1972) have not so far been confirmed by other workers (Russell et al 1971).

Differential diagnosis

The fetus found to have bone abnormalities by antenatal radio-graphy seldom presents a diagnostic problem but occasionally achondroplasia, cleido-cranial dysplasia and intra-uterine death need to be considered (Russell 1973a). The newborn infant with multiple fractures could have hypophosphatasia or osteopetrosis but these are readily identified by radiology and, in the case of hypophosphatasia, by the low serum alkaline phosphatase. Other causes of fractures in childhood include pycnodysostosis, hyperphosphatasia, homo-cystinuria and idiopathic juvenile osteoporosis (p. 238). Multiple wormian bones in the skull are found in cleido-cranial dysplasia, pycnodysostosis, progeria, Menkes kinky hair syndrome and Cheney syndrome (McKusick 1972). The Cheney syndrome resembles osteogenesis imperfecta in that it is characterised by thin bones with a tendency to fracture, wormian bones and an autosomal dominant inheritance. It differs in that there is hypoplasia of the mandible and bone loss from the terminal phalanges of fingers and toes.

Management

It is not surprising that many forms of treatment have been tried in this chronic distressing disorder. Properly controlled clinical trials have not been done and experience with individual patients is limited by the natural variability of the disease from time to time. However there have been reports suggesting a possible value of fluoride (Kuzemko 1970, Albright & Grunt 1971), ascorbic acid (Winterfeldt et al 1970) and calcitonin (Cannigia & Gennari 1972, Goldfield et al 1972, Castells et al 1972). There is an urgent need for well designed pro-spective clinical trials.

Surgical management of this disorder is proving of increasing value in children with repeated fractures and increasing deformity of leg bones. In the procedure originally described by Sofield and Millar (1959) the bone is fractured and wedges resected if necessary so that it can be realigned and a metal rod is then passed through the medullary cavity of the fragments (the 'shish-kebab' operation). With growth the intramedullary nails must be replaced at intervals, but despite this, the procedure prevents fractures and permits the child much more activity. The use of an extensible intramedullary rod which extends as growth proceeds may represent a further advance

(Rodriguez & Wickstrom 1971). Immobilisation after these operations and after fractures should be avoided as much as possible.

The general management of children with osteogenesis imperfecta is very demanding for the parents who have to steer a course between over- and under-protection. It is important that they should know that the condition tends to improve with age. In addition societies have recently formed in the United States and in Britain which can provide valuable information and mutual support for patients and their parents. These are The Osteogenesis Imperfecta Foundation, Inc. (1231, May Court, Burlington, North Carolina 27215) and the Brittle Bone Society (63, Byron Crescent, Dundee DD3 6SS, Scotland). Both societies issue regular newsletters.

OSTEOPETROSIS

This disorder was first described in 1904 by a German radiologist, Heinrich Albers-Schönberg in a 26-year old man with multiple fractures. It is characterised by the presence of an extensive or generalised increase in bone density, multiple fractures and anaemia. Some three hundred cases had been reported by 1968 (Johnston et al 1968) and they are divided approximately equally between a severe form which usually causes death in childhood and a benign form which is consistent with survival into old age. A probable case of the severe form of the disease was reported in a mandible dating from 350–550 AD (Nielsen & Alexandersen 1971) while Cawthorne (1970) has outlined evidence that Toulouse-Lautrec may have suffered from the benign form of osteopetrosis. Alternative names for osteopetrosis include Albers-Schönberg disease, marble bone disease and osteosclerosis fragilis generalisata.

Inheritance
The severe form of the disease is inherited in an autosomal recessive manner and a history of parental consanguinity is found in about one third of the cases. The benign form of the disease is inherited in an autosomal dominant manner but with instances of non-penetrance. The severity of the condition varies greatly within a family (Johnston et al 1968).

Clinical features

Severe form This condition usually presents in infancy, with leucoerythroblastic anaemia, infections, failure to thrive, blindness or fractures. The main physical signs are indicated in table 16.2. The optic atrophy and blindness result from local pressure of the bone on the optic nerves. The large spleens and livers are the site of erythropoiesis which cannot take place in bone marrow obliterated by the sclerotic bone. Haemolytic anaemia and thrombocytopaenia may be superimposed. Many children die within the first year of life from anaemia or infections; with the possible exception of the patient described by Denison et al (1971) none of these patients have survived for more than twenty years.

TABLE 16.2. Physical signs in 50 cases of the severe recessively-inherited form of osteopetrosis (Johnston et al 1968).

	Number affected
Optic atrophy	39
Splenomegaly	31
Hepatomegaly	24
Poor growth	18
Frontal bossing	17
Fractures	14
Loss of hearing	11
Mental retardation	11
Large head	11
Osteomyelitis	9
Genu valgum	8
Facial palsy	5
Deformities of chest	4

Benign form As many as half of these patients are symptomless and only discovered as a result of family studies or of x-rays for other purposes. The most common presenting problem is a fracture with little trauma. The other clinical consequences include cranial nerve defects, particularly blindness or tunnel vision due to optic atrophy, and defects of the occulomotor and facial nerves. Anaemia is uncommon in this form and hepato-splenomegaly is not seen.

An unusual proportion of patients develop osteomyelitis of the mandible; this often follows a dental extraction and patients may be left with a chronic discharging sinus. This complication is difficult to treat and may contribute to the early death of the patient. Other dental changes include underdevelopment of the maxilla and mandible, gross malocclusion, malformation of the roots, poor mineralisation of enamel and dentine and obliteration of the pulp cavity (Cangiano et al 1972, Dick & Simpson 1972).

Pathology and pathogenesis
The disturbance in osteopetrosis is usually described as a failure of bone resorption but the cause of this is quite unknown. Plasma levels of calcitonin and parathyroid hormone are normal as is the urinary cyclic AMP excretion after administration of PTH. Recent evidence suggests that there is a defect in the lysosomal response to parathyroid hormone, perhaps because of changes in the nature of the acid phosphatase (Rosen & Haymovits 1972).

The pathological changes in the bones have been outlined by Johnston et al (1968). The failure of the bone resorption means that there is usually little or no medullary cavity but in adults with the benign type of the disease a cellular marrow may be found in enlarged Haversian canals throughout the bone. There are persisting islands of unmineralised hyaline cartilage but most of the bone consists of Haversian systems. The bone matrix contains relatively few fibres, and these do not cross over from one system to another. Osteoblasts and osteoclasts can be seen. On the basis of the histological findings Johnston et al (1968) suggest that the basic defect is not the failure of bone resorption but the deposition of bone of abnormal structure. Further study of this subject is needed.

Radiology
There is no difference between the radiological appearances in the severe and benign forms of the disease, although in the most severe cases all the bones appear uniformly dense and featureless with no medullary cavities or trabecular bone. In milder cases the early changes are see in the thickening in the diaphyseal regions of long bones. Sometimes the trabecular bone is replaced by dense bone to give a 'bone within a bone' appearance (fig. 16.2); this is found especially in the carpus and tarsus, ribs, pelvis and vertebrae.

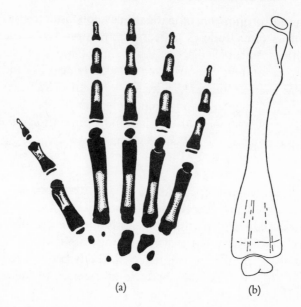

(a)   (b)

FIGURE 16.2. Osteopetrosis: (a) Dense bone to show the 'bone within a bone' appearance. (b) Failure of remodelling at the lower femoral metaphysis. From Wynne-Davies (1973) by permission.

Differential diagnosis of dense bones Table 16.3 lists the disorders which are associated with osteosclerosis. The radiological appearances which assist in distinguishing these conditions are discussed in standard texts such as those by Greenfield (1969) and Murray and Jacobson (1971). Several of these disorders are described elsewhere in this book. Bone sclerosis in myeloma was described by Brown and Paterson (1973) and skeletal fluorosis by Teotia et al (1971). Coccidioidmycosis as a cause of dense vertebrae was recorded by Eller and Siebert (1969). Melorheostosis is a very rare bone disorder characterised by well defined sclerotic areas in limb-bones (fig. 16.3). Its aetiology is unknown (Campbell et al 1968, Hoshino & Murakami 1971). The remaining bone disorders are described by McKusick (1972).

Clinical chemistry

The levels of calcium, phosphorus and alkaline phosphatase in the serum are normal, as is the urinary excretion of hydroxyproline. The only consistently recognised abnormality is a rise in the serum acid phosphatase, the non-prostatic fraction being involved (Johnston et al 1968).

TABLE 16.3. Causes of bone sclerosis.

Common

Paget's disease of bone
Uraemic osteodystrophy
Osteosclerotic metastases particularly from carcinomas of the prostate
   or breast

Uncommon

Myelosclerosis
Myelomatosis (rarely)
Sarcoidosis (rarely)
Primary hyperparathyroidism (rarely)
Infantile hypercalcaemia
Chronic vitamin D poisoning
Lead poisoning
Chronic fluoride excess
Cretinism and adult hypothyroidism
Coccidioidmycosis
Osteopetrosis
Hereditary hyperphosphatasia
Melorheostosis
Pycnodysostosis
Osteopoikilosis
Osteopathia striata
Diaphyseal dysplasia (Engelmann's disease)
Fibrogenesis imperfecta ossium

Management

Many methods of treatment have been tried in attempts to produce a negative calcium balance, including heparin, vitamin A, vitamin D, chelating agents and steroids. None of these has been of convincing value but there is a suggestion from a few cases that a low calcium diet augmented with cellulose phosphate may delay the progress of the bone sclerosis (Yu et al 1971b). The anaemia is often caused, in part, by haemolysis and thrombocytopaenia so that corticosteroids, and on occasion splenectomy, may be indicated. Despite the loss of the haematopoietic contribution of the spleen this procedure has been useful in most of the patients in whom it has been used (Moe & Skjaeveland 1969, Yu et al 1971b).

Surgical intervention is sometimes needed for progressive loss of vision. By relieving the pressure on the optic nerve further deterioration may be halted (Moe & Skjaeveland 1969, Utley 1970).

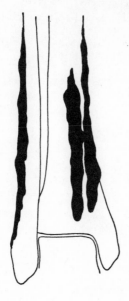

FIGURE 16.3. Melorheostosis: linear streaks of dense bone, the 'dripping candle' appearance. From Wynne-Davies (1973) by permission.

HYPOPHOSPHATASIA

This hereditary disorder which has some radiological resemblance to rickets was described by Chown in Winnipeg in 1935. In 1948 Rathbun noted that a patient had a low serum alkaline phosphatase activity and devised the name hypophosphatasia (Macpherson et al 1972). In most cases the pattern of inheritance suggests an autosomal recessive mode of transmission, and the disorder is particularly common in inbred communities as among Mennonites in Canada and in southern Hungary (Macpherson et al 1972, Méhes et al 1972).

Clinical features
Three main groups of patients can be distinguished according to the age of presentation. Although there is some overlap between the groups this classification is still useful in indicating prognosis. The most severe form of hypophosphatasia is that which occurs in neonates. These infants may have pathological fractures *in utero* and at birth are found to have bowed limb-bones, enlarged bone ends as in

rickets, a rachitic rosary and very deficient ossification in the skull. The very large fontanelles bulge, and the patients present with convulsions or failure to thrive or a bleeding tendency due to thrombocytopaenia. Most of these children die within the first year of life, often from chest infections related perhaps to the softness of the thoracic cage. The differential diagnosis is from osteogenesis imperfecta.

A less severe form of the disease is also recognised in infancy and childhood. These patients have milder symptoms which have a gradual onset. While fractures and rickets-like deformities occur, most patients come because of poor growth and failure to thrive. Physical examination shows a bulging fontanelle which results from the premature fusion of the sutures and the continuing growth of the brain. Later the head develops a remarkable brachycephalic shape. The differential diagnosis, depending on the age, is from vitamin D deficiency rickets, hypophosphataemic rickets, achondroplasia, congenital syphilis and from other conditions associated with premature fusion of the sutures. Most patients have little trouble apart from unduly frequent fractures in later life. One personal patient, a nineteen year-old boy developed weakness of the hands with invagination of the soft skull by the cervical spine (platybasia) a problem which occurs more often in Paget's disease.

A mild form of the disease may be detected in childhood or may not present until adult life. These patients mostly present because of fractures but one patient presented at the age of 51 having had an arthropathy, probably due to calcium pyrophosphate deposition, for 27 years (O'Duffy 1970). Many patients give a past history of fractures in childhood, delayed walking and a rickets-like disorder which healed spontaneously (Jardon et al 1970, Macpherson et al 1972).

The three main forms of hypophosphatasia probably do not represent different diseases. Several families have been described in which there have been marked differences in the severity of the disease in affected siblings.

Dental changes The characteristic dental problem is premature loss of deciduous teeth, delayed eruption of the permanent teeth and a liability to cavities. The dental disorder may be the only complaint in a patient with little or no skeletal changes. The teeth themselves show a lack of cementum at the roots (Casson 1969).

Pathology

The pathological changes in the bone in hypophosphatasia resemble those of rickets or osteomalacia. In the severely affected neonates large parts of the cranial vault consist of unmineralised osteoid; while the bones appear radiographically to be separated by wide sutures they are really in apposition. The ends of the long bones in children show a widened epiphyseal cartilage with strands of cartilage extending into the metaphysis. In both children and adults the trabecular bone surfaces are covered with osteoid. Numbers of osteoclasts or active osteoblasts are not increased.

Radiology

The radiological appearances of the long bones in hypophosphatasic children are not unlike those of rickets (fig. 16.4). The changes are however more severe and irregular than are commonly seen in rickets; there are wide epiphyses with irregular outlines and cupping. There are regular cyst-like defects in the metaphysis. The skull changes which are not found in rickets, consist of large areas apparently lacking in ossification.

In older children the premature fusion of the sutures is followed by a 'beaten copper' appearance perhaps resulting from increased intracranial pressure. In adults the radiological signs may include persisting deformity or pseudofractures and the apparent bone density is reduced (James & Moule 1966, Macpherson et al 1972).

Clinical chemistry

A low or very low serum alkaline phosphatase is a hallmark of this disease; the major source of such alkaline phosphatase as is present in the serum is the intestine (Warshaw et al 1971, Inglis et al 1972). The value for serum alkaline phosphatase does not correlate with the severity of the clinical disease. The serum calcium is usually normal except in severely affected neonates in whom it is often raised. The plasma inorganic phosphorus is usually normal.

Patients with hypophosphatasia excrete large amounts of phospho-ethanolamine in the urine. This amino-acid is not found in normal urine but it has occasionally been detected in coeliac disease, scurvy, hypothyroidism and magnesium deficiency (Fraser 1957, Hanna et al 1960). The plasma level of pyrophosphate and its excretion in the urine are both increased (Russell 1965, Russell et al 1971). The

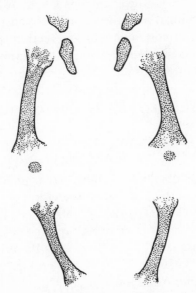

FIGURE 16.4. Hypophosphatasia: lower extremities of a three-week-old infant to show wide epiphyses and deep irregular defects in the metaphyses.

excretion of hydroxyproline in the urine is reduced (Teree & Klein 1968).

Heterozygotes for hypophosphatasia usually have a fairly low serum alkaline phosphatase activity. Many also excrete phosphoethanolamine in the urine. However the identification of heterozygotes is seldom needed in genetic counselling.

Pseudohypophosphatasia This term was applied by Scriver and Cameron (1969) to patients with convincing physical signs and phosphoethanolamine in the urine but who had a normal value for serum alkaline phosphatase. As these patients are found in the families known to include patients with hypophosphatasia (Méhes et al 1972), this must represent a form of the disease, but whether they are heterozygotes with unusual expression or homozygotes with an unusually high intestinal alkaline phosphatase is not known.

Management
Both phosphate supplements and corticosteroids have been tried in hypophosphatasia but neither influences the calcification defect

(Teree & Klein 1968). However there is a considerable spontaneous improvement in infants who survive the first year of life. In later life the fractures heal normally and intervention is only required in the few patients who develop neurological problems.

OTHER DISORDERS OF UNKNOWN CAUSE

HEREDITARY HYPERPHOSPHATASIA

This is a rare disease of childhood inherited in an autosomal recessive manner. It is characterised by fractures, deformity of long bones and enlargement of the skull. The radiographs resemble those of Paget's disease in adults with areas of resorption and sclerosis. The serum alkaline phosphatase level is very high as is the urinary excretion of hydroxyproline. In one case there was a prompt response to treatment with calcitonin (Woodhouse et al 1972).

PYCNODYSOSTOSIS

This is an uncommon disorder which is inherited as an autosomal recessive (Emami-Ahari et al 1969, McKusick 1972). It rivals osteopetrosis as a possible retrospective diagnosis for Toulouse-Lautrec's illness. It is characterised by bone sclerosis with a tendency to fracture, wide cranial fontanelles, a receding jaw caused by hypoplasia of the ramus of the mandible, hypoplasia of the clavicles and resorption of the terminal phalanges of the fingers.

FIBROUS DYSPLASIA

This curious disease, or group of diseases, is probably of developmental origin (Lichtenstein 1970, Gibson & Middlemiss 1971). It is characterised by fibrous tissue which spreads within the medullary space and erodes the cortex causing widened, distorted bones with a thin cortex. In the majority of cases it affects only one bone or a part of a bone (monostotic fibrous dysplasia). The femur, tibia and jaw are the most commonly affected bones. In a few cases it affects several bones (polyostotic fibrous dysplasia). The patients generally present in the second and third decades of life with painless swelling of a bone, especially in the jaw, or deformity or fracture of a long bone. The femur typically shows bending of the neck and proximal shaft into a 'Shepherd's crook' deformity while the tibia bends inwards. The polyostotic form is sometimes associated with skin pigmentation or endocrine problems such as precocious puberty or hyperthyroidism. This has been called the Albright syndrome or the McCune-Albright syndrome.

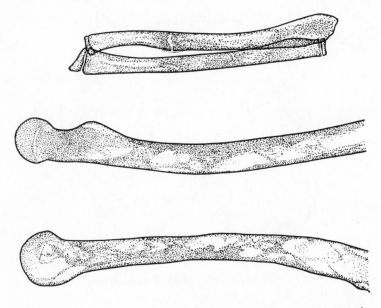

FIGURE 16.5. Polyostotic fibrous dysplasia. Typical appearances in long bones. There is patchy thinning of the cortex with expansion of the shaft best seen in the lower end of the humerus.

The differential diagnosis of the monostotic form is from many other benign lesions of bone including benign cysts, fibromas and enchondroma. Biopsy is usually needed to confirm the diagnosis. The polyostotic form usually has a sufficiently characteristic appearance on radiographs that biopsy is not needed. It must be distinguished from severe primary hyperparathyroidism; while the serum alkaline phosphatase is sometimes raised the serum calcium and phosphorus levels are normal. However there have been occasional reports of patients with both parathyroid adenomas and undoubted fibrous dysplasia (Ehrig & Wilson 1972).

The fibrous tissue proliferation ceases in adult life but the deformities and risk of fracture remain. Although sarcoma formation has been observed in affected bone, this is not common. There have been reports of a possible effect of calcitonin therapy on the raised serum alkaline phosphatase and urinary hydroxyproline excretion in this disease (Bell et al 1970, Morii et al 1971) but further study is needed to determine whether calcitonin has a place in management.

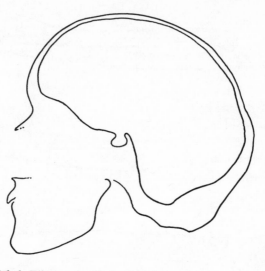

FIGURE 16.6. Fibrous dysplasia: Marked thickening of the occipital region but the remainder of the skull is normal.

Surgery may be needed for the disease affecting the maxilla or mandible. Persisting deformity and fracture in the femur or tibia calls for excision of the diseased tissue and correction of the deformity by osteotomy and internal fixation (Henry 1969).

Fibrogenesis Imperfecta Ossium

This is a disorder of unknown cause which presents in middle age with generalised bone pain and tenderness. Seven cases have been described (Frame et al 1971b, Swann & Cooke 1973, Henneman et al 1973). Radiographs show a general increase in bone density and a loss of the normal architecture; trabeculae are absent and the bones have a mottled appearance. Histologically there is an excess of osteoid but unlike that in osteomalacia the osteoid shows little birefringence under polarised light. It has been suggested that there is a defect in the maturation of collagen. In the serum the levels of calcium and phosphorus are normal but the alkaline phosphatase activity is increased.

In two reports there has been an apparent partial response to treatment with vitamin D_2 or dihydrotachysterol.

AXIAL OSTEOMALACIA

This disorder was first described by Frame and colleagues in 1961 and six cases have now been reported (Condon & Nassim 1971). The patients present in middle age with mild backache and radiology reveals an irregular coarse pattern in the trabecular bone of the spine and pelvis. Histologically there is an excess of osteoid in the affected bone but unlike that in fibrogenesis imperfecta ossium the lamellar pattern is normal. The serum calcium, phosphorus and alkaline phosphatase levels are generally normal.

This disorder, whose cause is quite unknown, appears to have a good prognosis without treatment. The relatively minor symptoms do not progress and fractures do not occur. Attempts have been made to treat patients with vitamin D but there has been no evidence of any response.

Chapter 17: Bone Changes in some Endocrine Disorders

Apart from parathyroid hormone and calcitonin, several hormones have direct actions on bone, notably growth hormone (Urist 1972), the thyroid hormones (Vaughan 1970) and the glucocorticoids (Silberberg & Silberberg 1971). This chapter is concerned with the effects of deficiency or excess of these hormones on the bone or on the metabolism of calcium and phosphorus.

ACROMEGALY

The clinical features of acromegaly are well known. They result from increased periosteal bone apposition (and in children increased epiphyseal bone formation as well).

Pathophysiology

In active acromegaly many kinetic studies have shown that there is an increased exchangeable calcium pool and increased rates both of bone formation and resorption. A few reports have suggested that patients with acromegaly have a negative calcium balance; this has not been confirmed in other studies and the limitations of this sort of evidence have already been outlined (p. 56). In general the total body calcium and therefore the total bone mass is a little more than would be expected from a patient's height (Aloia et al 1972).

Bone changes

Both histological and radiological studies indicate that in long bones the total bone width is increased while the cortical thickness is little changed and the cortical bone mass is normal or increased. The bone appearances of acromegaly were at one time thought to indicate osteoporosis and this is still mentioned in several current textbooks. While the appearances of the trabecular bone sometimes simulate those of age-related bone loss, there is no evidence of a reduced

274

bone mass and no evidence of an increased risk of fractures (Doyle 1967, Riggs et al 1972b).

The other radiological features of acromegaly are outlined by Doyle (1967) and by Murray and Jacobson (1971). Apart from changes in the sella turcica, the skull may be diffusely thickened, sometimes with frontal hyperostosis in addition. The mandible is frequently enlarged and prominent. In the thoracic spine there may be new bone formation on the anterior and lateral surfaces of the vertebral discs. The posterior surface of the bodies of the lumbar vertebrae may show a marked concavity. The overgrowth of the ribs leads to a chest with an increased antero-posterior diameter. Hypertrophy of the cartilage at the bone ends leads to an increase in length of bones particularly in the hands and feet and also to a greater risk of degenerative joint disorders. The tufts of the terminal phalanges are often enlarged and spade-like, while the sesamoid bone of the thumb is large.

Clinical chemistry

Many patients with active acromegaly have a high or high normal plasma phosphorus. This is related to an increase in the renal tubular reabsorption of phosphorus (TmP/GFR) and falls to normal when the acromegaly is treated (fig. 17.1). There is often a small rise in the serum calcium (Nadarajah et al 1968). While in some patients this is

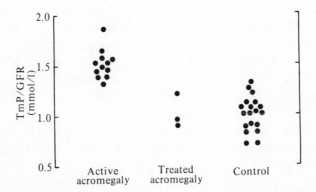

FIGURE 17.1. Ratio between tubular transport maximum for phosphorus and the glomerular filtration rate (TmP/GFR) in active acromegaly, treated acromegaly and adult controls. Data of Corvilain and Abramow (1972).

due to an associated hyperparathyroidism, in others it seems to be a feature of the acromegaly itself. Hypercalciuria is also common in acromegaly and may cause renal stones.

PITUITARY INSUFFICIENCY

In patients with pituitary insufficiency intestinal calcium absorption and urinary calcium excretion are reduced and both increase with the administration of growth hormone (Henneman et al 1960, Hanna et al 1961, Bryson et al 1972). Similar results can be obtained in rats with a hypophysectomy (Finkelstein & Schachter 1962). The plasma levels of calcium and phosphorus are generally normal for the patient's age in pituitary insufficiency. TmP/GFR is normal and not reduced as might be expected in growth hormone deficiency. It may be that associated lack of adrenal and thyroid hormones has a compensatory effect of the renal tubule (Corvilain & Abramow 1972).

Apart from the retardation of skeletal maturation in children with a deficiency of growth hormone, the bones in hypopituitarism are unremarkable.

HYPOTHYROIDISM

Pathophysiology
The mode of action of the thyroid hormones on bone is not known but they do appear to affect bone cells directly to permit bone resorption (Vaughan 1970). In hypothyroidism there is a reduction in bone blood flow and a reduction in both bone formation and bone resorption. The disturbance of remodelling in children leads to a delay in skeletal maturation and to other disorders of growth. In addition there is an increase in intestinal calcium absorption; this sometimes leads to hypercalcaemia and to metastatic calcification, for example in the kidneys.

Clinical and radiological features
Children The clinical features of cretins are well known. The retardation of growth depends on the severity and age of onset, but may be very severe especially when the illness begins in the first few years

of life. In minor degrees of hypothyroidism a retardation of growth
may be the only abnormality.

Radiological abnormalities include the delayed appearance and
fusion of all epiphyses. When ossification centres do appear they
may have a very irregular or stippled appearance or may be frag-
mented (fig. 17.2). In the head of the femur this disorder has its most

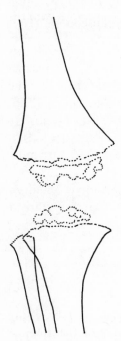

FIGURE 17.2. Knee joint in a cretin to show the
irregular development of the ossification centres.
(tracing from an x-ray).

serious effects and cretins may have epiphysiolysis and coxa vara or,
less commonly, dislocation of the hips. Symptoms from the hip joint
may be the cause for the presentation of a patient with juvenile
myxoedema. The hip changes must be distinguished from Perthe's
disease and dysplasia epiphysialis multiplex.

The vertebrae in cretins also show characteristic changes. The
upper lumber vertebrae are oval or wedge-shaped in lateral radiographs with tongue-like projections from the anterior surface fig.
17.3). This abnormality is first visible at six months of age and
progresses steadily. Many patients have a kyphosis or kyphoscoliosis.
Some have a spondylolysthesis.

In the skull the cretin has delayed closure of the fontanelles and sutures. The ossification of the base of the skull is delayed and the diploe and air sinuses do not develop normally (Fourman & Royer 1968, Murray & Jacobson 1971). Osteosclerosis of the skull has been described although some of these patients had also had large doses of vitamin D (Schmidt 1962).

The adult cretin It would be difficult to better Jackson's (1952) account of the clinical and radiological features of cretins first seen in adult life. They are severely dwarfed with a kyphoscoliosis. Their

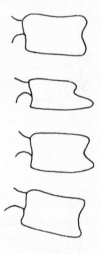

FIGURE 17.3. Lumbar vertebrae 1–4 in a cretin (tracing from an x-ray). From Fourman and Royer (1968) with permission.

radiographs may show persisting epiphyses, the vertebrae are irregular, the skull is long with thinning in the area of the anterior fontanelle and enlargement of the pituitary fossa. There is often severe damage to the femoral head and neck.

Adult hypothyroidism Hypothyroidism in adults does not give skeletal symptoms but there may be well marked diffuse or generalised osteosclerosis with unusually thick cortices in long bones (Bordier et al 1967).

Clinical chemistry
The serum calcium and phosphorus levels are usually normal in hypothyroidism but a few patients, both children and adults, have hypercalcaemia (Adams et al 1968, Pretorius & Potgieter 1971). The hypercalcaemia is probably not caused by any deficiency of

calcitonin because it responds to treatment with thyroxine alone. Calcitonin levels in serum cannot yet be determined with sufficient confidence to examine this question directly. The serum alkaline phosphatase activity is usually low or low-normal as is the urinary excretion of hydroxyproline.

HYPERTHYROIDISM

Pathophysiology

In hyperthyroidism there are increases both in bone formation and bone resorption but the increase in resorption is the greater. In addition the intestinal absorption of calcium is reduced (Shafer & Gregory 1972). Despite the negative calcium balance which this entails the predominant bone resorption means that the patients are normocalcaemic or, occasionally, hypercalcaemic. Deficiency of calcitonin does not appear to be a factor in the bone changes of hyperthyroidism (Lim et al 1969).

Bone changes

The principal change in the bone in hyperthyroidism is bone loss, or after maturity, an accelerated loss of bone (Smith et al 1973b). Radiologically this has been demonstrated very elegantly by Meema and Meema (1972) who used fine-grain industrial film with manual processing. With this technique abnormalities were found in 73% of hyperthyroid patients and consist of intracortical striation with very little decrease in the thickness of the cortex.

Although many patients appear to have normal bones on histological study, patients with active thyrotoxicosis may have excessive osteoclastic resorption with fibrosis or an excess of osteoid on bone surfaces (Follis 1953, Bordier et al 1967). There is no evidence that these changes are mediated by parathyroid hormone.

Clinical features

The disorder of calcium metabolism in hyperthyroidism seldom contributes to the clinical presentation of the disease. There may be an increased incidence of fractures in hyperthyroid patients compared with age-matched control subjects (Fraser et al 1971b) and fractures were common in hyperthyroidism in the early days before adequate treatment was available (Michie et al 1971). A few patients have hypercalcaemia severe enough to contribute to the symptoms (Buckle et al 1969, Twycross & Marks 1970). Despite the frequent occurrence of hypercalciuria urinary calculi are no more common than in the rest of the population (Walker 1971).

Clinical chemistry

As a group, patients with hyperthyroidism have higher serum calcium levels than control subjects, but only in a minority do the results exceed the normal range. Baxter and Bondy (1966) for example found hypercalcaemia in 17 out of 77 unselected patients with hyperthyroidism. Some patients with hypercalcaemia have coincidental hyperparathyroidism for there appears to be an increased incidence of hyperparathyroidism in patients with thyrotoxicosis (Heimann et al 1970a & b, Richards 1970, Rao 1970, Ghozlan et al 1973). The reason for the hypercalcaemia in the remaining patients is not entirely clear (Parfitt & Dent 1970) but it is corrected when the hyperthyroidism itself is corrected with carbimazole or even propranolol (Twycross & Marks 1970, Seedat et al 1970).

A few patients with hyperthyroidism have a high serum alkaline phosphatase activity. Some have a high urinary output of calcium, hydroxyproline and, in females, pyrophosphate (Bordier et al 1967, Russell & Hodgkinson 1969). The renal tubular transport maximum for phosphate (expressed as TmP/GFR) is generally increased in hyperthyroidism (Bijvoet 1969).

Effect of treatment on calcium metabolism

The incidence of permanent hypoparathyroidism after thyroidectomy for hyperthyroidism has already been mentioned in chapter 9 as has been the controversial question of partial hypoparathyroidism. After thyroid surgery a temporary hypocalcaemia is much more common than a permanent hypoparathyroidism. Until recently it was widely accepted that this temporary hypocalcaemia was caused by partial damage or ischaemia of parathyroid tissue which was able to recover or regenerate. However Michie et al (1971) have now suggested that an important factor in the temporary hypocalcaemia is an increased avidity of the bones for calcium after the hyperthyroidism is relieved. They advise that, in the absence of more precise tests to identify the patients most at risk, those with a high serum alkaline phosphatase preoperatively should be given oral calcium supplements before and after the operation.

Measurements of bone mass after treatment of the hyperthyroidism have suggested that the rate of loss of bone is diminished and the patients may show a modest improvement in the percentile value for bone mass (Smith et al 1973b).

ADRENAL INSUFFICIENCY

The clinical features and differential diagnosis of adrenocortical insufficiency have been reviewed by Irvine and Barnes (1972). Disorders of calcium metabolism can be demonstrated frequently in these patients but very seldom are the cause of the patient's presentation. An exception to this rule was provided by a recent personal case (Downie et al 1973). A married woman of 32 presented with listlessness, vomiting, confusion and dehydration. She had a serum calcium of 3·75 mmol/l and a serum phosphorus of 1·0 mmol/l. She was thought to have an acute hyperparathyroidism but a careful exploration of the neck revealed no abnormal parathyroid glands. During the postoperative period she failed to improve, again began to vomit and became confused and drowsy. A clinical diagnosis of adrenal insufficiency was then made and it was confirmed with the demonstration of a high titre of adrenal antibodies in the serum. This case was particularly remarkable in the extent to which her symptoms and blood chemistry resembled those of primary hyperparathyroidism. It illustrates the disturbance in calcium metabolism which occurs in adrenal insufficiency.

The association between adrenal insufficiency and hypoparathyroidism was described in chapter 9.

Pathophysiology
Adrenal insufficiency is associated with haemoconcentration and a rise in the total serum calcium could be a result only of a rise in the serum albumin. However this is not the whole explanation because there is a rise in the ionised fraction of the serum calcium after adrenalectomy in rats (Raman 1970b). Increased renal tubular reabsorption of calcium seems likely to be the principal cause of the hypercalcaemia in these cases (Walser et al 1963, Jørgensen 1973).

Bone changes
The histological and radiological appearances of the bone are usually normal.

Clinical chemistry
Several patients with adrenal insufficiency have been identified because of an unusually brisk and complete response to steroids in a steroid suppression test done because of hypercalcaemia. Hypercalcaemia is almost as frequently found in patients with adrenal insufficiency as is hyponatraemia (Walser et al 1963). The serum phosphorus is usually normal but values above the normal range are found in a minority of patients (Siegler 1970, Kasperlik-Zaluska 1971). In these patients increased renal tubular reabsorption appears to be responsible.

GLUCOCORTICOID EXCESS

Glucocorticoid excess may be caused by a tumour of the adrenal gland, by adrenal hyperplasia resulting from an excessive production of corticotrophin by the anterior pituitary or by therapy with corticosteroids, corticotrophin or its synthetic analogues. A similar syndrome is described as a result of the ectopic production of corticotrophin or a corticotrophin-like peptide by non-endocrine tumours notably carcinomas of the bronchus (Besser & Edwards 1972). If prolonged all these disorders can give rise to a disturbance of calcium metabolism.

Pathophysiology
Both in spontaneous and iatrogenic glucocorticoid excess there is microradiographic evidence of a decrease in bone formation and an increase in bone resorption (Thompson et al 1972). The mode of action of the steroid hormones is not fully understood but in tissue culture glucocorticoids have a direct action on bone to *inhibit* bone resorption (Raisz et al 1972c). It seems likely therefore that the effects of glucocorticoids on bone *in vivo* are secondary to actions on the intestine or kidney.

In the intestine there is good evidence that glucocorticoids reduce calcium absorption but a direct effect on vitamin D metabolism is unlikely (Gallagher et al 1973, Favus et al 1973). The effect of corticosteroids on the renal tubule is less well understood. Aldosterone seems to have no direct action on calcium reabsorption (Paunier et al 1972), but many patients with glucocorticoid excess have an increased urinary excretion of calcium in the presence of a normal serum calcium. It is likely therefore that tubular calcium reabsorption is diminished in this disorder.

Bone changes

Some patients present as a result of backache or fractures. Typical fractures are said to be painless and followed by abundant callus formation. In addition patients on long-term corticosteroid therapy sometimes develop collapse of the femoral head as a result of necrosis. The mechanism underlying this is not known (British Medical Journal 1972).

The main histological changes in the bone have been outlined by Birkenhäger et al (1967). There is a diminished amount of bone but different authors have found the numbers of osteoblasts to be diminished, normal or increased; in severe cases there are increased numbers of osteoclasts.

The radiological changes include bone rarefaction which is said to be more marked in the axial skeleton. Objective measurements of ulnar mineral content gave low values in one third of the patients studied by Doyle (1967) but some patients with normal values had fractures of the ribs or vertebrae. Cortical bone may be less affected in this condition than trabecular bone. Infants with glucocorticoid excess present with weight gain and severe growth impairment; radiographs show thin bones, often with fractures, and retarded bone maturation (Darling et al 1970). In infants and children new bone laid down after the disease has been treated is of normal appearance but the thin bone laid down previously persists. In adults there is no evidence that the bone loss is reversible.

Clinical chemistry

The serum calcium is generally normal perhaps because the effects of bone rarefaction are balanced by those of the diminished intestinal calcium absorption and increased urinary calcium excretion. Occasional patients have hypocalcaemia. One patient reported by

Schneider (1971) had borderline hypercalcaemia, but after an adrenal adenoma had been removed she developed severe hypercalcaemia and was found to have hyperparathyroidism. Schneider suggested that the symptoms and chemical changes of hyperparathyroidism had been masked by the glucocorticoid excess. The serum alkaline phosphatase and serum phosphorus are generally normal. The urinary excretion of calcium is often high even when the dietary calcium is normal.

Appendix: Commercially available and Standard Preparations for the Management of Metabolic Bone Disease

This list is not exhaustive and is even more liable to obsolescence than the remainder of the book. However, it is provided because commercial sources of many preparations are not widely known.

Aluminium hydroxide
Aludrox Wyeth (UK)
Amphojel Wyeth (USA & Australia)
Aluminium hydroxide tablets (BP)
Dried aluminium hydroxide gel tablets (USA)

Aluminium carbonate
Basaljel suspension Wyeth (USA)

Calcitonin (Porcine)
Calcitare Armour (UK and USA)

Calcium for oral use
Sandocal (Calcium-Sandoz effervescent tablets) Sandoz
Calcium-Sandoz syrup
Standard preparations of calcium gluconate and calcium lactate are found in most pharmacopoeias

Calcium for intravenous use
Calcium-Sandoz (calcium gluconoglactogluconate) Sandoz
Calcium gluconate BP (also USP and most other pharmacopoeias)

Cellulose phosphate
Whatman sodium cellulose phosphate (Whatman Biochemicals Ltd., Springfield Mill, Sandling Road, Maidstone, UK)

Dihydrotachysterol$_2$
AT10 Winthrop (UK)

Phosphate for oral use
Phosphate-Sandoz Sandoz (UK, Canada)
Hyper-Phos-K Davies Rose Hoyt (USA)
Neutraphos Willen Drug Co. (USA)
Phospho-Soda Fleet (USA)
(also anhydrous sodium phosphate (BPC, USNF and many other pharmacopoeias) but this is only Na_2HPO_4)

Phosphate for intravenous use

In Phos Davies Rose Hoyt (USA)

No standard preparation. The composition of a suitable infusion fluid was given on page 72.

Vitamin D for oral use

a. Small doses for nutritional rickets. Many standard and proprietary preparations are available. Preparations containing both calcium and vitamin D are sometimes unsatisfactory and are not recommended.

b. Large doses for hypoparathyroidism, etc.

Calciferol tablets BP, USP and other pharmacopoeias. These tablets have some limitations (Parfitt & Frame 1972) and preparations which are more precise and stable are available from the Chief Pharmacist, University College Hospital, London, WC1E 6AU.

Vitamin D for parenteral use

Large doses for the single-dose treatment of rickets and osteomalacia: Calciferol BP (made by Evans Medical Co., Speke, Liverpool, UK)

References

The order in which the references are placed is related to the manner in which they appear in the text. Thus *Jones* precedes *Jones & Williams* which precedes *Jones et al* irrespective of the date. Single author references are subclassified by date, two-author references by the second author's name and references with three or more authors by date. Initials are ignored throughout. Mac ... and Mc ... are classified as the authors have spelled their names (not as in British telephone directories) and ø has been treated as o (not as in the Danish convention.)

The numbers in parentheses after each entry indicate the page on which the reference is cited.

ÅBERG H JOHANSSON H WERNER I (1972a) Hyperparathyroidism and asthma *Lancet* **2** 381 (95)

ÅBERG H JOHANSSON H WERNER I WIMAN L-G (1972b) Sarcoidosis hypercalcemia and hyperparathyroidism *Scandinavian Journal of Respiratory Diseases* **53** 259–264 (120)

ACKERMAN NB WINER N (1971) Evaluation of methods for localizing parathyroid tumors *American Journal of Surgery* **122** 669–673 (103)

ADAMS PH CHALMERS TM (1965) Parathyroid function after ^{131}I therapy for hyperthyroidism *Clinical Science* **29** 391–395 (151)

ADAMS P CHALMERS TM RIGGS BL JONES JD (1968) Parathyroid function in spontaneous primary hypothyroidism *Journal of Endocrinology* **40** 467–475 (278)

ADAMS P DAVIES GT SWEETMAN P (1970a) Osteoporosis and the effects of ageing on bone mass in elderly men and women *Quarterly Journal of Medicine* NS **39** 601–615 (230)

ADAMS P CHALMERS TM HILL LF TRUSCOTT BMcN (1970b) Idiopathic hypercalciuria and hyperparathyroidism *British Medical Journal* **4** 582–585 (Read with the subsequent correspondence: *British Medical Journal* (1971) **1** pages 47 108 and 109 and **2** page 108) (101, 134)

ADIE R TAYLOR S (1973) The surgery of hyperparathyroidism *Medical Journal of Australia* **1** 688–691 (104)

AGNOLETTO A (1971) Blue sclerotics in iron deficiency *Lancet* **2** 1160 (258)

AGRAWAL JR SHETH SC TIBREWALA NS (1969) Rickets—a study of 300 cases *Indian Pediatrics* **6** 792–798 (168)

AGUS ZS PUSCHETT JB SENESKY D GOLDBERG M (1971) Mode of action of parathyroid hormone and cyclic adenosine 3′,5′-monophosphate on renal tubular phosphate reabsorption in the dog *Journal of Clinical Investigation* **50** 617–626 (16)

287

AITKEN JM LINDSAY R (1973) Mithramycin in Paget's disease *Lancet* **1** 1177–1178 (251)

AITKEN JM HART DM ANDERSON JB LINDSAY R SMITH DA SPEIRS CF (1973) Osteoporosis after oophorectomy for non-malignant disease in premenopausal women *British Medical Journal* **2** 325–328 (236)

AKSOY M CAMLI N DINCOL K ERDEM S AKGÜN T (1972) Osseous changes in Wilson's disease *Radiology* **102** 505–509 (209)

ALBRIGHT F (1970) Hyperparathyroidism: Some early patients *Archives of Internal Medicine* **126** 558–566 (79)

ALBRIGHT JA GRUNT JA (1971) Studies of patients with osteogenesis imperfecta *Journal of Bone and Joint Surgery* **53A** 1415–1425 (260)

ALBRIGHT F REIFENSTEIN EC (1948) *The parathyroid glands and metabolic bone disease* Baltimore: Williams and Wilkins (28)

ALBRIGHT F AUB JC BAUER W (1934) Hyperparathyroidism A common and polymorphic condition as illustrated by seventeen proved cases from one clinic *Journal of the Americal Medical Association* **102** 1276–1287 (91)

ALBRIGHT F BURNETT CH SMITH PH PARSON W (1942) Pseudo-hypoparathyroidism an example of the "Seabright-Bantam" syndrome *Endocrinology* **30** 922–932 (161)

ALBRIGHT F FORBES AP HENNEMAN PH (1952) Pseudo-pseudohypoparathyroidism *Transactions of the Association of American Physicians* **65** 337–350 (164)

ALOIA JF ROGINSKY MS JOWSEY J DOMBROWSKI CS SHUKLA KK COHN SH (1972) Skeletal metabolism and body composition in acromegaly *Journal of Clinical Endocrinology and Metabolism* **35** 543–551 (274)

ALPERS DH LEE SW AVIOLI LV (1972) Identification of two calcium-binding proteins in human small intestine *Gastroenterology* **62** 559–571 (26)

ALTENÄHR E (1972) Ultrastructural pathology of parathyroid glands *Current Topics in Pathology* **56** 1–54 Berlin: Springer Verlag (71, 80, 81, 110)

ALTENÄHR E LEONHARDT F (1972) Suppression of parathyroid gland activity by magnesium *Virchows Archiv Abteilung A: Pathologische Anatomie* **355** 297–308 (15)

ALTERMAN SL LIEBER AK (1965) Albright's hereditary osteodystrophy *Annals of Internal Medicine* **63** 140–146 (163)

ALVERYD A (1968) Parathyroid glands in thyroid surgery *Acta Chirurgica Scandinavica* Suppl 389 (13, 79)

AMBLER J GREEN AG PULVERTAFT CN (1970) A study of total serum alkaline phosphatase activity in men following partial gastrectomy *Gut* **11** 255–257 (172)

AMENT ME (1972) Malabsorption syndromes in infancy and childhood *Journal of Pediatrics* **81** 685–697 867–884 (169)

AMERICAN ACADEMY OF PEDIATRICS (Dr D Fraser) (1967) The relation between infantile hypercalcemia and vitamin D—public health implications in North America *Pediatrics* **40** 1050–1061 (125)

ANAST CS CONAWAY HH (1972) Calcitonin *Clinical Orthopaedics* **84** 207–262 (17, 220)

ANAST CS MOHS JM KAPLAN SL BURNS TW (1972) Evidence for parathyroid failure in magnesium deficiency *Science* **177** 606–608 (146)

ANDERSEN DA (1969) Historical and geographical differences in the pattern of incidence of urinary stones considered in relation to possible aetiological factors In *Renal stone research symposium* ed Hodgkinson A Nordin BEC pp 7–31 London: Churchill (129)

ANDERSON J BANNISTER DW TOMLINSON RWS (1965) Total urinary hydroxy-proline excretion in normal human subjects *Clinical Science* **29** 583–587 (Among the 74 normal adults reported in this paper the coefficient of variation of the hydroxyproline excretion results was 31.4% for results expressed in mg/24 hours and 30.9% for results expressed as mg/m²/24 hours) (54, 55)

ANDERSON DC STEWART WK PIERCY DM (1968) Calcifying panniculitis with fat and skin necrosis in a case of uraemia with autonomous hyperparathyroidism *Lancet* **2** 323–325 (201)

ANDERSON DC PETERS TJ STEWART WK (1969) Association of hypo-kalaemia and hypophosphataemia *British Medical Journal* **4** 402–403 (See also the subsequent letter by Dr JR Condon and Dr R Nassim *ibid* (1970) **1** 110) (40)

ANNING ST DAWSON J DOLBY DE INGRAM JT (1948) The toxic effects of calciferol *Quarterly Journal of Medicine* **17** 203–228 (116, 118)

ANTIA AU (1970) Observations on nutritional rickets in childhood *West African Medical Journal* **19** 169–172 (168)

ARDAILLOU R PAILLARD F SAVIER C BERNIER A (1971) Renal uptake of radioiodinated human calcitonin in man *Revue Européene d'Etudes Cliniques et Biologiques* **16** 1031–1036 (20)

ARNAUD CD TENENHOUSE A (1970) Parathyroid hormone In *International encyclopedia of pharmacology and therapeutics Section 51 Vol 1 Parathyroid hormone thyrocalcitonin and related drugs* ed Rasmussen H pp 197–235 Oxford: Pergamon (15, 16, 17)

ARNAUD CD LITTLEDIKE T TSAO HS (1970a) Calcium homeostasis and the simultaneous measurement of calcitonin and parathyroid hormone in the pig In *Calcitonin 1969* ed Taylor S pp 95–101 London: Heinemann (19)

ARNAUD C MAIJER R READE T SCRIVER CR WHELAN DT (1970b) Vitamin D dependency: an inherited postnatal syndrome with secondary hyperparathyroidism *Pediatrics* **46** 871–880 (176)

ARNAUD C GLORIEUX F SCRIVER C (1971) Serum parathyroid hormone in X-linked hypophosphatemia *Science* **173** 845–847 (211)

ARNAUD C GLORIEUX F SCRIVER CR (1972) Serum parathyroid hormone levels in acquired vitamin D deficiency of infancy *Pediatrics* **49** 837–840 (47, 186)

ARNAUD CD GOLDSMITH RS SIZEMORE GW OLDHAM SB BISCHOFF J LARSEN JA BORDIER P (1973) Studies on characterization of human parathyroid hormone in hyperparathyroid serum: practical considerations In *Clinical aspects of metabolic bone disease* ed Frame B Parfitt AM Duncan H pp 281–290 Amsterdam: Excerpta Medica (47, 63))

290 REFERENCES

ARNSTEIN AR ROSENBERG IK BELAMARIC J PIERCE JM McCANN D PRUNTY J
(1971) Palpable calcified parathyroid gland in primary chief-cell hyperplasia
New England Journal of Medicine **285** 1365–1366 (103)

ASANTI R HULTIN H VISAKORPI JK (1966) Serum alkaline phosphatase in
healthy infants. Occurence of abnormally high values without known cause.
Annales Paediatriae Fenniae **12** 139–142 (42)

ASHKAR FS MILLER R KATIMS RB (1971) Effects of corticosteroids on hypercalcaemia of malignant disease *Lancet* **1** 41 (64)

ASK-UPMARK E (1939) Osteomalacia hepatica *Acta Medica Scandinavica* **101**
138–210 (173)

ATKINS D ZANELLI JM PEACOCK M NORDIN BEC (1972) The effect of oestrogens
on the response of bone to parathyroid hormone *in vitro*. *Journal of Endocrinology* **54** 107–117 (16, 77, 236)

ATKINSON PJ WEST RR (1970) Loss of skeletal calcium in lactating women
Journal of Obstetrics and Gynaecology of the British Commonwealth **77** 555–560
(238)

ATKINSON M NORDIN BEC SHERLOCK S (1956) Malabsorption and bone disease
in prolonged obstructive jaundice *Quarterly Journal of Medicine* NS **25**
299–312 (173)

ATKINSON PJ WEST RR PARSONS FM REED GW (1970) Loss of skeletal calcium by
patients on maintenance dialysis *British Medical Journal* **3** 490–492 (223)

AURBACH GD MARCUS R WINICKOFF RN EPSTEIN EH NIGRA TP (1970) Urinary
excretion of 3′,5′-AMP in syndromes considered refractory to parathyroid
hormone *Metabolism* **19** 799–808 (157)

AURBACH GD MARCUS R HEERSCHE J MARX S NIALL H TREGEAR GW KEUTMANN
HT POTTS JT (1971) Hormones and other factors regulating calcium metabolism *Annals of the New York Academy of Sciences* **185** 386–394 (15, 21)

AURELL M HANSSON G JAGENBURG R NILSSON O (1971) Hyperparathyroidism and
maximal glucose reabsorption *Acta Medica Scandinavica* **190** 445–449 (91)

AVIOLI LV (1972) Intestinal absorption of calcium *Archives of Internal Medicine*
129 345–355 (8, 26)

AVIOLI LV McDONALD JE SINGER RA HENNEMAN PH (1965) A new oral isotopic
test of calcium absorption *Journal of Clinical Investigation* **44** 128–139 (16, 96)

BAGUET J-C RAMPON S BUSSIÈRE J-L SAUVEZIE B GONTIER Y FLORI B DOLY J
NEURY N JANNY P (1972) Traitement de l'hypercalcémie aiguë par le
furosémide *Revue du Rhumatisme* **39** 531–535 (74)

BAILEY JA (1971) Forms of dwarfism recognizable at birth *Clinical Orthopaedics*
76 150–159 (256)

BAILEY CB (1972) The precipitation of polymerized silicic acid by urine protein:
a possible mechanism in the etiology of silica urolithiasis *Canadian Journal of
Biochemistry* **50** 305–311 (135)

BAKER WH (1956) Abnormalities in calcium metabolism in malignancy: effects
of hormone therapy *American Journal of Medicine* **21** 714–720 (114)

BAKKE JL (1970) Is medical management of hyperparathyroidism ever justified? *Northwest Medicine* **69** 854–855 (102)

BALL MF CANARY JJ HOUCK JC (1972) Studies of the hydroxyprolinuria of fasting *Journal of Clinical Endocrinology and Metabolism* **35** 416–424 (54)

BALLARD HS FRAME B HARTSOCK RJ (1964) Familial multiple endocrine adenoma-peptic ulcer complex *Medicine* **43** 481–516 (94)

BALSAN S GARABEDIAN M (1972) 25-hydroxycholecalciferol: a comparative study in deficiency rickets and different types of resistance rickets *Journal of Clinical Investigation* **51** 749–759 (211)

BALSAN S GARABEDIAN M (1974) 1,25 dihydroxycholecalciferol: effect in rachitic children In *Endocrinology 1973* ed Taylor S London: Heinemann (176)

BANK N AYNEDJIAN HS (1965) On the mechanism of hyposthenuria in hypercalcemia *Journal of Clinical Investigation* **44** 681–693 (69)

BANK S BARBEZAT GO MARKS IN (1966) Post-gastrectomy steatorrhoea due to intestinal lactase deficiency *South African Medical Journal* **40** 597–599 (173)

BARAK Y (1970) Osteoblasts and osteoclasts in bone marrow aspirated from children with rickets *Acta Paediatrica Scandinavica* **59** 363–368 (179)

BARLTROP D OPPÉ TE (1970) Dietary factors in neonatal calcium homeostasis *Lancet* **2** 1333–1335 (147, 148)

BARNETT E NORDIN BEC (1960) The radiological diagnosis of osteoporosis: a new approach *Clinical Radiology* **11** 116–174 (224)

BARNHART J (1967) Hyperparathyroidism in the orthopedic patient *American Journal of Orthopedics* **9** 8–13 (86)

BARNICOT NA (1948) The local action of the parathyroid and other tissues on bone in intracerebral grafts *Journal of Anatomy* **82** 233–248 (16)

BARNICOT NA DATTA SP (1972) Vitamin A and bone, In *The Biochemistry and Physiology of bone* 2nd edition Vol 2 pp 197–229 ed Bourne GH New York: Academic Press (128)

BARR DGD FORFAR JO (1969) Oral calcium-loading test in infancy with particular reference to idiopathic hypercalcaemia *British Medical Journal* **1** 477–480 (123)

BARR DGD PRADER A ESPER U RAMPINI S MARRIAN VJ FORFAR JO (1971) Chronic hypoparathyroidism in two generations *Helvetica Paediatrica Acta* **26** 507–521 (152, 160, 161)

BARRANCO VP (1971) Cutaneous ossification in pseudohypoparathyroidism *Archives of Dermatology* **104** 643–647 (163)

BARRY HC (1969) *Paget's disease of bone* Edinburgh: Livingstone (240, 241, 243, 244, 245, 246)

BARTOS HR HENNEMAN PH (1965) Parathyroid hyperplasia in osteomalacia *Journal of Clinical Endocrinology and Metabolism* **25** 1522–1523 (179)

BARZEL US (1969) Systemic alkalosis in hypoparathyroidism *Journal of Clinical Endocrinology* **29** 917–918 (67, 156)

BARZEL US (1971) Parathyroid hormone, blood phosphorus and acid-base metabolism *Lancet* **1** 1329–1331 (156)

BASTIS-MAOUNIS B MATSANIOTIS N MAOUNIS F (1973) Serum alkaline phosphatase in infants with obstructive jaundice: relation to vitamin D supplementation *Journal of Pediatrics* **82** 68–72 (173)

BAUER JM FREYBERG RH (1946) Vitamin D intoxication with metastatic calcification *Journal of the American Medical Association* **130** 1208–1215 (118)

BAUME PE RADCLIFF FJ REEVE TS (1969) The detection and significance of small degrees of hypercalcaemia *Medical Journal of Australia* **2** 543–545 (36)

BAXTER JD BONDY PK (1966) Hypercalcemia of thyrotoxicosis *Annals of Internal Medicine* **65** 429–442 (280)

BAYARD F BEC P LOUVET JP (1972) Measurement of plasma 25-hydroxy-cholecalciferol in man *European Journal of Clinical Investigation* **2** 195–198 (185)

BELCHETZ PE LLOYD MH JOHNS RGS COHEN RD (1973) Effect of late night calcium supplements on overnight urinary calcium excretion in premenopausal and postmenopausal women *British Medical Journal* **2** 510–512 (234)

BELFIELD A GOLDBERG DM (1969) Application of a continuous spectro-photometric assay for 5′ nucleotidase activity in normal subjects and patients with liver and bone disease *Clinical Chemistry* **15** 931–939 (46)

BELFIELD A GOLDBERG DM (1971) Normal ranges and diagnostic value of serum 5′ nucleotidase and alkaline phosphatase activities in infancy *Archives of Disease in Childhood* **46** 842–846 (43, 44)

BELL NH BARTTER FC (1967) Studies of ⁴⁷Ca metabolism in sarcoidosis: evidence for increased sensitivity of bone to vitamin D *Acta Endocrinologica* **54** 173–180 (120)

BELL NH GILL JR BARTTER FC (1964) On the abnormal calcium absorption in sarcoidosis *Americal Journal of Medicine* **36** 500–513 (120)

BELL NH AVERY S JOHNSTON CC (1970) Effects of calcitonin in Paget's disease and polyostotic fibrous dysplasia *Journal of Clinical Endocrinology and Metabolism* **31** 283–290 (272)

BELL NH AVERY S SINHA T CLARK CM ALLEN DO JOHNSTON C ((1972) Effects of dibutyryl cyclic adenosine 3′,5′-monophosphate and parathyroid extract on calcium and phosphorous metabolism in hypoparathyroidism and pseudo-hypoparathyroidism *Journal of Clinical Investigation* **51** 816–823 (161)

BELLIN DE GERSHWIN BS (1935) Hyperparathyroidism with renal insufficiency *American Journal of Medical Sciences* **190** 519–525 (70, 85)

BENNETT RC HUGHES ESR (1972) Urinary calculi and ulcerative colitis *British Medical Journal* **2** 494–496 (136)

BERENS JJ POTTER DJ NICKAS GM (1970) Parathyroidectomy: Treatment for secondary hyperparathyroidism and azotemic osteodystrophy *Archives of Surgery* **100** 338–342 (206)

BERGMAN L (1972) Plasma calcium fractions during the first days of life with special reference to neonatal hypocalcaemia *Biology of the Neonate* **20** 346–359 (28)

BERGMAN L HAGBERG S (1972) Primary hyperparathyroidism in a child investigated by determination of ultrafiltrable calcium *Americal Journal of Diseases of Children* **123** 174–176 (97)

BERGMAN L ISAKSSON B (1971) Plasma calcium fractions in normal subjects from birth to adult ages *Acta Paediatrica Scandinavica* **60** 630–636 (39)

BERLYNE GM (1968) Microcrystalline conjunctival calcifications in renal failure *Lancet* **2** 366–370 (201)

BERLYNE GM BEN-ARIE J EPSTEIN N BOOTH EM YAGIL R (1973) Rarity of renal osteodystrophy in Israel due to low phosphorous intake *Nephron* **10** 141–156 (205)

BERNICK S (1971) Histochemical study of bone in parathyroidectomized rats *Calcified Tissue Research* **6** 316–328 (155)

BERNIER JJ RAMBAUD JC CATTAN D PROST A (1969) Diarrhoea associated with medullary carcinoma of the thyroid *Gut* **10** 980–985 (218)

BERNSTEIN DS SADOWSKY N HEGSTED DM GURI CD STARE FJ (1966) Prevalence of osteoporosis in high and low fluoride areas in North Dakota *Journal of the American Medical Association* **198** 499–504 (231)

BERNSTEIN DS WACHMAN A HATTNER RS (1970) Acid-base balance in metabolic bone disease. In *Osteoporosis* ed Barzel U.S. pp 207–216 New York: Grune and Stratton (15)

BERTHAUX P LAURENT M BECK H (1970) Fréquence et causes de l'hypo-vitaminose D chez les personnes âgées à l'hospice *Internationale Zeitschrift für Vitaminforschung* **40** 489–496 (169)

BESSER GM EDWARDS CRW (1972) Cushing's syndrome *Clinics in Endocrinology and Metabolism* **1** 451–490 (282)

BETRO MG PAIN RW (1972) Hypophosphataemia and hyperphosphataemia in a hospital population *British Medical Journal* **1** 273–276 (40, 41)

BICKEL H HARRIS H (1952) The genetics of Lignac-Fanconi disease *Acta Paediatrica* Suppl. **90** 22–26 (208)

BIJVOET OLM (1969) Relation of plasma phosphate concentration to renal tubular reabsorption of phosphate *Clinical Science* **37** 23–36 (50, 51, 156, 280)

BIJVOET OLM MORGAN DB (1971) The tubular reabsorption of phosphate in man. In *Phosphate et Métabolisme Phosphocalcique* ed. Hioco DJ pp 153–180 Paris: Sandoz (52)

BIJVOET OLM VAN DER SLUYS VEER J JANSEN AP (1968) Effects of calcitonin on patients with Paget's disease, thyrotoxicosis or hypercalcaemia *Lancet* **1** 876–881 (250)

BIJVOET OLM MORGAN DB FOURMAN P (1969) The assessment of phosphate reabsorption *Clinica Chimica Acta* **26** 15–24 This subject is discussed further in a leading article in *Lancet* (1970) **1** 820–822 and in the subsequent correspondence *Lancet* (1970) **1** 1345–1346 and **2** 212 (51, 52, 53)

BIJVOET OLM VAN DER SLUYS VEER J DE VRIES HR VAN KOPPEN AJT (1971) Natriuretic effect of calcitonin in man *New England Journal of Medicine* **284** 681–688 (Read with the subsequent correspondence: **285** 463–464 (21)

BILEZIKIAN JP AURBACH GD CONNOR TB PACHAS WN APTEKAR R WELLS SA FRIEJANES J DECKER JL (1973) Pseudogout after parathyroidectomy *Lancet* **1** 445–447 (89)

BIRGE SJ AVIOLI LV (1969) Glucagon-induced hypocalcemia in man *Journal of Clinical Endocrinology and Metabolism* **29** 213–218 (144)

BIRKENHÄGER JC (1970) The urinary excretion of hydroxyproline in metabolic disorders of connective tissue and bone *Folia Medica Neerlandica* **13** 79–87 (54)

BIRKENHÄGER JC VAN DER HEUL RO SMEENK D VAN DER SLUYS VEER J VAN SETERS AP (1967) Bone changes associated with glucocorticoid excess *Proceedings of the Royal Society of Medicine* **60** 1134–1136 (283)

BIRTWELL WM MAGSAMEN BF FENN PA TORG JS TOURTELLOTTE CD MARTIN JH (1970) An unusual hereditary osteomalacic disease: pseudo-vitamin-D deficiency *Journal of Bone and Joint Surgery* **52-A** 1222–1228 (176)

BISHOP MC SMITH R (1971) Non-protein-bound hydroxyproline in plasma in renal bone disease *Clinica Chimica Acta* **33** 403–408 (202)

BISHOP MC WOODS CG OLIVER DO LEDINGHAM JGG SMITH R TIBBUTT DA (1972) Effects of haemodialysis on bone in chronic renal failure *British Medical Journal* **3** 664–667 (200)

BJERNULF A HALL K SJOGREN I WERNER I (1970) Primary hyperparathyroidism in children *Acta Paediatrica Scandinavica* **59** 249–258 (110)

BLACK WC (1969) Correlative light and electron microscopy in primary hyperparathyroidism *Archives of Pathology* **88** 225–241 (82)

BLACK BM (1971a) Primary hyperparathyroidism and peptic ulcer *Surgical Clinics of North America* **51** 955–960 (93)

BLACK BM (1971b) Hyperparathyroidism: Some aspects of current surgical interest *American Surgeon* **37** 130–134 (104)

BLACK WC SLATOPOLSKY E ELKAN I HOFFSTEN P (1970a) Parathyroid morphology in suppressible and nonsuppressible renal hyperparathyroidism *Laboratory Investigation* **23** 497–509 (200)

BLACK MM SHUSTER S BOTTOMS E (1970b) Osteoporosis skin collagen and androgen *British Medical Journal* **4** 773–774 (232)

BLACKLOCK NJ (1969) The pattern of urolithiasis in the Royal Navy In *Renal stone research symposium* ed. Hodgkinson A Nordin BEC pp 33–47 London: Churchill (136)

BLACKMAN JE GIBSON GR LAVAN JN LEAROYD HM POSEN S (1967) Urinary calculi and the consumption of analgesics *British Medical Journal* **2** 800–802 (136)

BLAIR A HAWKER CD UTIGER RD (1973) Ectopic hyperparathyroidism in a patient with metastatic hypernephroma *Metabolism* **22** 147–154 (116)

BLALOCK JB (1971) Surgical treatment of hyperparathyroidism *Surgery, Gynecology and Obstetrics* **133** 627–628 (104)

BLIZZARD RM CHEE D DAVIS W (1966) The incidence of parathyroid and other antibodies in the sera of patients with idiopathic hypoparathyroidism *Clinical and Experimental Immunology* **1** 119–128 (152)

BLOCK MB PACHMAN LM WINDHORST D GOLDFINE ID (1971) Immunological findings in familial juvenile endocrine deficiency syndrome associated with mucocutaneous candidiasis *Americal Journal of the Medical Sciences* **261** 213–218 (154)

BLOOM WL FLINCHUM D (1960) Osteomalacia with pseudofractures caused by the ingestion of aluminum hydroxide *Journal of the American Medical Association* **174** 1327–1330 (210)

BLÜMCKE S NIEDORF H-R THEIL H-J LANGNESS U (1972) Histochemical and fine structural studies on the cornea with osteogenesis imperfecta congenita *Virchows Archiv: Abteilung B: Zellpathologie* **11** 124–132 (255)

BODANSKY A JAFFE HL (1934) Phosphatase studies: V Serum phosphatase as a criterion of the severity and rate of healing of rickets *American Journal of Diseases of Children* **48** 1268–1278 (190)

BOELENS PA NORWOOD W KJELLSTRAND C BROWN DM (1970) Hypophosphatemia with muscle weakness due to antacids and hemodialysis *American Journal of Diseases of Children* **120** 350–353 (210, 212)

BOEN ST LEIJNSE B GERBRANDY J (1962) Influence of serum calcium concentration on QT-interval and circulation *Clinica Chimica Acta* **7** 432–436 (143)

BOHRER SP (1970) Osteitis deformans in Nigerians *African Journal of Medical Science* **1** 109–113 (241)

BOLD AM (1970) Determination of calcium in plasma: a review of some modern methods *Annals of Clinical Biochemistry* **7** 131–135 (36)

BONE JM DAVISON AM ROBSON JS (1972) Role of dialysate calcium concentration in osteoporosis in patients on haemodialysis *Lancet* **1** 1047–1049 (196)

BONNET M MOULIN J BIARD L (1969) Maladie de Lobstein associée à des anomalies de l'angle irido-cornéen *Bulletin des Sociétés D'Ophtalmologie de France* **69** 581–583 (258)

BOONSTRA CE JACKSON CE (1965) Hyperparathyroidism detected by routine serum calcium analysis *Annals of Internal Medicine* **63** 468–474 (62)

BOONSTRA CE JACKSON CE (1971) Serum calcium survey for hyperparathyroidism: Results in 50,000 clinic patients *American Journal of Clinical Pathology* **55** 523–526 (79)

BORDIER PJ TUN CHOT S (1972) Quantitative histology of metabolic bone disease *Clinics in Endocrinology and Metabolism* **1** 197–215 (59, 178)

BORDIER P MATRAJT H MIRAVET L HIOCO D (1964) Mesure histologique de la masse et de la résorption des travées osseuses *Pathologie et Biologie* **12** 1238–1243 (58)

BORDIER P MIRAVET L MATRAJT H HIOCO D RYCKEWAERT A (1967) Bone changes in adult patients with abnornal thyroid function (with special reference to ^{45}Ca kinetics and quantitative histology) *Proceedings of the Royal Society of Medicine* **60** 1132–1134 (278, 279, 280)

BORDIER P HIOCO D ROUQUIER M HEPNER GW THOMPSON GR (1969) Effects of intravenous vitamin D on bone and phosphate metabolism in osteomalacia *Calcified Tissue Research* **4** 78–83 (191)

BORDIER PJ TUN CHOT S EASTWOOD JB FOURNIER A DE WARDENER HE (1973a) Lack of histological evidence of vitamin D abnormality in the bones of anephric patients *Clinical Science* **44** 33–41 (27, 193)

BORDIER PJ ARNAUD C HAWKER C TUN CHOT S HIOCO D (1973b) Relationship between serum immunoreactive parathyroid hormone, osteoclastic and osteocytic bone resorptions and serum calcium in primary hyperparathyroidism and osteomalacia. In *Clinical aspects of metabolic bone disease*, ed. Frame B Parfitt AM Duncan H pp 222–228 Amsterdam: Excerpta Medica. (87, 186)

BORGSTEDT AD BRYSON MF YOUNG LW FORBES GB (1972) Long-term administration of antiepileptic drugs and the development of rickets *Journal of Pediatrics* **81** 9–15 (174)

BOSTRÖM H ALVERYD A (1972) Stroke in hyperparathyroidism *Acta Medica Scandinavica* **192** 299–308 (96)

BOURNE GH (ed) (1972) *The Biochemistry and Physiology of Bone* (2nd Edition) New York: Academic Press (1)

BOVILL EG (1972) Analogies between the defects characteristic of osteogenesis imperfecta and aberrations in vitamin A metabolism *Clinical Orthopaedics* **83** 292–299 (256)

BOWDEN TE WHELAN TJ NELSON TG (1971) Sudden death after phosphorus burns *Annals of Surgery* **174** 779–784 (146)

BOYLE IT GRAY RW OMDAHL JL DE LUCA HF (1972) Calcium control of the *in vivo* biosynthesis of 1,25 dihydroxyvitamin D_3. Nicolaysen's endogenous factor In *Endocrinology 1971* ed Taylor S pp 468–476 London: Heinemann (10, 26)

BREIDAHL HD HAMILTON NT (1970) Parathyroid intoxication *Australian and New Zealand Journal of Surgery* **39** 244–249 (107, 108)

BRESNIHAN B (1971) Hypercalcaemia with sarcoidosis and hyperparathyroidism *Journal of the Irish Medical Association* **64** 581–582 (120)

BRETLAU P JORGENSEN MB (1969) Otosclerosis and osteogenesis imperfecta *Acta Oto-Laryngologica* **67** 269–276 (258)

BREWER HB FAIRWELL T RONAN R SIZEMORE GW ARNAUD CD (1972) Human parathyroid hormone: amino-acid sequence of the amino-terminal residues 1–34 *Proceedings of the National Academy of Sciences of the United States of America* **69** 3585–3588 (14)

BRIARD-GUILLEMOT M-L RAVERDY E BALSAN S REY J FRÉZAL J (1972) Etude critique de l'hypophosphatemie pour l'etude genetique de rachitisme vitamino-resistant hypophosphataemique familial *Archives Françaises de Pediatrie* **29** 1059–1068 (208)

BRICKER N (1970) Renal osteodystrophy: therapy based on mechanism *Journal of the American Medical Association* **211** 97–101 (194)

BRICKMAN AS MASSRY SG COBURN JW (1972a) Changes in serum and urinary calcium during treatment with hydrochlorothiazide: studies on mechanism *Journal of Clinical Investigation* **51** 945–954 (127)

BRICKMAN AS COBURN JW NORMAN AW (1972b) Action of 1,25 dihydroxycholecalciferol, a potent kidney-produced metabolite of vitamin D_3, in uremic man *New England Journal of Medicine* **287** 891–895 (193, 194, 195, 203)

BRIGGS WA KOMINAMI N WILSON RE MERRILL JP (1972) Kidney transplantation in Fanconi syndrome *New England Journal of Medicine* **286** 25 (214)

BRITISH MEDICAL JOURNAL (1969) Bone and joint changes in haemochromatosis *British Medical Journal* **3** 191–192 (236)

BRITISH MEDICAL JOURNAL (1971) Mineral metabolism of astronauts *British Medical Journal* **4** 696 (235)

BRITISH MEDICAL JOURNAL (1972) Corticosteroid-induced bone collapse *British Medical Journal* **1** 581–582 (283)

BRITISH MEDICAL JOURNAL (1973) Compression of cord by Paget's disease *British Medical Journal* **2** 321–322 (247)

BRITISH PAEDIATRIC ASSOCIATION (Dr T E Oppé) (1964) Infantile hypercalcaemia, nutritional rickets, and infantile scurvy in Great Britain *British Medical Journal* **1** 1659–1661 (121, 125)

BRITTON DC JOHNSTON IDA THOMPSON MH FLEMING LB (1971) Renal function following parathyroid surgery in primary hyperparathyroidism *Lancet* **2** 74–75 (Read with subsequent correspondence, pages 428 and 429) (92, 106)

BRONSKY D (1970) Hyperparathyroidism with Albright's osteodystrophy: case report and a proposed new classification of parathyroid disease *Journal of Clinical Endocrinology and Metabolism* **31** 271–276 (164)

BRONSKY D KUSHNER DS DUBIN A SNAPPER I (1958) Idiopathic hypoparathyroidism and pseudohypoparathyroidism: case reports and review of the literature *Medicine* **37** 317–352 (154)

BRONSKY D WEISBERY MG GROSS MC BARTON JJ (1970) Hyperparathyroidism and acute postpartum pancreatitis with neonatal tetany in the child *American Journal of the Medical Sciences* **260** 160–164 (108)

BROOK CGD VALMAN HB (1971) Osteoma cutis and Albright's hereditary osteodystrophy *British Journal of Dermatology* **85** 471–475 (163, 164)

BROOKE RI (1970) Giant-cell tumor in patients with Paget's disease *Oral Surgery Oral Medicine and Oral Pathology* **30** 230–241 (246)

BROWN TS PATERSON CR (1973) Osteosclerosis in myeloma *Journal of Bone and Joint Surgery* **55B** 621–623 (264)

BROWN OT WIGZELL FW (1964) The significance of span as a clinical measurement. In *Current achievements in geriatrics*, ed. Anderson WF and Isaacs B London: Cassell (32)

BROWN P THIN CG MALONE DNS ROSCOE P STRONG JA (1970) Metabolic studies with porcine calcitonin in osteoporosis *Scottish Medical Journal* **15** 207–212 (234)

BROWN HP LAROCCA H WICKSTROM JK (1971) Paget's disease of the atlas and axis *Journal of Bone and Joint Surgery* **53A** 1441–1444 (247)

BRUBAKER RF WONG VG SCHULMAN JD SEEGMILLER JE KUWABARA T (1970) Benign cystinosis *American Journal of Medicine* **49** 546–550 (209)

BRUNETTE MG (1972) La physiologie rénale du phosphore *Union Médicale du Canada* **101** 2669–2671 (50)

BRYSON MF FORBES GB AMIRHAKIMI GH REINA JC (1972) Metabolic response to growth hormone administration with particular reference to the occurrence of hypercalcuria *Pediatric Research* **6** 743–751 (276)

BUCKERFIELD JP (1971) Primary hyperparathyroidism causing bony swelling in the endentulous jaw: A case report *British Dental Journal* **131** 497–499 (87)

BUCKLE RM (1970) Hyperparathyroidism in chronic renal failure *Lancet* **2** 234–257 (195)

BUCKLE RM MASON AMS MIDDLETON JE (1969) Thyrotoxic hypercalcaemia treated with porcine calcitonin *Lancet* **1** 1128–1130 (77, 280)

BUCKLE RM GAMLEN TR PULLEN IM (1972) Vitamin D intoxication treated with porcine calcitonin *British Medical Journal* **3** 205–207 (76)

BULLAMORE JR (1970) The estimation of calcium 47 in faeces *International Journal of Applied Radiation and Isotopes* **21** 677–678 (56)

BULLAMORE JR GALLAGHER JC WILKINSON R NORDIN BEC MARSHALL DH (1970) Effect of age on calcium absorption *Lancet* **2** 535–537 (56, 232)

BULUSU L HODGKINSON A NORDIN BEC PEACOCK N (1970) Urinary excretion of calcium and creatinine in relation to age and body weight in normal subjects and patients with renal calculus *Clinical Science* **38** 601–612 (48, 49)

BURDEN RP (1971) Familial hyperparathyroidism *Proceedings of the Royal Society of Medicine* **64** 1067–1068 (180)

BURKE BS (1947) The dietary history as a tool in research *Journal of the American Dietetic Association* **23** 1041–1046 (61)

BURKHARDT R (1971) *Bone marrow and bone tissue* Berlin: Springer Verlag (58)

BURNETT CH COMMONS RR ALBRIGHT F HOWARD JE (1949) Hypercalcemia without hypercalcuria or hypophosphatemia, calcinosis and renal insufficiency *New England Journal of Medicine* **240** 787–794 (126)

BURWOOD RJ (1972) Personal communication (88)

BUTLER TJ (1961) The effect of gastrectomy on pancreatic secretion in man *Annals of the Royal College of Surgeons* **29** 300–327 (173)

BUTLER ML (1970) Hypercalcemia and leukemia *Southern Medical Journal* **63** 591–592 (115)

BUXTON RL WEBSTER D JOHNSTON IDA HALL R (1970 Further assessment of the venous-compression test in hyperparathyroidism *Lancet* **2** 498–499 (101)

BYERS PD SMITH R (1971) Quantitative histology of bone in hyperparathyroidism *Quarterly Journal of Medicine* NS **40** 471–486 (87)

BYWATERS EGL DIXON AStJ SCOTT JT (1963) Joint lesions of hyperparathyroidism *Annals of Rheumatic Diseases* **22** 171–187 (89)

CAFFEY J (1951) Chronic poisoning due to excess of vitamin A *Americal Journal of Roentgenology and Radium Therapy* **65** 12–26 (128)

CALDWELL JG WEBBER BL AVIOLI LV (1971) Calcified parathyroids in a case of renal osteodystrophy *Journal of Clinical Endocrinology and Metabolism* **33** 105–109 (200)

CALLIS L CASTELLO F FORTUNY G VALLO A BALLABRIGA A (1970) Effect of hydrochlorothiazide on rickets and on renal tubular acidosis in two patients with cystinosis *Helvetica Paediatrica Acta* **25** 602–619 (214)

CALLOW RK KODICEK E THOMPSON GA (1966) Metabolism of tritiated vitamin D *Proceedings of the Royal Society B* **164** 1–20 (26)

CAMERON J (1972a) The battered baby syndrome *Practitioner* **209** 302–310 (31)

CAMERON DA (1972b) The ultrastructure of bone. In *The Biochemistry and Physiology of Bone* ed Bourne G H (2nd edition) Vol 1 pp 191–236a New York: Academic Press (2, 7).

CAMP JD MCCULLOUGH JAL (1941) Pseudofractures in diseases affecting the skeletal system *Radiology* **36** 651–663 (182)

CAMPBELL CJ PAPADEMETRIOU T BONFIGLIO M (1968) Melorheostosis *Journal of Bone and Joint Surgery* **50A** 1281–1304 (264)

CANGIANO R MOONEY J STRATIGOS GT (1972) Osteopetrosis *Journal of Oral Surgery* **30** 217–222 (263)

CANIGGIA A GENNARI C (1972) Calcitonin treatment in Ekman-Lobstein disease *Calcified Tissue Research* **9** 243–244 (260)

CANIGGIA A GENNARI C BORRELLO G BENCINI M CESARI L POGGI C ESCOBAR S (1970) Intestinal absorption of calcium-47 after treatment with oral oestrogen-gestogens in senile osteoporosis *British Medical Journal* **4** 30–32 (233)

CANTERBURY JM LEVEY GS REISS E (1973) Activation of renal cortical adenylate cyclase by circulating immunoreactive parathyroid hormone fragments *Journal of Clinical Investigation* **52** 524–527 (14)

CARE AD BATES RFL GITELMAN HJ (1970) A possible role for the adenyl cyclase system in calcitonin release *Journal of Endocrinology* **48** 1–15 (20)

CARE AD BATES RFL SWAMINATHAN R GANGULI PC (1971) The role of gastrin as a calcitonin secretagogue *Journal of Endocrinology* **51** 735–744 (20)

CASSON MH (1969) Oral manifestations of primary hypophosphatasia *British Dental Journal* **127** 561–566 (267)

CASTELLS S INAMDAR S BAKER RK WALLACH S (1972) Effects of porcine calcitonin in osteogenesis imperfecta tarda *Journal of Pediatrics* **80** 757–762 (260)

CAWTHORNE T (1970) Toulouse Lautrec—triumph over infirmity *Proceedings of the Royal Society of Medicine* **63** 800–805 (261)

CHAIMOVITZ C ABINADER E BENDERLY A BETTER OS (1972) Hypocalcemic hypotension *Journal of the American Medical Association* **222** 86–87 (143)

CHAKMAKJIAN ZH BETHUNE JE (1966) Sodium sulfate treatment of hypercalcaemia *New England Journal of Medicine* **265** 862–869 (73)

CHALMERS J (1968) Osteomalacia: a review of 93 cases *Journal of the Royal College of Surgeons of Edinburgh* **13** 255–275 (182)

CHALMERS J (1970) Subtrochanteric fractures in osteomalacia *Journal of Bone and Joint Surgery* **52B** 509–513 (178)

CHALMERS J CONACHER WDH GARDNER DL SCOTT PJ (1967) Osteomalacia—a common disease in elderly women *Journal of Bone and Joint Surgery* **49B** 403–423 (169, 172, 177, 178, 182, 183, 185)

CHAN AM LYNCH MJG BAILEY JD EZRIN C FRASER D (1970) Hypothyroidism in cystinosis *American Journal of Medicine* **48** 678–692 (208)

CHAPLIN H CLARK LD ROPES MW (1951) Vitamin D intoxication *American Journal of the Medical Sciences* **221** 369–378 (117)

CHAPMAN K (1971) Osteomalacia in Iran *Journal of Obstetrics and Gynaecology of the British Commonwealth* **78** 857–860 (169)

CHARBON GA PIEPER EEM (1972) Effect of calcitonin on parathyroid hormone-induced vasodilation *Endocrinology* **91** 828–831 (17)

CHASE LR MELSON GL AURBACH GD (1969) Pseudohypoparathyroidism: defective excretion of 3′,5′-AMP in response to parathyroid hormone *Journal of Clinical Investigation* **48** 1832–1844 (157, 161, 163)

CHAUSMER AB SHERMAN BS WALLACH S (1972) The effect of parathyroid hormone on hepatic cell transport of calcium *Endocrinology* **91** 663–672 (17)

CHISHOLM C (1933) The incidence of rickets in Manchester *British Journal of Children's Diseases* **30** 83–97 (23)

CHISWICK ML (1971) Association of oedema and hypomagnesaemia with hypocalcaemic tetany of the newborn *British Medical Journal* **3** 15–18 (148)

CHITTAL SM OREOPOULOS DG DE VEBER GA THOMAS P RABINOVICH S LLOYD GJ KUMAR MA RAPOPORT A (1971) Plasma calcitonin in renal osteodystrophy *Canadian Medical Association Journal* **104** 1098–1100 and 1091 (196)

CHODACK P ATTIE JN GRODER MG (1965) Hypercalcemic crisis coincidental with hemorrhage in parathyroid adenoma *Archives of Internal Medicine* **116** 416–423 (82, 108)

CHOLOD EJ HAUST MD HUDSON AJ LEWIS FN (1970) Myopathy in primary familial hyperparathyroidism *American Journal of Medicine* **48** 700–707 (90)

CHRISTENSEN WR LIEBMAN C SOSMAN MC (1951) Skeletal and periarticular manifestations of hypervitaminosis D *American Journal of Roentgenology and Radium Therapy* **65** 27–41 (119)

CHRISTENSEN MF NIELSEN JA HENRIKSEN O (1970) Treatment of cystinosis with a diet poor in cystine and methionine *Acta Paediatrica Scandinavica* **59** 613–620 (214)

CHRISTENSEN J AAGAARD P (1971) Gastric secretion of calcium and inorganic phosphorus in patients with primary hyperparathyroidism *Scandinavian Journal of Gastroenterology* **6** 569–572 (93)

CHRISTIENSEN J AAGAARD P (1972a) Parathyroid adenoma and gastric acid secretion *Scandinavian Journal of Gastroenterology* **7** 445–449 (93)

CHRISTIANSEN J AAGAARD P (1972b) Gastric secretion of calcium in patients with primary hyperparathyroidism before and after removal of parathyroid adenomas *Scandinavian Journal of Gastroenterology* **7** 639–641 (93)

CHRISTIANSEN C RØDBRO P LUND M (1973) Effect of vitamin D on bone mineral mass in normal subjects and in epileptic patients on anticonvulsants: a controlled therapeutic trial *British Medical Journal* **2** 208–209 (174)

CHRISTIE AC (1967) The parathyroid oxyphil cells *Journal of Clinical Pathology* **20** 591–602 (110)

CLARK CG (1963) Malabsorption following partial gastrectomy *Journal of the Royal College of Surgeons of Edinburgh* **9** 52–60 (173)

CLARK L (1971) Hypervitaminosis A: a review *Australian Veterinary Journal* **47** 568–571 (128)

CLARK LC BECK E (1950) Plasma "alkaline" phosphatase activity: I Normative data for growing children *Journal of Paediatrics* **36** 335–341 (43)

CLARK I RIVERA-CORDERO F (1971) Effect of parathyroid function on absorption and excretion of calcium magnesium and phosphate by rats *Endocrinology* **88** 302–308 (16)

CLARK O TAYLOR S (1972) Persistent and recurrent hyperparathyroidism *British Journal of Surgery* **59** 555–558 (103, 105)

CLARK F SIMPSON W YOUNG JR (1972) Osteomalacia in immigrants from the Indian Subcontinent in Newcastle-upon-Tyne *Proceedings of the Royal Society of Medicine* **65** 478–480 (168, 169)

CLARKSON B KOWLESSAR OD HORWITH M SLEISENGER MH (1960) Clinical and metabolic study of a patient with malabsorption and hypoparathyroidism *Metabolism* **9** 1093–1106 (154)

CLARKSON EM LUCK VA HYNSON WV BAILEY RR EASTWOOD JB WOODHEAD JS CLEMENTS VR O'RIORDAN JLH DE WARDENER HE (1972) The effect of aluminium hydroxide on calcium, phosphorus and aluminium balances, the serum parathyroid hormone concentration and the aluminium content of bone in patients with chronic renal failure *Clinical Science* **43** 519–531 (205)

CLUNIE GJA GUNN A ROBSON JS (1967) Hyperparathyroid crisis *British Journal of Surgery* **54** 538–541 (108)

COBURN JW MASSRY SG GORDON S RUBINI ME (1969a) Spurious hypocalcemia in patients undergoing maintenance hemodialysis *American Journal of Clinical Pathology* **52** 572–576 (144)

COBURN JW MASSRY SG DEPALMA JR SHINABERGER JH (1969b) Rapid appearance of hypercalcemia with initiation of hemodialysis *Journal of the American Medical Association* **210** 2276–2278 (202)

COBURN JW BRICKMAN AS KUROKAWA K MASSRY SG BETHUNE JE HARRISON HE NORMAN AW (1974) Action of 1,25 (OH)₂ cholecalciferol in normal man and patients with hypophosphataemic resistant rickets, pseudohypoparathyroidism and uraemia In *Endocrinology 1973* ed Taylor S London: Heinemann (176, 211)

COCHRAN M NORDIN BEC (1969) Role of acidosis in renal osteomalacia *British Medical Journal* **2** 276–279 (196)

COCHRAN M NORDIN BEC (1971) The causes of hypocalcaemia in chronic renal failure *Clinical Science* **40** 305–315 (194, 195)

COCHRAN M HODGKINSON A ZAREMBSKI PM ANDERSON CK (1968) Hyperoxaluria in adults *British Journal of Surgery* **55** 121–128 (134)

COCHRAN M PEACOCK M SACHS G NORDIN BEC (1970) Renal effects of calcitonin *British Medical Journal* **1** 135–137 (76, 77)

COE FL RAISEN L (1973) Allopurinol treatment of uric-acid disorders in calcium-stone formers *Lancet* **1** 129–131 (135, 140)

COE FL CANTERBURY J REISS E (1971) Hyperparathyroidism in idiopathic hypercalciuria: primary or secondary? *Transactions of the American Association of American Physicians* **84** 152–161 (134)

COHANIM M DE LUCA HF YENDT ER (1972) Effects of prolonged treatment with 25-hydroxycholecalciferol in hypophosphatemic (vitamin D refractory) rickets and osteomalacia *Johns Hopkins Medical Journal* **131** 118–132 (211)

COHEN RD VINCE FP (1969) Pseudohypoparathyroidism with raised plasma alkaline phosphatase *Archives of Disease in Childhood* **44** 96–101 (163, 164)

COLEMAN EN (1965) Infantile hypercalcaemia and cardiovascular lesions *Archives of Disease in Childhood* **40** 535–540 (122)

COLLINS DH (1956) Paget's disease of bone: incidence and subclinical forms *Lancet* **2** 51–57 (240, 243)

COLLINS D (1966) *Pathology of bone* London: Butterworths (31, 60, 86, 240, 241, 242)

CONDON JR NASSIM JR (1971) Axial osteomalacia *Postgraduate Medical Journal* **47** 817–820 (273)

CONDON JR NASSIM JR MILLARD FJC HILBE A STAINTHORPE EM (1970) Calcium and phosphorus metabolism in relation to lactose tolerance *Lancet* **1** 1027–1029 (237)

CONDON JR REITH SBM NASSIM JR MILLARD FJC HILB A STAINTHORPE EM (1971a) Treatment of Paget's disease of bone with mithramycin *British Medical Journal* **1** 421–423 (251)

CONDON JR NASSIM JR RUTTER A (1971b) Pathogenesis of rickets and osteomalacia in familial hypophosphataer iia *Archives of Disease in Childhood* **46** 269–272 (211)

CONNOR TB TOSKES P MAHAFFEY J MARTIN LG WILLIAMS JB WALSER M (1972) Parathyroid function during chronic magnesium deficiency *Johns Hopkins Medical Journal* **131** 100–117 (145, 146)

COOKE BED (1956) Paget's disease of the jaws: fifteen cases *Annals of the Royal College of Surgeons of England* **19** 223– 240 (247)

COOKE SAR (1973) Calcium concentration within the nephron, and calcium stone formation. In *Proceedings of the International Symposium on Renal Stone Research, Madrid 1972*, ed. Delatte L.C. Basle: Karger (132)

COOPER RR MILGRAM JW ROBINSON RA (1966) Morphology of the osteon: an electron microscopic study *Journal of Bone and Joint Surgery* **48A** 1239–1271 (1)

COPE CL (1935) Base changes in the alkalosis produced by the treatment of gastric ulcer with alkalies *Clinical Science* **2** 287–300 (126)

COPE O (1960) Hyperparathyroidism: Diagnosis and management *American Journal of Surgery* **99** 394–403 (84)

COPE O (1966) The story of hyperparathyroidism at the Massachusetts General Hospital *New England Journal of Medicine* **274** 1174–1182 (81)

COPE O KEYNES WM ROTH SI CASTLEMAN B (1958) Primary chief-cell hyperplasia of the parathyroid glands: A new entity in the surgery of hyperparathyroidism *Annals of Surgery* **148** 375–388 (82)

COPP DH (1969) Endocrine control of calcium homeostasis *Journal of Endocrinology* **43** 317–161 (17)

COPP DH CAMERON EC CHENEY BA DAVIDSON AGF HENZE KG (1962) Evidence for calcitonin—a new hormone from the parathyroid that lowers blood calcium *Endocrinology* **70** 638–649 (17)

CORTESE AF GLENN F (1968) Hypocalcemia and tetany with steroid-induced acute pancreatitis *Archives of Surgery* **96** 119–122 (144)

CORVILAIN J ABRAMOW M (1972) Growth and renal control of plasma phosphate *Journal of Clinical Endocrinology* **34** 452–459 (40, 52, 275, 276)

COSTANZA DJ SMOLLER M (1963) Multiple myeloma with the Fanconi syndrome *American Journal of Medicine* **34** 125–133 (210)

COSTELLO JM DENT CE (1963) Hypo-hyperparathyroidism *Archives of Disease in Chidhood* **38** 397–407 (112, 164)

COX EV WILLIAMS JA JONES CT (1963) Anaemia and the post gastrectomy state In *Partial gastrectomy* ed. Stammers FAR and Williams JA pp 148–189 London: Butterworth (172)

CRAVEN RE GOODMAN AD CARTER JH (1972) Familial multiple endocrine adenomatosis *Archives of Internal Medicine* **129** 567–569 (94)

CRAWHALL JC WATTS RWE (1968) Cystinuria *American Journal of Medicine* **45** 736–755 (135)

CREAMER B (1974) *The small intestine* London: Heinemann (169)

CREERY RDG NEILL DW (1954) Idiopathic hypercalcaemia in infants with failure to thrive *Lancet* **2** 110–114 (123)

CROPP GJA MYERS DN (1972) Physiological evidence of hypermetabolism in osteogenesis imperfecta *Pediatrics* **49** 375–391 (256, 259)

CRUESS RL CLARK I (1965) Alterations in the lipids of bone caused by hyper-vitaminosis A and D *Biochemical Journal* **96** 262–265 (119)

CUISINIER-GLEIZES P DELORME A DULAC H MATHIEU H (1972) Parathyroid glands and bone calcium mobilization by 25-hydroxycholecalciferol *Revue Euro-péenne d'Etudes Cliniques et Biologiques* **17** 903–905 (25)

CUSHARD WG (1971) Hypocalcemia and carbohydrate intolerance *Annals of Internal Medicine* **74** 299–300 (156)

CUSHARD WG SIMON AB CANTERBURY JM REISS E (1972a) Parathyroid function in sarcoidosis *New England Journal of Medicine* **286** 395–398 (120)

CUSHARD WG CREDITOR MA CANTERBURY JM REISS E (1972b) Physiologic hyperparathyroidism in pregnancy *Journal of Clinical Endocrinology and Metabolism* **34** 767–771 (28)

CUSWORTH DC DENT CE SCRIVER CR (1972) Primary hyperparathyroidism and hyperaminoaciduria *Clinica Chimica Acta* **41** 355–361 (91)

DARLING DB LORIDAN L SENIOR B (1970) The roentgenographic manifestations of Cushing's syndrome in infancy *Radiology* **96** 503–508 (283)

DARMADY EM STRANACK F (1957) Microdissection of the nephron in disease *British Medical Bulletin* **13** 21–26 (208)

DASTUR FD KAJI DM (1971) Paget's disease of bone *Journal of Postgraduate Medicine* **17** 43–46 (241)

DAUNCEY MJ WIDDOWSON EM (1972) Urinary excretion of calcium, magnesium sodium and potassium in hard and soft water areas *Lancet* **1** 711–715 (48)

DAVIDSON ET JOHNSON JH COLLINS JP (1971) Age and primary hyperparathyroidism *Southern Medical Journal* **64** 760–761 (80)

DAVIES DR FRIEDMAN M (1966) Complications after parathyroidectomy fractures from low calcium and magnesium convulsions *Journal of Bone and Joint Surgery* **48B** 117–126 (105)

DAVIES DR DENT CE WATSON L (1968) Tertiary hyperparathyroidism *British Medical Journal* **3** 395–399 (110)

DAVIES DR DENT CE WATSON L (1971) Idiopathic hypercalciuria and hyperparathyroidism *British Medical Journal* **1** 108 (36)

DAVIES DR DENT CE IVES DR (1973a) Successful removal of single metastasis in recurrent parathyroid carcinoma *British Medical Journal* **1** 397–398 (112)

DAVIES DR SHAW DG IVES DR THOMAS BM WATSON L (1973b) Selective venous catheterisation and radioimmunoassay of parathyroid hormone in the diagnosis and localisation of parathyroid tumours *Lancet* **1** 1079–1082 (103)

DAVIS RH MORGAN DB RIVLIN RS (1970) The excretion of calcium in the urine and its relation to calcium intake, sex and age *Clinical Science* **39** 1–12 (48, 49)

DAWIDSON I JAMESON S (1972) Sarcoidosis with hypercalcemia, reversible uremia and hyperparathyroidism *Scandinavian Journal of Urology and Nephrology* **6** 308–311 (120)

DAY EA MALCOM GT BEELER MF (1969) Tumor sterols *Metabolism* **18** 646–651 (114)

DEBRÉ R (1948) Toxic effects of overdosage of vitamin D_2 in children *American Journal of Diseases of Children* **75** 787–791 (117)

DEBRÉ R BRISSAUD H-E (1949) Action toxique de la vitamine D_2 administrée a doses trop fortes chez l'enfant *Annales de Médecine* **50** 417–489 (117)

DEFTOS LJ (1971) Immunoassay for human calcitonin: I Method *Metabolism* **20** 1122–1128 (47)

DEFTOS LJ BURY AE HABENER JF SINGER FR POTTS JT (1971) Immunoassay for human calcitonin: II Clinical studies *Metabolism* **20** 1129–1137 (47, 217, 219)

DELATTE LC (1973) ed. *Proceedings of international symposium on renal stone research, Madrid 1972* Basel: Karger (129)

DELATTE LC HIDALGO A BELLANATO J SANTOS M (1973) Interpretacion de imagenes cristalinas de calculos con microscopio de polarizacion y espectroscopia infra-roja. In *Proceedings of the International Symposium on Renal Stone Research, Madrid 1972* ed Delatte LC Basle: Karger (131)

DELLER DJ (1965) Functional and metabolic results of partial gastrectomy *Medical Journal of Australia* **1** 405–410 (173)

DE LUCA HF (1972) Parathyroid hormone as a trophic hormone for 1,25-dihydroxyvitamin D_3, the metabolically active form of vitamin D *New England Journal of Medicine* **287** 250–251 (See also correspondence **287** 1152 **288** 471) (25, 158)

DE LUCA HF STEENBOCK H (1972) 1,25-dihydroxycholcaleciferol: isolation, identification, regulation and mechanism of action In *Endocrinology 1971* ed. Taylor S pp. 452–467 London: Heinemann (24)

DE LUCA K MASOTTI RE PARTINGTON MW (1972) Altered calcium metabolism due to anticonvulsant drugs *Developmental Medicine and Child Neurology* **14** 318–321 (174)

DENISON EK PETERS RL REYNOLDS TB (1971) Portal hypertension in a patient with osteopetrosis *Archives of Internal Medicine* **128** 279–283 (262)

DENT CE (1962) Some problems of hyperparathyroidism *British Medical Journal* **2** 1419–1425 1495–1500 (72, 105, 107)

DENT CE (1969) Osteoporosis In *Aging of connective and skeletal tissue* ed. by Engel A and Larsson T pp. 261–269 Stockholm: Nordiska Bokhandelns Förlag (234, 238, 239)

DENT CE (1970) Rickets (and osteomalacia), nutritional and metabolic (1919–69) *Proceedings of the Royal Society of Medicine* **63** 401–408 (165, 173, 207, 208)

DENT CE (1971) The problem of osteoporosis *Practitioner* **206** 793–794 (234, 236)

DENT CE HARPER CM (1962) Plasma-alkaline-phosphatase in normal adults and in patients with primary hyperparathyroidism *Lancet* **1** 559–563 (97)

DENT CE SMITH R (1969) Nutritional osteomalacia *Quarterly Journal of Medicine* N.S. **38** 195–209 (169)

DENT CE STAMP TCB (1970) Theoretical renal phosphorus threshold in investigation and treatment of osteomalacia *Lancet* **1** 857–860 (53, 186, 190)

DENT CE STAMP TCB (1971) Hypophosphataemic osteomalacia presenting in adults *Quarterly Journal of Medicine* N.S. **40** 303–329 (209, 210, 212, 214)

DENT CE SUTOR DJ (1971) Presence or absence of inhibitor of calcium-oxalate crystal growth in urine of normals and of stoneformers *Lancet* **2** 775–778 (84, 132, 133)

DENT CE WATSON L (1965) Metabolic studies in a patient with idiopathic hypercalciuria *British Medical Journal* **2** 449–452 (139)

DENT CE WATSON L (1968) The hydrocortisone test in primary and tertiary hyperparathyroidism *Lancet* **2** 662–664 (63, 64)

DENT CE NORRIS TSTM SMITH R SUTTON RAL TEMPERLEY JM (1968) Steatorrhoea with striking increase of plasma-alkaline-phosphatase of intestinal origin *Lancet* **1** 1333–1336 (45)

DENT CE RICHENS A ROWE DJF STAMP TCB (1970) Osteomalacia with long-term anticonvulsant therapy in epilepsy *British Medical Journal* **4** 69–72 (174, 189)

DENT RI JAMES JH WANG C-A DEFTOS LJ TALAMO R FISCHER JE (1972) Hyperparathyroidism: gastric acid secretion and gastrin *Annals of Surgery* **176** 360–369 (93)

DENT CE ROUND JM ROWE DJF STAMP TCB (1973) Effect of chapattis and ultraviolet irradiation on nutritional rickets in an Indian immigrant *Lancet* **1** 1282–1284 (168, 188)

DEQUEKER JV (1970) Parathyroid activity and postmenopausal osteoporosis *Lancet* **2** 211–212 (223, 224)

DEQUEKER J (1972) *Bone Loss in Normal and Pathological Conditions* Leuven: Leuven University Press (32, 224)

DEQUEKER J FRANSSENS R BORREMANS A (1971a) Relationship between peripheral and axial osteoporosis and osteoarthrosis *Clinical Radiology* **22** 74–77 (227)

DEQUEKER J REMANS J FRANSSENS R WAES J (1971b) Ageing patterns of trabecular and cortical bone and their relationship *Calcified Tissue Research* **7** 23–30 (228)

DEREN JJ WILLIAMS LA MUENCH H CHALMERS T ZAMCHECK N (1964) Comparative study of four methods of determining alkaline phosphatase *New England Journal of Medicine* **270** 1277–1283 (42, 43)

DE ROSE J AVRAMIDES A BAKER RK WALLACH S (1972) Treatment of Paget's disease with calcitonin *Seminars in Drug Treatment* **2** 51–55 (250, 251)

DEUIL R PUECH H TUGAYE A DULAC DE FUGERES Y BOUTELIER D DUPUY R (1963) Ostéomalacie douloureuse de Looser-Milkman-Debray apres gastroentérostomie et dénutrition *Archives des Maladies de l'Appareil Digestif* **52** 1027–1031 (172)

DE WARDENER HE (1972) Some fresh observations on calcium and phosphate metabolism in chronic renal failure In *Scientific basis of medicine Annual Review 1972* London: Athlone Press (192, 201, 205)

DE WIJN JF (1966) Changing levels of blood constituents during growth. In *Somatic growth of the child* Ed. van der Werff ten Bosch JJ Haak A pp. 99–118 Leiden: Stenfert Kroese (40, 43)

DE WIND LT (1961) Hypervitaminosis D with osteosclerosis *Archives of Disease in Childhood* **36** 373–380 (119)

DICK HM SIMPSON WJ (1972) Dental changes in osteopetrosis *Oral Surgery Oral Medicine Oral Pathology* **34** 408–416 (263)

DICKSTEIN SS FRAME B (1973) Urinary tract calculi after intestinal shunt operations for the treatment of obesity *Surgery Gynecology and Obstetrics* **136** 257–260 (134)

DI GIULIO W LINDENAUER SM (1970) Use of tolonium chloride in localization of parathyroid tissue *Journal of the American Medical Association* **214** 2302–2306 (103)

DI GIULIO W MORALES JO (1969) The value of the selenomethionine Se 75 scan in preoperative localization of parathyroid adenomas *Journal of the American Medical Association* **209** 1873–1880 (103)

DIREKZE M MILNES JN (1970) Spinal cord compression in Paget's disease *British Journal of Surgery* **57** 239–240 (247)

DODDS WJ STEINBACH HK (1966) Gout associated with calcification of cartilage *New England Journal of Medicine* **275** 745–749 (89)

DONOHOE JF FREANEY R MULDOWNEY FP (1969) Osteomalacia in ureterosigmoidostomy *Irish Journal of Medical Science* **8** 523–530 (215, 216)

DOUGLAS WR (1970) The calcium metabolism problem in space medical science *Space Life Sciences* **2** 151–157 (235)

DOWLING RH ROSE GA SUTOR DJ (1971) Hyperoxaluria and renal calculi in ileal disease *Lancet* **1** 1103–1106 (134)

DOWNIE WW GUNN A HOWIE GH BROWNING MCK (1973) Personal communication (281)

DOYLE FH (1966) Some quantatitive radiological observations in primary and secondary hyperparathyroidism *British Journal of Radiology* **39** 161–167 (89)

DOYLE FH (1967) Radiologic assessment of endocrine effects on bone *Radiologic Clinics of North America* **5** 289–302 (275, 283)

DOYLE FH (1972) Radiological patterns of bone disease associated with renal glomerular failure in adults *British Medical Bulletin* **28** 220–224 (198)

DRACH GW KING JS (1970) Estimating aberrant homeostasis: Variance in serum calcium concentration as an aid in diagnosis of hyperparathyroidism *Clinical Chemistry* **16** 792–796 (96)

DRAGOO MR IRWIN RK (1972) A method of procuring cancellous iliac bone utilizing a trephine needle *Journal of Periodontology* **43** 82–87 (58)

DRUMMOND KN MICHAEL AF ULSTROM RA GOOD RA (1964) The blue diaper syndrome: Familial hypercalcemia with nephrocalcinosis and indicanuria *American Journal of Medicine* **37** 928–948 (126)

DRURY MI O'LOUGHLIN S SWEENEY EC MERRIMAN A TIMONEY FJ (1971) Idiopathic hypoparathyroidism: a report of four cases *Irish Journal of Medical Science* **140** 513–522 (154)

D'SOUZA A FLOCH MH (1973) Calcium metabolism in pancreatic disease *American Journal of Clinical Nutrition* **26** 352–361 (144)

DUBÉ WJ GOLDSMITH RS ARNAUD SB ARNAUD CD (1972) Hyperparathyroidism secondary to long-term therapy of Paget's disease of bone with calcitonin. In *Calcium, parathyroid hormone and the calcitonins.* ed. Talmage RV Munson PL pp. 113–115 Amsterdam: Excerpta Medica (219)

DUBÉ WJ GOLDSMITH RS ARNAUD SB ARNAUD CD (1973) Development of antibodies to porcine calcitonin during treatment of Paget's disease of bone *Mayo Clinic Proceedings* **49** 43–46 (77)

DUBOST C (1973) Risques de la localisation des adénomes parathyroïdiens par l'artériographie et ses risques *Nouvelle Press Médicale* **2** 722 (103)

DUDLEY NE (1971) Methylene blue for rapid identification of the parathyroids *British Medical Journal* **3** 680–681 (103)

DUDLEY FJ BLACKBURN CRB (1970) Extraskeletal calcification complicating oral neutral-phosphate therapy *Lancet* **2** 628–630 (72)

DUDLEY HR RITCHIE AC SCHILLING A BAKER WH (1955) Pathologic changes associated with the use of sodium ethylene diamine tetra-acetate in the treatment of hypercalcemia *New England Journal of Medicine* **252** 331–337 (75)

DUDRICK SJ MACFADYEN BV VAN BUREN CT RUBERG RL MAYNARD AT (1972) Parental hyperalimentation: metabolic problems and solutions *Annals of Surgery* **176** 259–264 (40)

DUPONT B DUPONT A BLIDDAL J HOLST E MELCHIOR JC OTTESEN OE (1970) Idiopathic hypercalcaemia of infancy: The elfin face sydrome *Danish Medical Bulletin* **17** 33–46 (121, 122, 124, 126)

DUURSMA SA VISSAR WJ NJIO L (1972) A quantitative histological study of bone in 30 patients with renal insufficiency *Calcified Tissue Research* **9** 216–225 (197)

DYER NH DAWSON AM (1968) Malabsorption *British Medical Journal* **2** 161–163 225–227 (169)

EDE MCM FAULKNER MH TREDRE BE (1972) An intrinsic rhythm of urinary calcium excretion and the specific effect of bedrest on the excretory pattern *Clinical Science* **42** 433–445 (48)

EHRIG U WILSON DR (1972) Fibrous dysplasia of bone and primary hyperparathyroidism *Annals of Internal Medicine* **77** 234–238 (272)

EICHOLTZ W MÜLLER D (1972) Elektronenmikroskopische Befunde an der Hornhaut und Sklera bei Osteogenesis imperfecta *Klinische Monatsblätter für Augenheilkunde* **161** 646–653 (255)

EIGLER JOC SALASSA RM BAHN RC OWEN CA (1962) Renal distribution of sodium in potassium-depleted and vitamin D-intoxicated rats *American Journal of Physiology* **202** 1115–1120 (69)

EILERT JB CASEY D DEL GRECO F CONN J (1971) Experience with subtotal parathyroidectomy for "tertiary" hyperparathyroidism *Archives of Surgery* **103** 303–307 (206)

EISENBERG E (1968) Effects of varying phosphate intake in primary hyperparathyroidism *Journal of Clinical Endocrinology and Metabolism* **28** 651–660 (72, 100)

EISENBERG E GOTCH FA (1968) Normocalcemic hyperparathyroidism culminating in hypercalcemic crisis *Archives of Internal Medicine* **122** 258–264 (78)

ELIAS EG EVANS JT (1972) Hypercalcemic crisis in neoplastic diseases: Management with mithramycin *Surgery* **71** 631–635 (76)

ELIAS EG REYNOSO G MITTELMAN A (1972) Control of hypercalcemia with mithramycin *Annals of Surgery* **175** 431–435 (76)

ELLER JL SIEBERT PE (1969) Sclerotic vertebral bodies: an unusual manifestation of disseminated coccidioidomycosis *Radiology* **93** 1099–1100 (264)

ELLIOT JS (1954) Vitamin A and urolithiasis *California Medicine* **80** 462–464 (137)

ELLIOT JS (1973) The structure and composition of ureteral calculi In *Proceedings of the International Symposium on Renal Stone Research Madrid 1972* ed. Delatte LC Basle: Karger (131)

ELLIOT JS RIBEIRO ME EUSEBIO E (1970) The effect of oral phosphate upon the urinary excretion of oxalic acid *Investigative Urology* **7** 528–531 (139)

ELLIS C NICOLOFF DM (1968) Hyperparathyroidism and peptic ulcer disease *Archives of Surgery* **96** 114–118 (93)

ELLIS HA PEART KM (1972) Quantitative observations on mineralized and non-mineralized bone in the iliac crest *Journal of Clinical Pathology* **25** 277–286 (60, 226, 227, 228)

ELLIS HA PEART KM (1973) Azotaemic renal osteodystrophy: a quantitative study on iliac bone *Journal of Clinical Pathology* **26** 83–101 (197)

ELLIS FR HOLESH S ELLIS JW (1972) Incidence of osteoporosis in vegetarians and omnivores *American Journal of Clinical Nutrition* **25** 555–558 (231)

ELVEBACK LR GUILLIER CL KEATING RF (1970) Health normality and the ghost of Gauss *Journal of the American Medical Association* **211** 69–75 (43)

EMAMI-AHARI Z ZARABI M JAVID B (1969) Pycnodysostosis *Journal of Bone and Joint Surgery* **51B** 307–312 (270)

ENGFELDT B HJERTQUIST S-O (1960) Vitamin-D deficiency and bone and tooth structure *World Review of Nutrition and Dietetics* **2** 185–208 (179, 211)

EPSTEIN S PIMSTONE B BAKER G MODLIN M JACKSON WPU (1970) The clinical syndrome and investigation of primary hyperparathyroidism at Groote Schuur Hospital *South African Medical Journal* **44** 1047–1053 (84, 97)

EPSTEIN S SAGEL J JACKSON WPU (1971) A case of pseudohypoparathyroidism *South African Medical Journal* **45** 115–117 (163)

ERTEL NH REISS JS SPERGEL G (1969) Hypomagnesemia in neonatal tetany associated with maternal hyperparathyroidism *New England Journal of Medicine* **280** 260–263 (108)

ESSELSTYN CB POPOWNIAK KL (1971) Parathyroid surgery in the treatment of renal osteodystrophy and tertiary hyperparathyroidism *Surgical Clinics of North America* **51** 1211–1217 (206)

ESTEP H SHAW WA WATLINGTON C HOBE R HOLLAND W TUCKER StG (1969) Hypocalcemia due to hypomagnesemia and reversible parathyroid hormone unresponsiveness *Journal of Clinical Endocrinology and Metabolism* **29** 842–848 (145, 146)

ETHERIDGE JE GRABOW JD (1971) Hypercalcemia without EEG abnormalities *Diseases of the Nervous System* **32** 479–483 (70)

EUGENIDIS N OLAH AJ HAAS HG (1972) Osteosclerosis in hyperparathyroidism *Radiology* **105** 265–275 (89)

EVANS NAP (1971) Osteogenesis imperfecta in a child presenting with neurological features *Postgraduate Medical Journal* **47** 512–514 (259)

EVANS DJ AZZOPARDI JG (1972) Distinctive tumours of bone and soft tissue causing acquired vitamin-D-resistant osteomalacia *Lancet* **1** 353–354 (210)

ÉVREUX R (1962) Le rachitisme dans les grands ensembles *Revue d'hygiène et de médicine sociale* **10** 175–180 (168)

EYRE WG REED WB (1971) Albright's hereditary osteodystrophy with cutaneous bone formation *Archives of Dermatology* **104** 635–642 (163)

EXTON-SMITH AN MILLARD PH PAYNE PR WHEELER EF (1969) Pattern of development and loss of bone with age *Lancet* **2** 1154–1157 (227)

FACCINI JM (1970) The ultrastructure of parathyroid glands removed from patients with primary hyperparathyroidism: A report of 40 cases, including four carcinomata *Journal of Pathology* **102** 189–199 (81, 111)

FAIRNEY A WEIR AA (1970) The effect of abnormal maternal plasma calcium levels on the offspring of rats *Journal of Endocrinology* **48** 337–345 (109)

FANCONI G DE CHASTONAY E (1950) Die D-hypervitaminose im Säuglingsalter *Helvetica Paediatrica Acta* **5** 5–36 (119)

FANCONI A ROSE GA (1958) The ionized complexed and protein-bound fractions of calcium in plasma *Quarterly Journal of Medicine* NS **27** 463–494 (37, 97)

FARESE G MAGER M BLATT WF (1970) A membrane ultrafiltration procedure for determining diffusible calcium in serum *Clinical Chemistry* **16** 226–228 (39)

FAVUS MJ (1970) Treatment of vitamin D intoxication *New England Journal of Medicine* **283** 1468–1469 (75)

FAVUS MJ KIMBERG DV MILLAR GN GERSHON E (1973) Effects of cortisone administration on the metabolism and localization of 25-hydroxychole-calciferol in the rat. *Journal of Clinical Investigation* **52** 1328–1335 (283)

FEINBERG SB FISCH RO (1972) Bone changes in untreated neonatal phenylketo-nuric patients *Journal of Pediatrics* **81** 540–543 (180)

FIENBLATT J BÉLANGER LF RASMUSSEN H (1970) Effect of phosphate infusion on bone metabolism and parathyroid hormone action *American Journal of Physiology* **218** 1624–1631 (73)

FELTON DJC STONE WD (1966) Osteomalacia in Asian immigrants during pregnancy *British Medical Journal* **1** 1521–1522 (169)

FENNELLY JJ HOGAN A (1972) Pseudouridine excretion—a reflection of high RNA turnover in Paget's disease *Irish Journal of Medical Science* **141** 103–107 (249)

FERRIS T KASHGARIAN M LEVITIN H BRANDT I EPSTEIN FH (1961) Renal tubular acidosis and renal potassium wasting acquired as a result of hypercalcemic nephropathy *New England Journal of Medicine* **265** 924–928 (118)

FINE RN ROSOFF L GRUSHKIN CM DONNELL GN LIEBERMAN E (1970) Total parathyroidectomy in the treatment of renal osteodystrophy *Journal of Pediatrics* **76** 32–40 (206)

FINKELSTEIN JD SCHACHTER D (1962) Active transport of calcium by intestine: effects of hypophysectomy and growth hormone *American Journal of Physiology* **203** 873–880 (276)

FINLAYSON B HENCH LL SMITH LH (ed). (1972) *Urolithiasis: Physical Aspects* Washington: National Academy of Sciences (129)

FISCHER JA BINSWANGER U SCHENK RK MERZ W (1970) Histological observations on bone in intestinal malabsorption and vitamin D deficiency *Hormone and Metabolic Research* **2** 110–115 (191)

FLANAGAN TA GOODWIN DW ALDERSON P (1970) Psychiatric illness in a large family with familial hyperparathyroidism *British Journal of Psychiatry* **117** 693–698 (85)

FLEISCH H (1973) Diphosphonates and urinary stone formation. In *Proceedings of the International Symposium on Renal Stone Research Madrid 1972* ed Delatte LC Basle: Karger (139)

FLEISCH H BONJOUR J-P MORGAN DB REYNOLDS JJ SCHENK R SMITH R RUSSELL RGG (1972) Diphosphonates. In *Endocrinology* 1971 ed Taylor S 430–443 London: Heinemann (7)

FLETCHER RF JONES JH MORGAN DB (1963) Bone disease in chronic renal failure *Quarterly Journal of Medicine* N.S. **32** 321–339 (204)

FOLLIS RH (1953) Skeletal changes associated with hyperthyroidism *Johns Hopkins Hospital Bulletin* **92** 405–421 (279)

FONSECA OA CALVERLEY JR (1967) Neurological manifestations of hypoparathyroidism *Archives of Internal Medicine* **120** 202–206 (153)

FORBES GB BRYSON MF MANNING J AMIRHAKIMI GH REINA JC (1972) Impaired calcium homeostasis in the infantile hypercalcemic syndrome *Acta Paediatrica Scandinavica* **61** 305–309 (123)

FORD JA COLHOUN EM MCINTOSH WB DUNNIGAN MG (1972a) Rickets and osteomalacia in the Glasgow Pakistani Community 1961–71 *British Medical Journal* **2** 677–680 (167, 168)

FORD JA COLHOUN EM MCIINTOSH WB DUNNIGAN MG (1972b) Biochemical response of late rickets and osteomalacia to a chupatty-free diet *British Medical Journal* **3** 446–447 (168, 188)

FORD JA DAVIDSON DC MCINTOSH WB FYFE WM DUNNIGAN MG (1973) Neonatal rickets in Asian immigrant population *British Medical Journal* **3** 211–212 (167)

FORFAR JO TOMPSETT SL FORSHALL W (1959) Biochemical studies in idiopathic hypercalcaemia of infancy *Archives of Disease in Childhood* **34** 525–537 (123)

FOSTER GV (1973) Calcitonin. In *Recent Advances in Clinical Pathology Series 6* ed Dyke SC 43–60 Edinburgh: Churchill Livingstone (17)

FOURMAN P (1954) Experimental observations on the tetany of potassium deficiency *Lancet* **2** 525–528 (34)

FOURMAN P (1967) Magnesium in therapeutics. In *Modern Trends in Pharmacology and Therapeutics* ed Fulton WFM London: Butterworths (145)

FOURMAN P LEESON PM (1959) Thirst and polyuria with a note on the effects of potassium deficiency and calcium excess *Lancet* **1** 268–271 (69, 91)

FOURMAN P ROYER P (1968) Calcium metabolism and the bone Oxford: Blackwell (13, 22, 29, 31, 34, 56, 79, 102, 118, 126, 161, 164, 165, 181, 199, 207, 226, 231, 257, 278)

FOURMAN P DAVIS RH JONES KH MORGAN DB SMITH JWG (1963) Parathyroid insufficiency after thyroidectomy *British Journal of Surgery* **50** 608–619 (143, 160)

FOURNIER AE JOHNSON WJ TAVES DR BEABOUT JW ARNAUD CD GOLDSMITH RS (1971a) Etiology of hyperparathyroidism and bone disease during chronic hemodialysis *Journal of Clinical Investigation* **50** 592–598 (196)

FOURNIER AE ARNAUD CD JOHNSON WJ TAYLOR WF GOLDSMITH RS (1971b) Etiology of hyperparathyroidism and bone disease during chronic hemodialysis *Journal of Clinical Investigation* **50** 599–605 (196)

FRAME B (1965) Parkinsonism in postoperative hypoparathyroidism *Archives of Internal Medicine* **116** 424–427 (154, 155)

FRAME B HAUBRICH WS (1960) Peptic ulcer and hyperparathyroidism *Archives of Internal Medicine* **105** 536–541 (93)

FRAME B FOROOZANFAR F PATTON RB (1970) Normocalcemic primary hyperparathyroidism with osteitis fibrosa *Annals of Internal Medicine* **73** 253–257 (101)

FRAME B GUIANG HL FROST HM REYNOLDS WA (1971a) Osteomalacia induced by laxative (phenolphthalein) ingestion *Archives of Internal Medicine* **128** 794–796 (170)

FRAME B FROST HM PAK CYC REYNOLDS W ARGEN RJ (1971b) Fibrogenesis imperfecta ossium *New England Journal of Medicine* **285** 769–772 (272)

FRAME B HANSON CA FROST HM BLOCK M ARNSTEIN AR (1972) Renal resistance to parathyroid hormone with osteitis fibrosa *American Journal of Medicine* **52** 311–321 (164)

FRANCIS MJO SMITH R MACMILLAN DC (1973) Polymeric collagen of skin in normal subjects and in patients with inherited connective tissue disorders *Clinical Science* **44** 429–438 (255)

FRANK M LAZEBNIK J DE VRIES A (1970) Uric acid lithiasis—a study of six hundred and twenty-two patients *Urologia Internationalis* **25** 32–46 (91, 135)

FRASER D (1957) Hypophosphatasia *American Journal of Medicine* **22** 730–746 (269)

FRASER D (1971) Rickets In *Current therapy*, ed. Conn HF 358–363 Philadelphia: Saunders (188)

FRASER DR KODICEK E (1973) Regulation of 25-hydroxycholecalciferol-1-hydroxylase activity in kidney by parathyroid hormone *Nature New Biology* **241** 163–166 (25)

FRASER D KIDD BSL KOOH SW PAUNIER L (1966) A new look at infantile hypercalcemia *Pediatric Clinics of North America* **13** 503–525 (121, 124)

FRASER D KOOH SW SCRIVER CR (1967) Hyperparathyroidism as the cause of hyperaminoaciduria and phosphaturia in human vitamin D deficiency *Pediatric Research* **1** 425–435 (186)

FRASER P HEALEY M ROSE N WATSON L (1971a) Discriminant functions in differential diagnosis of hypercalcaemia *Lancet* **1** 1314–1319 (There is a printing error in this article: see *British Medical Journal* (1972) **2** 151) (68)

FRASER SA ANDERSON JB SMITH DA WILSON GM (1971b) Osteoporosis and fracture following thyrotoxicosis *Lancet* **1** 981–983 (279)

FRECH RS MCALISTER WH (1970) Pseudohypoparathyroidism (infant) and pseudopseudohypoparathyroidism (mother) *American Journal of Diseases of Children* **119** 447–448 (164)

FREEDMAN AP JURKOWITZ L (1971) Hypercacemia of malignancy: Ethics of treatment *Annals of Internal Medicine* **75** 481 (113)

FREEDOM RM ROSEN FS NADAS AS (1972) Congenital cardiovascular disease and anomalies of the third and fourth pharyngeal pouch *Circulation* **46** 165–172 (160)

FREMLIN JH (1972) Determination of whole-body calcium by neutron activation analysis *in vivo. Nuclear Medicine* **2** 86–93 (57)

FRENSILLI JA STONER RE HINRICHS EH (1971) Dental changes of idiopathic hypoparathyroidism *Journal of Oral Surgery* **29** 727–731 (155)

FRETHEIM B GARDBORG O (1965) Primary hyperparathyroidism in an infant *Acta Chirurgica Scandinavica* **129** 557–566 (109)

FREIDMAN P SKLAVER P KLAWANS HL (1971) Neurologic manifestations of Paget's disease of the skull *Diseases of the Nervous System* **32** 809–817 (246–247)

FREIDMAN Z HANLEY WB RADDE IC (1972) Ionized calcium in exchange transfusion with THAM-buffered ACD blood *Canadian Medical Association Journal* **107** 742–745 (147)

FROMM GA LITVAK J DEGROSSI OJ (1970) Intestinal absorption of calcium in fasting patients *Lancet* **1** 616–617 (144)

FRYE H CHAN P (1972) Analysis of urinary calculi with attenuated total reflectance infrared spectrophotometry *Investigative Urology* **10** 144–146 (131)

FUCHS C PASCHEN K (1972) Determination of ionized calcium in serum by means of an ion-sensitive electrode *German Medicine* **2** 7–8 (39)

FUJITA T ORIMO H YOSHIKAWA M (1970) Parathyroid hormono-hydrolyzing enzymes in human kidney *Endocrinologia Japonica* **17** 203–206 (15)

FUJITA T OKUYAMA Y HANDA N ORIMO H OHATA M YOSHIKAWA M AKIYAMA H KOGURE T (1971) Age-dependent bone loss after gastrectomy *Journal of the American Geriatrics Society* **19** 840–846 (237)

FULMER DH DIMICH AB ROTHSCHILD EO MYERS WPL (1972) Treatment of hypercalcemia. Comparison of intravenously administered phosphate sulphate and hydrocortisone *Archives of Internal Medicine* **129** 923–930 (72, 73, 75, 108)

GABRIEL R JOEKES AM ORTON E (1970) Hypervitaminosis D anaemia and renal failure *Postgraduate Medical Journal* **46** 455–457 (118)

GACA A HARTJE B OTTO J (1973) Analisis estructural de calculos urinarios en cortes finos y microscopio de polarizacion. In *Proceedings of the International Symposium on Renal Stone Research Madrid 1972* ed Delatte LC Basle: Karger (131)

GAILLARD PJ (1965) Observations on the effect of parathyroid products on explanted mouse limb-bone rudiments. In *The parathyroid glands* ed Gaillard PJ Talmage RV Budy AM Chicago: University of Chicago Press (16)

GALANTE L GUDMUNDSSON TV MATTHEWS EW TSE A WILLIAMS ED WOODHOUSE NJY MACINTYRE I (1968) Thymic and parathyroid origin of calcitonin in man *Lancet* **2** 537–539 (17)

GALANTE L JOPLIN GF MACINTYRE I WOODHOUSE NJY (1973) The calcium lowering effect of synthetic human porcine and salmon calcitonin in patients with Paget's disease *Clinical Science* **44** 605–610 (251)

GALASKO CSB BURN JI (1971) Hypercalcaemia in patients with advanced mammary cancer *British Medical Journal* **3** 573–577 (113)

GALE TC OWENS CWI (1972) Hyperfunctioning carcinoma of the parathyroid gland *Postgraduate Medical Journal* **48** 626–631 (111)

GALLAGHER JC NORDIN BEC (1972) Treatment with oestrogens of primary hyperparathyroidism in post-menopausal women *Lancet* **1** 503–507 (77)

GALLAGHER JC AARON J HORSMAN A WILKINSON R NORDIN BEC (1973) Corticosteroid osteoporosis *Clinics in Endocrinology and Metabolism* **2** 355–368 (283)

GALLINA AM WOLKE RE FRIER HI EATON HD HELMBOLDT CF (1971) Bone lesions in mild chronic bovine hypervitaminosis A. *Archiv für Experimentelle Veterinär Medezin* **24** 1091–1100 (128)

GALTON DAG AND OTHERS (1970) A case of chronic lymphocytic leukaemia *British Medical Journal* **1** 546–551 (115)

GAMBLE WS (1970) Hypercalcemia in hyperparathyroidism: Response to prednisone *New York State Journal of Medicine* **70** 427–429 (64)

GARDNER LI (1970) Pseudo-pseudohypoparathyroidism due to unequal crossing-over *Lancet* **2** 879–880 (162)

GARN SM ROHMANN CG WAGNER B (1967) Bone loss as a general phenomenon in man *Federation Proceedings* **26** 1729–1736 (228, 229, 231)

GARN SM POZNANSKI AK NAGY JM (1971) Bone measurement in the differential diagnosis of osteopenia and osteoporosis *Radiology* **100** 509–518 (224)

GARNETT J GARNETT ES MARDELL RJ BARNARD DL (1970) Urinary calcium excretion during ketoacidosis of prolonged total starvation *Metabolism* **19** 502–508 (48)

GAULT MH KINSELLA TD (1965) Carcinoma of lung with adrenal hyperfunction and hypercalcemia treated by parathyroidectomy *Canadian Medical Association Journal* **92** 317–324 (69)

GAY JDL GRIMES JD (1972) Idiopathic hypoparathyroidism with impaired vitamin B_{12} absorption and neuropathy *Canadian Medical Association Journal* **107** 54–58 (154)

GAYLER BW BROGDON BG (1965) Soft tissue calcifications in the extremities in systematic disease *American Journal of the Medical Sciences* **249** 590–605 (70)

GEKLE D STRÖDER J ROSTOCK D (1969) The effect of vitamin D on the inorganic phosphate reabsorption in the proximal convolution of the rat kidney *Klinische Wochenschrift* **47** 1177–1178 (27)

GENUTH SM KLEIN L (1972) Hypoparathyroidism and Paget's disease: the effect of parathyroid hormone administration *Journal of Clinical Endocrinology and Metabolism* **35** 693–699 (241)

GENUTH SM SHERWOOD LM VERTES V LEONARDS JP (1970) Plasma parathormone calcium and phosphorus in patients with renal osteodystrophy undergoing chronic hemodialysis *Journal of Clinical Endocrinology and Metabolism* **30** 15–23 (196)

GENUTH SM KLEIN L RABINOVICH S KING KC (1972) Osteomalacia accompanying chronic anticonvulsant therapy *Journal of Clinical Endocrinology and Metabolism* **35** 378–386 (174)

GHOZLAN R BROCHERIOU C CATZ G GODEAU P (1973) Hyperthyroïdie avec hypercalcémie *Nouvelle Presse Médicale* **2** 771–773 (280)

GIBBERD FB (1965) Idiopathic hypoparathyroidism with unusual bone changes and spastic paraplegia *Acta Endocrinologica* **48** 23–30 (155)

GIBSON MJ MIDDLEMISS JH (1971) Fibrous dysplasia of bone *British Journal of Radiology* **44** 1–13 (270)

GINSBERG DS KAPLAN EL KATZ AI (1973) Hypercalcaemia after oral calcium-carbonate therapy in patients on chronic haemodialysis *Lancet* **1** 1271–1274 (202, 205)

GLORIEUX F SCRIVER CR (1972) Loss of a parathyroid hormone-sensitive component of phosphate transport in X-linked hypophosphatemia *Science* **175** 997–1000 (211)

GLORIEUX FH SCRIVER CR READE TM GOLDMAN H ROSEBOROUGH A (1972) Use of phosphate and vitamin D to prevent dwarfism and rickets in X-linked hypophosphataemia *New England Journal of Medicine* **287** 481–487 (214)

GLORIEUX F SCRIVER C HOLICK M DE LUCA HF (1974) The response to 1,25 dihydroxycholecalciferol (1,25 DHCC) in X-linked hypophosphataemia In *Endocrinology 1973*, ed. Taylor S London: Heinemann (211)

GLYNNE A HUNTER IP THOMSON JA (1972) Pseudohypoparathyroidism with paradoxical increase in hypocalcaemic seizures due to long-term anticonvulsant therapy *Postgraduate Medical Journal* **48** 632–636 (163)

GOEBELL H STEFFEN C BALTZER G SCHLOTT KA BODE C (1972) Stimulation of enzyme secretion in the pancreas by acute hypercalcaemia *German Medicine* **2** 16–18 (85)

GOLDBERG LD (1972) Transmission of a vitamin-D metabolite in breast milk *Lancet* **2** 1258–1259 (160)

GOLDBLOOM RB GILLIS DA PRASAD M (1972) Hereditary parathyroid hyperplasia: A surgical emergency of early infancy *Pediatrics* **49** 514–523 (109)

GOLDFIELD EB BRAIKER BM PRENDERGAST JJ KOLB FO (1972) Synthetic salmon calcitonin: treatment of Paget's disease and osteogenesis imperfecta *Journal of the American Medical Association* **221** 1127–1129 (250, 260)

GOLDFINGER P (1969) Hypokalemia metabolic acidosis and hypocalcemic tetany in a patient taking laxatives *Journal of Mount Sinai Hospital* **36** 113–116 (146)

GOLDSMITH RS (1972) Treatment of Paget's disease with phosphate *Seminars in Drug Treatment* **2** 69–75 (250)

GOLDSMITH RS INGBAR SH (1966) Inorganic phosphate treatment of hypercalcemia of diverse etiologies *New England Journal of Medicine* **274** 1–7 (72)

GOLDSMITH RS BARTOS H HULLEY SB INGBAR SH MOLONEY WC (1968a) Phosphate supplementation as an adjunct in the therapy of multiple myeloma *Archives of Internal Medicine* **122** 128–133 (72, 73)

GOLDSMITH RE KING LR ZALME E BAHR GK (1968b) Serum calcium homeostasis in radio-iodine treated thyrotoxic subjects as measured by ethylenediamine tetra-acetate infusion *Acta Endocrinologica* **58** 565–577 (151)

GOLDSMITH NF JOHNSTON JO URY H VOSE G COLBERT C (1971) Bone-mineral estimation in normal and osteoporotic women *Journal of Bone and Joint Surgery* **53-A** 83–100 (227)

GOLDSMITH RS FURSZYFER J JOHNSON WJ FOURNIER AE SIZEMORE GW ARNAUD CD (1973) Etiology of hyperparathyroidism and bone disease during chronic hemodialysis *Journal of Clinical Investigation* **52** 173–180 (196)

GOLDSTEIN RA ISRAEL HL BECKER KL MOORE CF (1971) The infrequency of hypercalcemia in sarcoidosis *American Journal of Medicine* **51** 21–30 (120)

GOODENDAY LS GORDAN GS (1971) No risk from vitamin D in pregnancy *Annals of Internal Medicine* **75** 805–808 (160)

GOODHUE WW DAVIS JN PORRO RS (1972) Ischemic myopathy in uremic hyperparathyroidism *Journal of the American Medical Association* **221** 911–912 (200)

GORDAN GS GOLDMAN L (1970) Hyperparathyroidism *Modern Treatment* **7** 649–661 (104)

GORDAN GS CANTINO TJ ERHARDT L HANSEN J LUBICH W (1966) Osteolytic sterol in human breast cancer *Science* **151** 1226–1228 (114)

GORDON HE COBURN JW PASSARO E (1972) Surgical management of secondary hyperparathyroidism *Archives of Surgery* **104** 520–526 (206)

GÖRGÉNYI Á (1969) Idiopathic juvenile osteoporosis *Acta Paediatrica Academiae Scientiarum Hungaricae* **10** 315–321 (238)

GORODISCHER R ACETO T TERPLAN K (1970) Congenital familial hypoparathyroidism *American Journal of Diseases of Children* **119** 74–78 (160, 161)

GOUGH KR LLOYD OC WILLS MR (1964) Nutritional osteomalacia *Lancet* **2** 1261–1264 (169)

GOUGH MH SMITH R BISHOP MC (1971) Parathyroidectomy for symptomless hyperparathyroidism: A surgical dilemma *Lancet* **1** 1178 (See also the subsequent letter **2** 49) (102)

GRAHAME R SUTOR DJ MITCHENER MB (1971) Crystal deposition in hyperparathyroidism *Annals of the Rheumatic Diseases* **30** 597–604 (89)

GRANT ME PROCKOP DJ (1972) The biosynthesis of collagen *New England Journal of Medicine* **286** 194–199 242–249 291–300 (4)

GRAVELLE IH (1970) Articular manifestations of hyperparathyroidism. In *Symposium Ossium* ed. Jelliffe AM and Strickland B 105–108 Edinburgh: Livingstone (89)

GRAY PHK (1969) A case of osteogenesis imperfecta, associated with dentinogenesis imperfecta, dating from antiquity *Clinical Radiology* **20** 106–108 (253)

GREAVES JP HOLLINGSWORTH DF (1966) Trends in food consumption in the United Kingdom *World Review of Nutrition and Dietetics* **6** 34–89 (23)

GREENBERG BG WINTERS RW GRAHAM JB (1960) The normal range of serum inorganic phosphorus and its utility as a discriminant in the diagnosis of congenital hypophosphataemia *Journal of Clinical Endocrinology and Metabolism* **20** 364–379 (41)

GREENBERG SR KARABELL S SAADE GA (1972) Pseudohypoparathyroidism: a disease of the second messenger (3′-5′-Cyclic AMP) *Archives of Internal Medicine* **129** 633–637 (161)

GREENE ML FUJIMOTO WY SEEGMILLER JE (1969) Urinary xanthine stones—a rare complication of allopurinol therapy *New England Journal of Medicine* **280** 426–427 (135)

GREENFIELD GB (1969) *Radiology of bone diseases* Philadelphia: Lippincott (88, 120, 179, 180, 243, 264)

GREENWOOD RH PRUNTY FTG SILVER J (1973) Osteomalacia after prolonged glutethimide administration *British Medical Journal* **1** 643–645 (174)

GREGORY DH MESSNER RP (1969) Studies on the reliability of the isotopic calcium absorption test in patients with chronic renal disease *Journal of Laboratory and Clinical Medicine* **74** 464–471 (195)

GREIG A FAUCHALD P OVERSKEID K (1970) Venous-compression test in hyperparathyroidism *Lancet* **1** 835–836 (101)

GRIEVE J ZAREMBSKI PM (1973) Infra-red spectroscopy in the clinical analysis of renal stones. In *Proceedings of the International Symposium on Renal Stone Research, Madrid 1972* ed. Delatte LC Basle: Karger (131)

GRIFFITH DP (1971) Immobilization hypercalciuria: treatment and a possible pathophysiologic mechanism *Aerospace Medicine* **42** 1322–1324 (235)

GRIFFITH GC NICHOLS G ASHER JD FLANAGAN B (1965) Heparin osteoporosis *Journal of the American Medical Association* **193** 91–94 (see also the subsequent annotation: *Lancet* (1965) **2** 376) (237)

GRIMELIUS L JOHANSSON H LINDQUIST B WIBELL L (1972) Tertiary hyperparathyroidism occurring during a renal transplantation programme: report and discussion of three cases *Journal of Pathology* **108** 23–33 (200, 203, 206)

GRIMELIUS L JOHANSSON H LINDQUIST B THORÉN L WERNER I (1973) Normocalcemic primary hyperparathyroidism *Acta Chirurgica Scandinavica* **139** 42–44 (101)

GROEN JJ ESCHAR J BEN-ISHAY D ALKAN WJ BEN ASSA BI (1965) Osteomalacia among the Bedouin of the Negev Desert *Archives of Internal Medicine* **116** 195–204 (169)

GROTH CG POPOVTZER M HAMMOND WS CASCARDO S IWATSUKI S HALGRIMSON CG STARZL TE (1973) Survival of a homologous parathyroid implant in an immunosuppressed patient *Lancet* **1** 1082–1085 (159)

GRUNDY M (1970) Fractures of the femur in Paget's disease of bone *Journal of Bone and Joint Surgery* **52B** 252–263 (244, 245)

GRUNDY M PATTON JT (1969) The hand in Paget's disease (osteitis deformans) *British Journal of Radiology* **42** 748–752 (244)

GRÜNFELD J-P GANEVAL D CHARNARD J FARDEAU M DREYFUS J-C (1972) Acute renal failure in McArdle's disease *New England Journal of Medicine* **286** 1237–1241 (128)

GRYFE CI EXTON-SMITH AN PAYNE PR WHEELER EF (1971) Pattern of development of bone in childhood and adolescence *Lancet* **1** 523–526 (224)

GÜLLER R KAYASSEH L HAAS HG (1973) Osteoporose und Laktoseintoleranz *Schweizerische Medizinische Wochenschrift* **103** 107–109 (237)

HAAS HG DAMBACHER MA GUNČAGA J LAUFFENBURGER T (1971) Renal effects of calcitonin and parathyroid extract in man *Journal of Clinical Investigation* **50** 2689–2702 (21)

HABENER JF KEMPER B (1972) Pro-parathyroid hormone *Annals of Internal Medicine* **77** 151–152 (15)

HADDAD JG AVIOLI LV (1970) Comparative effects of phosphate and thyrocalcitonin on skeletal turnover *Endocrinology* **87** 1245–1250 (73, 77)

HADDAD JG COURANZ S AVIOLI LV (1970a) Nondialyzable urinary hydroxy-proline as an index of bone collagen formation *Journal of Clinical Endocrinology and Metabolism* **30** 282–287 (54, 55)

HADDAD JG BIRGE SJ AVIOLI LV (1970b) Effects of prolonged thyrocacitonin administration on Paget's disease of bone *New England Journal of Medicine* **283** 549–555 (250)

HADDAD JG BOISSEAU V AVIOLI LV (1972) Phosphorus deprivation: the metabolism of vitamin D_3 and 25-hydroxycholecalciferol in rats *Journal of Nutrition* **102** 269–282 (211)

HADDAD JG CHYU KJ HAHN TJ STAMP TCB (1973) Serum concentration of 25-hydroxyvitamin D in sex-linked hypophosphatemic vitamin D-resistant rickets *Journal of Laboratory and Clinical Medicine* **81** 22-27 (211)

HAFF RC BALLINGER WF (1971) Causes of recurrent hypercalcemia after para-thyroidectomy for primary hyperparathyroidism *Annals of Surgery* **173** 884–891 (82, 105)

HAFF RC BLACK WC BALLINGER WF (1970) Primary hyperparathyroidism: changing clinical surgical and pathologic aspects *Annals of Surgery* **171** 85–92 (104)

HAHN TJ HENDIN BA SCHARP CR HADDAD JG (1972a) Effect of chronic anticon-vulsant therapy on serum 25-hydroxycalciferol levels in adults *New England Journal of Medicine* **287** 900–904 (174, 175)

HAHN TJ BIRGE SJ SCHARP CR AVIOLI LV (1972b) Phenobarbital-induced alterations in vitamin D metabolism *Journal of Clinical Investigation* **51** 741–748 (174)

HALL RF REYNOLDS RA (1972) Concentrations of magnesium and calcium in plasma of Hereford cows during and after hypomagnesemic tetany *American Journal of Veterinary Research* **33** 1711–1713 (35)

HALLICK RB DE LUCA HF (1972) Metabolites of dihydrotachysterol₃ in target tissues *Journal of Biological Chemistry* **247** 91–97 (25)

HAMBURGER J RICHET G GROSNIER J FUNCK-BRENTANO JL ANTOINE B DUCROT H MERY JP DE MONTERA H (1968) *Nephrology* Philadelphia: Saunders (70, 91)

HAMPERS CL KATZ AI WILSON RE MERRILL JP (1969) Calcium metabolism and osteodystrophy after renal transplantation *Archives of Internal Medicine* **124** 282–291 (197)

HANCOX NM (1972a) The osteoclast. In *The Biochemistry and Physiology of Bone* ed Bourne GH (2nd edition) Vol 1 45–67 New York: Academic Press (2)

HANCOX NM (1972b) *Biology of bone* Cambridge: Cambridge University Press (1, 3)

HANNA S HARRISON M MACINTYRE I FRASER R (1960) The syndrome of magnesium deficiency in man *Lancet* **2** 172–175 (269)

HANNA S HARRISON MT MACINTYRE I FRASER R (1961) Effects of growth hormone on calcium and magnesium metabolism *British Medical Journal* **2** 12–15 (276)

HANSEN SO THEODORSEN L (1971) The usefulness of an improved calcium elec-trode in the measurement of ionized calcium in serum *Clinica Chimica Acta* **31** 119–122 (39)

HARDT AB (1972) Early metabolic responses of bone to immobilization *Journal of Bone and Joint Surgery* **54A** 119–124 (235)

HARGIS GK YAKULIS VJ WILLIAMS GA WHITE AA (1964) Cytological detection of parathyroid hormone by immunofluorescence *Proceedings of the Society for Experimental Biology and Medicine* **117** 836–839 (80)

HARRELL GT FISHER S (1939) Blood chemical changes in Boeck's sarcoid with particular reference to protein, calcium and phosphatase values *Journal of Clinical Investigation* **18** 687–693 (119)

HARRIS PWR (1969) An unusual case of calcinosis due to vitamin D intoxication *Guy's Hospital Reports* **118** 533–541 (70, 118)

HARRIS WH HEANEY RP (1969) Skeletal renewal and metabolic bone disease *New England Journal of Medicine* **280** 193–202 253–259 303–311 (11, 57, 96, 186)

HARRIS WH HEANEY RP (1970) *Skeleton Renewal and Metabolic Bone Disease* Boston: Little, Brown (11, 57, 96, 186)

HARRISON AR (1973) Results of parathyroidectomy In *Proceedings of the International Symposium on Renal Stone Research Madrid 1972* ed Delatte LC Basle: Karger (102)

HARRISON HE HARRISON HC (1963) Sodium, potassium and intestinal transport, of glucose, 1-tyrosine, phosphate and calcium *American Journal of Physiology* **205** 107–111 (29)

HARTENSTEIN H GARDNER LI (1966) Tetany of the newborn associated with maternal parathyroid adenoma *New England Journal of Medicine* **274** 266–268 (108)

HASKELL CM DE VITA VT CANELLOS CP (1971) Hypercalcemia in chronic granulocytic leukemia *Cancer* **27** 872–880 (115)

HATHAWAY WE SOLOMONS CC OTT JE (1972) Platelet function and pyrophosphates in osteogenesis imperfecta *Blood* **39** 500–509 (54, 259)

HATTNER RS BERNSTEIN DS ALIAPOULIOS MA GEORGE B ROSE E (1970) The hypocalcaemic activity of glucagon: demonstration of independence from endogenous calcitonin secretion in the rat *Acta Endocrinologica* **64** 726–736 (144)

HAZARD J MODAÏ J DOMART A (1969) Hypoparathyroïdie après thyroïdectomie; hypercalcémie thérapeutique par déficit en thyroïcalcitonine *Annales de Médecine Interne* **120** 305–308 (217)

HEANEY RP SKILLMAN TG (1971) Calcium metabolism in normal human pregnancy *Journal of Clinical Endocrinology and Metabolism* **33** 661–670 (27)

HEATH DA WILLS MR (1971) Normocalcaemic primary hyperparathyroidism with osteitis fibrosa *Postgraduate Medical Journal* **47** 815–817 (101)

HEATH H EARLL JM SCHAAF M PIECHOCKI JT LI T-K (1972a) Serum ionized calcium during bed rest in fracture patients and normal men *Metabolism* **21** 633–640 (127)

HEATH DA PALMER JS AURBACH GD (1972b) The hypocalcemic action of colchicine *Endocrinology* **90** 1589–1593 (147)

HEATON FW (1973) Magnesium requirement for enzymes and hormones *Biochemical Society Transactions* **1** 67–70 (145)

HEATON FW FOURMAN P (1965) Magnesium deficiency and hypocalcaemia in intestinal malabsorption *Lancet* **2** 50–52 (145, 146)

HEATON KW LEVER JV BARNARD D (1972) Osteomalacia associated with cholestyramine therapy for postileectomy diarrhoea *Gastroenterology* **62** 642–646 (24, 170)

HEBERT LA LEMANN J PETERSEN JR LENNON EJ (1966) Studies of the mechanism by which phosphate infusion lowers serum calcium concentration *Journal of Clinical Investigation* **45** 1886–1894 (73)

HECKMAN BA WALSH JH (1967) Hypernatremia complicating sodium sulfate therapy for hypercalcemic crisis *New England Journal of Medicine* **276** 1082–1083 (74)

HEDBERG CA MELNYK CS JOHNSON CF (1966) Gluten enteropathy appearing after gastric surgery *Gastroenterology* **50** 796–804 (173)

HEGSTED DM MOSCOSO I COLLAZOS C (1952) A study of the minimum calcium requirements of adult men *Journal of Nutrition* **46** 181–201 (9)

HEIMANN P NILSSON O (1970) Postoperative acute hyperparathyroidism *Acta Chirurgica Scandinavica* **136** 467–469 (107, 108)

HEIMANN P MORTENSEN A NILSSON O HANSSON G (1970a) Parathyroid and thyroid disease: I parathyroid disease discovered during surgical exploration of the thyroid *Acta Chirurgica Scandinavica* **136** 139–141 (280)

HEIMANN P NILSSON O HANSSON G (1970b) Parathyroid and thyroid disease: II thyroid disease connected with hyperparathyroidism *Acta Chirurgica Scandinavica* **136** 143–146 (280)

HEIMANN P NILSSON O ROSENGREN K (1971) Per-operative marking of the parathyroid glands with silver-clips *Acta Chirurgica Scandinavica* **137** 217–219 (13)

HELLSTRÖM J IVEMARK BI (1962) Primary hyperparathyroidism: Clinical and structural findings in 138 cases *Acta Chirurgica Scandinavica* Suppl. 294 (83, 92, 98)

HELLSTRÖM J BIRKE G EDVALL CA (1958) Hypertension in hyperparathyroidism *British Journal of Urology* **30** 13–24 (92, 106)

HEMET J CHLEQ C (1973) Les calcifications métastatiques des hyperparathyroïdies primitives *Semaine des Hôpitaux* **49** 495–500 (70)

HENKIN RI LIFSCHITZ MD LARSON AL (1972) Hearing loss in patients with osteoporosis and Paget's disease of bone *American Journal of Medical Sciences* **263** 383–392 (246)

HENNEMAN PH FORBES AP MOLDAWER M DEMPSEY EF CARROLL EL (1960) Effects of human growth hormone in man *Journal of Clinical Investigation* **39** 1223–1238 (276)

HENNEMAN DH PAK CYC BARTTER FC (1973) Collagen composition, solubility and biosynthesis in fibrogenesis imperfecta ossium In *Clinical aspects of metabolic bone disease* ed Frame B Parfitt AM Duncan H 469–472 Amsterdam: Excerpta Medica (272)

HENRY A (1969) Monostotic fibrous dysplasia *Journal of Bone and Joint Surgery* **51B** 300–306 (272)

HERRING LC (1962) Observations on the analysis of ten thousand urinary calculi *Journal of Urology* **88** 545–562 (130, 131)

HERRING GM (1972) The organic matrix of bone In *The Biochemistry and Physiology of Bone* ed. Bourne GH (2nd edition) Vol 1 127–189 New York: Academic Press (4, 5)

HESCH R-D HÜFNER M PASCHEN K VON ZUR MÜHLEN A (1971) Akute Behandlung des hypercalcämischen Hyperparathreoidismus mit Calcitonin *Deutsche Medizinische Wochenschrift* **96** 764–767 (76)

HESCH R-D GERLACH W HENNING HV EMRICH D SCHELER F KATTERMANN R (1972) Untersuchungen zur intestinalen ^{47}Ca-Absorption bei Gesunden und Patienten mit chronischer Niereninsuffzienz *Deutsche Medizinische Wochenschrift* **97** 1735–1742 (195)

HIGGINS PM PRIDIE RB (1966) Postgastrectomy osteomalacia: incidence after the no-loop and other types of gastrectomy *British Journal of Surgery* **53** 881–885 (172)

HIGGINS CB BRAUNWALD E (1972) The prostaglandins: biochemical, physiologic and clinical considerations *American Journal of Medicine* **53** 93–112 (218)

HIGHMAN JH SANDERSON PH SUTCLIFFE MML (1970) Vitamin-D-resistant osteomalacia as a cause of cord compression *Quarterly Journal of Medicine* NS **39** 529–537 (212)

HILL PG SAMMONS HG (1967) An assessment of 5'-nucleotidase as a liver-function test *Quaterly Journal of Medicine* NS 36 457–468 (46)

HILL CS OUAIS SG LEISER AE (1972) Long-term administration of calcitonin for hypercalcemia secondary to recurrent parathyroid carcinoma *Cancer* **29** 1016–1020 (76)

HILLEGAS J EVANS WE (1971) Hyperparathyroidism: A review of 45 cases *Wisconsin Medical Journal* **70** 89–92 (84)

HILLEMAND P MIALERET J BOUTELIER D (1961) Exclusion duodenale et osteomalacie des gastrectomisés *Presse médicale* **69** 627–630 (173)

HILLMAN DA SCRIVER CR PEDVIS S SHRAGOVITCH I (1964) Neonatal familial primary hyperparathyroidism *New England Journal of Medicine* **270** 483–490 (80)

HINKLE JE COOPERMAN LH (1971) Serum ionized calcium changes following citrated blood transfusion in anaesthetized man *British Journal of Anaesthesia* **43** 1108–1112 (147)

HIOCO D DORFMANN H TUN CHOT S BORDIER P DE SÈZE S (1972) Anomalies du métabolisme phosphocalcique dans l'insuffisance rénale *Revue du Rhumatisme* **39** 617–625 (201, 202)

HIRSCH PF GAUTHIER GF MUNSON PL (1963) Thyroid hypocalcemic principle and recurrent laryngeal nerve injury as factors affecting the response to parathyroidectomy in rats *Endocrinology* **73** 244–252 (17)

HOCKADAY TDR KEYNES WM MCKENZIE JK (1966) Catatonic stupor in elderly women with hyperparathyroidism *British Medical Journal* **1** 85–87 (85)

HODGKINSON A (1971) A combined qualitative and quantitative procedure for the chemical analysis of urinary calculi *Journal of Clinical Pathology* **24** 147–151 (131)

HODGKINSON A EDWARDS NA (1963) Total and ultrafilterable serum calcium in primary hyperparathyroidism *British Journal of Urology* **35** 445–456 (97)

HODGKINSON A NORDIN BEC (1969) ed *Renal stone research symposium* London: Churchill (129)

HODGKINSON A PYRAH LN (1958) The urinary excretion of calcium and inorganic phosphate in 344 patients with calcium stone of renal origin *British Journal of Surgery* **46** 10–18 (48)

HOEHN JG BEAHRS OH WOOLNER LB (1969) Unusual surgical lesions of the parathyroid gland *American Journal of Surgery* **118** 770–778 (81)

HOFFMAN E (1958) The Chvostek sign *American Journal of Surgery* **96** 33–37 (34)

HOLICK MF DE LUCA HF (1971) A new chromatographic system for vitamin D_3 and its metabolites: resolution of a new vitamin D_3 metabolite *Journal of Lipid Research* **12** 460–465 (26)

HOLICK MF GARABEDIAN M DE LUCA HF (1972) 1,25-dihydroxycholecalciferol: metabolite of vitamin D_3 active on bone in anephric rats *Science* **176** 1146–1147 (27)

HOLLANDER D ROSENSTREICH SJ VOLWILER W (1971) Role of the duodenum in vitamin D_3 absorption in man *American Journal of Digestive Diseases* **16** 145–149 (24, 170)

HOLMAN CB (1952) Roentgenologic manifestations of vitamin D intoxication *Radiology* **59** 805–816 (119)

HOLMES G (1971) Urinary calculi in Fiji Indians—the curry kidney *Medical Journal of Australia* **2** 755–756 (137)

HOLMES GE TUCKER V (1972) Oculo-cerebro-renal syndrome *Clinical Pediatrics* **11** 119–124 (216)

HOLMES EC MORTON DL KETCHAM AS (1969) Parathyroid carcinoma: A collective review *Annals of Surgery* **169** 631–640 (111, 112)

HOLMES AM ENOCH BA TAYLOR JL JONES ME (1973) Occult rickets and osteomalacia amongst the Asian immigrant population *Quarterly Journal of Medicine* NS **42** 125–149 (167, 168, 188)

HORNUM I (1971) Post-transplant hypercalcemia due to mobilization of metastatic calcification *Acta Medica Scandinavica* **189** 199–205 (203)

HORNUM I TRANSBØL I HAHNEMANN S HALVER B (1968) An endocrine and metabolic study of idiopathic hyperabsorption hypercalcemia in the adult. In *Les Tissus Calcifiés (Proceedings of the 5th European Symposiun on Calcified Tissues)* ed Milhaud G Owen M and Blackwood HJJ 307–312 Paris: Societé d'edition d'enseignement supérieur (128)

HORWITZ CA MYERS WPL FOOTE FW (1972) Secondary malignant tumors of the parathyroid glands: Report of two cases with associated hypoparathyroidism *American Journal of Medicine* **52** 797–808 (152)

HOSHINO T MURAKAMI Y (1971) Melorheostosis *Acta Orthopaedica Scandinavica* **42** 28–34 (264)

HOSKIN DJ CHAMBERLAIN MJ FREMLIN JH JAMES H (1972) Changes in total body calcium and sodium in osteomalacia *British Medical Journal* **1** 19–22 (186)

HOSSAIN M (1970) Neurological and psychiatric manifestations in idiopathic hypoparathyroidism: response to treatment *Journal of Neurology, Neurosurgery and Psychiatry* **33** 153–156 (153)

HOWARD JE (1961) Adventures in clinical research on bone and stones *Journal of Clinical Endocrinology and Metabolism* **21** 1254–1259 (132)

HOWARD JE MEYER RJ (1948) Intoxication with vitamin D *Journal of Clinical Endocrinology* **8** 895–910 (118, 119)

HOWARD JE FOLLIS RH YENDT ER CONNOR TB (1953) Hyperparathyroidism: Case report illustrating spontaneous remission due to necrosis of adenoma, and a study of the incidence of necroses in parathyroid adenomas *Journal of Clinical Endocrinology and Metabolism* **13** 997–1008 (82)

HOWELL A (1972) Occult hyperparathyroidism presenting as a parathyroid cyst *Proceedings of the Royal Society of Medicine* **65** 881–882 (83)

HUBAY CA GONZALEZ-BARCENA D KLEIN L FRANKEL V ECKEL RE PEARSON OH (1970) Parathyroidectomy in the treatment of renal osteodystrophy *Archives of Surgery* **101** 181–192 (the discussion on pages 197 and 198 is also valuable) (206)

HULLEY SB VOGEL JM DONALDSON CL BAYERS JH FREIDMAN RJ ROSEN SN (1971) The effect of supplemental oral phosphate on the bone mineral changes during prolonged bed rest *Journal of Clinical Investigation* **50** 2506–2518 (233, 235)

HUMBERT G FILLASTRE J-P LEROY J ROBERT M DELAUNAY P (1972) Les hypercalcémies aiguës: Traitement par le furosémide *Nouvelle Presse Médicale* **1** 2025–2029 (See also the subsequent letter by Dr. M Fiorentino **2** 245) (74)

HUNDER GG KELLY PJ (1971) Bone scans in transient osteoporosis *Annals of Internal Medicine* **75** 134 (239)

HUNT G MORGAN DB (1970) The early effects of dihydrotachysterol on calcium and phosphorus metabolism in patients with hypoparathyroidism *Clinical Science* **38** 713–725 (158)

HUNT DD STEARNS G McKINLEY JB FRONING E HICKS P BONFIGLIO M (1966) Long-term study of family with Fanconi syndrome without cystinosis (De Toni-Débre-Fanconi syndrome) *American Journal of Medicine* **40** 492–510 (209)

HUNTER R (1972) Rickets, ruckets, rekets or rackets? *Lancet* **1** 1176–1177 (165)

HUNTER J MAXWELL JD STEWART DA PARSONS V WILLIAMS R (1971) Altered calcium metabolism in epileptic children on anticonvulsants *British Medical Journal* **4** 202–204 (See also the subsequent correspondence on page 684) (174)

HURXTHAL LM VOSE GP (1969) The relationship of dietary calcium intake to radiographic bone density in normal and osteoporotic persons *Calcified Tissue Research* **4** 245–256 (231)

HYMAN LR BONER G THOMAS JC SEGAR WE (1972) Immobilization hypercalcemia *American Journal of Diseases of Children* **124** 723–727 (127)

INGHAM JP STEWART JH POSEN S (1973) Quantitative skeletal histology in untreated end-stage renal failure *British Medical Journal* 2 745–748 (197, 198)

INGLIS NR FISHMAN L STOLBACH LL WARSHAW JB FISHMAN WH (1972) A comparison of chyle isoenzymes of alkaline phosphatase in chyle and hypophosphatasemic sera *Clinica Chimica Acta* 38 67–73 (269)

IRELAND AW CLUBB JS NEALE FC POSEN S REEVE TS (1968) The calciferol requirements of patients with surgical hypoparathyroidism *Annals of Internal Medicine* 69 81–89 (159)

IRNELL L (1969) Metastatic calcification of soft tissue on overdosage of vitamin D *Acta Medica Scandinavica* 185 147–152 (118)

IRVIN GL COHEN MS MOEBUS R MINTZ DH (1972) Primary hyperparathyroidism: current diagnosis, treatment and results *Archives of Surgery* 105 738–740 (96, 103)

IRVINE WJ (1971) Adrenalitis hypoparathyroidism and associated diseases In *Immunological diseases* ed Samter M 2nd ed Vol 2 1214–1227 Boston: Little Brown (152)

IRVINE WJ BARNES EW (1972) Adrenocortical insufficiency *Clinics in Endocrinology and Metabolism* 1 549–594 (152, 281)

ISAKSSON B SJÖGREN B (1967) A critical evaluation of the mineral and nitrogen balances in man *Proceedings of the Nutrition Society* 26 106–116 (56)

ISAKSSON B LINDHOLM B SJÖGREN B (1967) A critical evaluation of the calcium balance technic: II Dermal calcium losses *Metabolism* 16 303–313 (11)

IVANHOE F (1970) Was Virchow right about Neandertal? *Nature* 227 577–579 (166)

IVES DR THOMPSON DM (1973) Urticaria pigmentosa with spinal osteoporosis *Proceedings of the Royal Society of Medicine* 66 175–176 (237)

JACKSON WPU (1952) Studies of adult cretins *South African Medical Journal* 26 605–607 631–633 645–647 (278)

JACKSON WPU (1967) *Calcium metabolism and bone disease* London: Arnold (9, 30)

JACKSON CE BOONSTRA CE (1967) The relationship of hereditary hyperparathyroidism to endocrine adenomatosis *American Journal of Medicine* 43 727–734 (80)

JACKSON WPU HARRIS F (1965) Gout with hyperparathyroidism: Report of case with examination of synovial fluid *British Medical Journal* 2 211 (98)

JACOB HS AMSDEN T (1971) Acute hemolytic anemia with rigid red cells in hypophosphatemia *New England Journal of Medicine* 285 1446–1450 (41)

JAFFE N KIM BS VAWTER GF (1972) Hypocalcemia—a complication of childhood leukemia *Cancer* 29 392–398 (147)

JAMES W MOULE B (1966) Hypophosphatasia *Clinical Radiology* 17 368–376 (269)

JARDON OM BURNEY DW FINK RL (1970) Hypophosphatasia in an adult *Journal of Bone and Joint Surgery* 52A 1477–1484 (267)

JELLIFFE AM STRICKLAND B (ed.) (1970) *Symposium Ossium* Edinburgh: Livingstone (particularly sessions 10, 16 & 18) (223)

JELONEK A BARYLAK H DOMOSLAWSKI W (1971) Hereditary pseudo-deficiency rachitis with hypocalcaemia (in Polish) *Przeglad Lekarski* **28** 427–430 (176)

JENNIS F LAVAN JN NEALE FC POSEN S (1970) Staghorn calculi of the kidney: clinical bacteriological and biochemical features *British Journal of Urology* **42** 511–518 (136)

JEWELEWICZ R NACHTIGALL LE (1971) Pseudo-pseudohypoparathyroidism and pregnancy *Obstetrics and Gynecology* **37** 396–401 (164)

JIMENEA CV FRAME B CHAYKIN LB SIGLER JW (1971) Spondylitis of hypoparathyroidism *Clinical Orthopaedics* **74** 84–89 (155)

JOEKES AM ROSE GA SUTOR J (1973) Multiple renal silica calculi *British Medical Journal* **1** 146–147 (135)

JOFFE BI HACKENG WHI SEFTEL HC HARTDEGEN RG (1972) Parathyroid hormone concentrations in nutritional rickets *Clinical Science* **42** 113–116 (186)

JOHANSSON H THORÉN L WERNER I (1973) Pernicious hyperparathyroidism *Acta Chirurgica Scandinavica* **139** 37–41 (107)

JOHNSON RD CONN JW (1969) Hyperparathyroidism with a prolonged period of normocalcemia *Journal of the Anerican Medical Association* **210** 2063–2066 (101)

JOHNSON KA RIGGS BL KELLY PJ JOWSEY J (1971a) Osteoid tissue in normal and osteoporotic individuals *Journal of Clinical Endocrinology and Metabolism* **33** 745–751 (60)

JOHNSON JW HATTNER RS HAMPERS CL BERNSTEIN DS MERRILL JP SHERWOOD LM (1971b) Secondary hyperparathyroidism in chronic renal failure *Journal of the American Medical Association* **215** 478–480 (197, 203)

JOHNSTON CC LAVY N LORD T VELLIOS F MERRITT AD DEISS WP (1968) Osteopetrosis: a clinical, genetic, metabolic and morphologic study of the dominantly inherited benign form *Medicine* **47** 149–167 (261, 262, 263, 264)

JOHNSTONE RE KREINDLER T JOHNSTONE RE (1972) Hyperparathyroidism during pregnancy *Obstetrics and Gynecology* **40** 580–585 (108)

JONES KH FOURMAN P (1966) Effects of infusions of magnesium and of calcium in parathyroid insufficiency *Clinical Science* **30** 139–150 (156)

JORDAN WM (1972) Bone disease after gastrectomy *British Medical Journal* **2** 113 (177)

JØRGENSEN H (1973) Hypercalcemia in adrenocortical insufficiency *Acta Medica Scandinavica* **193** 175–179 (281)

JOSEPH MC PARROTT D (1958) Severe infantile hypercalcaemia with special reference to the facies *Archives of Disease in Childhood* **33** 385–395 (122)

JOWSEY J BALASUBRAMANIAM P (1972) Effect of phosphate supplements on soft-tissue calcification and bone turnover *Clinical Science* **42** 289–299 (73)

JOWSEY J JOHNSON KA (1972) Juvenile osteoporosis: bone findings in seven patients *Journal of Pediatrics* **81** 511–517 (238)

JOWSEY J RIGGS BL KELLY PJ HOFFMAN DL BORDIER P (1971) The treatment of osteoporosis with disodium ethane-l-hydroxy-l,l-diphosphonate *Journal of Laboratory and Clinical Medicine* **78** 574–584 (233)

JOWSEY J RIGGS BL KELLY PJ HOFFMAN DL (1972) Effect of combined therapy with sodium fluoride, vitamin D and calcium in osteoporosis *American Journal of Medicine* **53** 43–49 (See also the subsequent letters *British Medical Journal* (1973) **1** 551 613) (233)

JUBIZ W CANTERBURY JM REISS E TYLER FH (1972) Circadian rhythm in serum parathyroid hormone concentration in human subjects: correlation with serum calcium, phosphate, albumin and growth hormone levels *Journal of Clinical Investigation* **51** 2040–2046 (37, 40)

KALLIO DM GARANT PR MINKIN C (1972) Ultrastructural effects of calcitonin on osteoclasts in tissue culture *Journal of Ultrastructure Research* **39** 205–216 (20)

KAMINSKI DL WILLMAN VL (1972) Acute hyperparathyroidism *American Surgeon* **38** 307–311 (107)

KAPLAN E (1942) The parathyroid gland in infancy *Archives of pathology* **34** 1042–1049 (179)

KAPLAN MM (1972) Alkaline phosphatase *Gastroenterology* **62** 452–468 (42, 45)

KAPLAN EL ARNAUD CD HILL BJ PESKIN GW (1970) Adrenal medullary calcitonin-like factor: A key to multiple endocrine neoplasia, type 2? *Surgery* **68** 146–149 (95, 218)

KAPLAN L KATZ AD BEN-ISAAC C MASSRY SG (1971) Malignant neoplasms and parathyroid adenoma *Cancer* **28** 401–407 (95, 113)

KAPLAN EL PESKIN GW JAFFE BM (1972) The effects of acute metabolic acid-base changes on secretion of gastrin and parathyroid hormone *Surgery* **72** 53–59 (15)

KARPATI G FRAME B (1964) Neuropsychiatric disorders in primary hyperparathyroidism *Archives of Neurology* **10** 387–397 (69, 85)

KASPERLIK-ZALUSKA A (1971) Urinary phosphates excretion in hyper- and hypoadrenalism (in Polish) *Polskie Archiwum Medycyny Wewnetrznej* **47** 507–518 (282)

KATZ CM TZAGOURNIS M (1972) Chronic adult hypervitaminosis A with hypercalcemia *Metabolism* **21** 1171–1176 (128)

KATZ AI HAMPERS CL MERRILL JP (1969) Secondary hyperparathyroidism and renal osteodystrophy in chronic renal failure *Medicine* **48** 333–374 (192, 198, 200, 202)

KATZ A KAPLAN L MASSRY SG HELLER R PLOTKIN D KNIGHT I (1970) Primary hyperparathyroidism in patients with breast carcinoma *Archives of Surgery* **101** 582–585 (113)

KAYE M (1971) Recognition of osteodystrophy in chronic uraemia *American Journal of the Medical Sciences* **261** 183–187 (198, 202)

KAYE M SAGAR S (1972) Effect of dihydrotachysterol on calcium absorption in uremia *Metabolism* **21** 815–824 (204)

KAYE M JUST G WILSON M (1971) Comparison of dihydrotachysterol and calciferol *Canadian Journal of Physiology and Pharmacology* **49** 857–861 (158)

KEELING DH TODD-POKROPEK AE (1969) Computer-assisted parathyroid scanning In *Medical Radioisotope Scintigraphy* 745–757 Vienna: International Atomic Energy Agency (103)

KEEN JH (1969) Significance of hypocalcaemia in neonatal convulsions *Archives of Disease of Childhood* **44** 356–361 (147)

KEENE JE CORREA RJ (1971) Pheochromocytoma associated with parathyroid adenoma Report of a case and review of literature *Journal of Urology* **106** 443–447 (95)

KEIPERT JA (1970) Rickets with multiple fractured ribs in a premature infant *Medical Journal of Australia* **1** 672–675 (167)

KEISER HR BEAVEN MA DOPPMAN J WELLS S BUJA LM (1973) Sipple's syndrome: medullary thyroid carcinoma, pheochromocytoma and parathyroid disease *Annals of Internal Medicine* **78** 561–579 (95, 218, 219)

KELLY TR (1970) Relationship of hyperparathyroidism to peptic ulcer *Archives of Surgery* **101** 193–197 (93)

KELLY S LEIKHIM E DESJARDINS L (1972) A qualitative spot test for cystinuria *Clinica Chimica Acta* **39** 469–471 (137)

KEMPE CH (1971) Paediatric implications of the battered baby syndrome *Archives of disease in childhood* **46** 28–37 (31)

KENDALL AC (1972) Rickets in the tropics and sub-tropics *Central African Journal of Medicine* **18** 47–49 (168)

KENNETT S POLLICK H (1971) Jaw lesions in familial hyperparathyroidism *Oral Surgery Oral Medicine and Oral Pathology* **31** 502–510 (87)

KESSINGER A LEMON HM FOLEY JF (1972) Hypercalcemia of malignancy *Geriatrics* **27** 97–106 (75 113 114 115 116)

KEUTMANN HT DAWSON BF AURBACH GD POTTS JT (1972) A biologically active amino-terminal fragment of bovine parathyroid hormone prepared by dilute acid hydrolysis *Biochemistry* **11** 1973–1979 (14)

KEYNES M (1961) Primary hyperparathyroidism In *British Surgical Practice: Surgical Progress 1961* 255–291 Ed Rock-Carling E Paterson-Ross J London: Butterworths (104)

KEYNES WM CAIRD FI (1970) Hypocalcaemic primary hyperparathyroidism *British Medical Journal* **1** 208–211 (101)

KEYNES WM TILL AS (1971) Medullary carcinoma of the thyroid gland *Quarterly Journal of Medicine* NS **40** 443–456 (95, 217, 218, 219)

KING JS (1971) Currents in renal stone research *Clinical Chemistry* **17** 971–982 (129)

KING RG STANBURY SW (1970) Magnesium metabolism in primary hyperparathyroidism *Clinical Science* **39** 281–303 (98, 105)

KIRKWOOD JR OZONOFF MB STEINBACH HL (1972) Epiphyseal displacement after metaphyseal fracture in renal osteodystrophy *American Journal of Roentgenology Radium Therapy and Nuclear Medicine* **115** 547–554 (198)

KISTLER HJ NEUBAUER W (1970) Phosphatbehandlung bei Hypercalcämie *Klinische Wochenschrift* **48** 741–752 (72)

KIVIRIKKO KI LAITINEN O (1965) Clinical significance of urinary hydroxyproline determinations in children *Annales Paediatriae Fenniae* **11** 148–153 (55)

KLEEMAN CR MASSRY SG COBURN JW POPOVTZER MM (1970) Calcium and phosphorus metabolism and bone disease in uremia *Clinical Orthopaedics* **68** 210–237 (196, 201, 202, 203)

KLEEMAN CR MASSRY SG COBURN JW (1971) The clinical physiology of calcium homeostasis, parathyroid hormone and calcitonin *California Medicine* **114** No 3 16–43 (3)

KLEIN L TEREE TM (1966) Skeletal metabolism in early infancy: urinary hydroxyproline *Journal of Pediatrics* **68** 266–273 (55)

KLENERMAN L (1966) Cauda equina and spinal cord compression in Paget's disease *Journal of Bone and Joint Surgery* **48B** 365–370 (247)

KNUCKEY T O'HALLORAN MT YU JS (1971) Hypocalcaemia in infancy: a retrospective study *Australian Paediatric Journal* **7** 187–192 (149)

KNUDSEN A BENFORD F (1938) Quantitative studies of the effectiveness of ultra-violet radiation of various wavelengths in rickets *Journal of Biological Chemistry* **124** 287–299 (23)

KODICEK E (1972) The intermediary metabolism of vitamin D: 1,25-dihydroxy-cholecalciferol, a kidney hormone affecting calcium metabolism In *Endocrinology 1971* ed Taylor S 444–451 London: Heinemann (24)

KOSOY J MADDOX HE (1971) Surgical findings in van der Hoeve's syndrome *Archives of Otolaryngology* **93** 115–122 (258)

KRAMER F (1936) Die relative Nebenschilddrüseninsuffizienz und ihre Behandlung *Fortschritte der Therapie* **12** 521–526 (151)

KRAMER WM (1970) Association of parathyroid hyperplasia with neoplasia *American Journal of Clinical Pathology* **53** 275–283 (81, 104)

KRANE SM (1970) Serum phosphorus in uremia *New England Journal of Medicine* **283** 264 (194)

KRANE SM MUÑOZ AJ HARRIS ED (1970) Urinary polypeptides related to collagen synthesis *Journal of Clinical Investigation* **49** 716–729 (54)

KRAWITT EL BLOOMER HA (1965) Increased cerebrospinal-fluid protein secondary to hypercalcemia of the milk-alkali syndrome *New England Journal of Medicine* **273** 154 (69)

KRETSCHMER R SAY B BROWN D ROSEN FS (1968) Congenital aplasia of the thymus gland (Di George's Syndrome) *New England Journal of Medicine* **279** 1295–1301 (160)

KŘIŽEK V (1971) Urolithiasis and prostatolithiasis in alcaptonuria with ochronosis *International Urology and Nephrology* **3** 245–250 (137)

KROLL W LICHTE K-H LUTZ P MAURER R (1973) Cystinosis: quantitative assay of cystine accumulation of homozygotes and heterozygotes *Humangenetik* **17** 337–340 (209)

KRULL GH MULLER H LEIJNSE B GERBRANDY J (1969) Venous-compression test in hyperparathyroidism *Lancet* **2** 174–177 (101)

KUMAR R STEEN P MCGEOWN MG (1972) Chronic renal failure or simple starvation? *Lancet* **2** 1005 (144)

KUZEMKO JA (1970) Osteogenesis imperfecta tarda treated with sodium fluoride *Archives of Disease in Childhood* **45** 581–582 (260)

LA DU B GJESSING LR (1972) Tyrosinosis and tyrosinaemia. In *The metabolic Basis of Inherited Disease* ed Stanbury J B Wyngaarden J B Fredrickson D S New York: McGraw-Hill (209)

LACHMAN E (1955) Osteoporosis: the potentialities and limitations of its roentgenologic diagnosis *American Journal of Roentgenology* **74** 712–715 (221)

LAFFERTY FW (1966) Pseudohyperparathyroidism *Medicine* **45** 247–260 (115)

LANCET (1971) Cadmium pollution and Itai-itai disease *Lancet* **1** 382–383 (176)

LANDING BH KAMOSHITA S (1970) Congenital hyperparathyroidism secondary to maternal hypoparathyroidism *Journal of Pediatrics* **5** 842–847 (109, 160)

LANGMAN MJS LEUTHOLD E ROBSON EB HARRIS J LUFFMAN JE HARRIS H (1966) Influence of diet on the 'intestinal' component of serum alkaline phosphatase in people of different ABO blood groups and secretor status *Nature* **212** 41–43 (42)

LANGNESS U BEHNKE H (1970) Biochemische Untersuchungen zur Osteogenesis imperfecta *Deutsche Medizinische Wochenschrift* **95** 213–221 (259)

LANGNESS U BEHNKE H (1971) Collagen metabolites in plasma and urine in osteogenesis imperfecta *Metabolism* **20** 456–463 (259)

LAPATSANIS P KAVADIAS A VRETOS K (1971) Juvenile osteoporosis *Archives of Disease in Childhood* **46** 66–71 (238)

LAURENCE DJR NEVILLE AM (1972) Foetal antigens and their role in the diagnosis and clinical management of human neoplasms *British Journal of Cancer* **26** 335–355 (44)

LAVAN JN NEALE FC POSEN S (1971) Urinary calculi: clinical, biochemical and radiological studies in 619 patients *Medical Journal of Australia* **2** 1049–1061 (129, 133, 134)

LAVENGOOD RW MARSHALL VF (1972) The prevention of renal phosphatic calculi in the presence of infection by the Shorr regimen *Journal of Urology* **108** 368–371 (139)

LAVERTY CR MUNRO VF ATKINSON KH (1971) Osteogenesis imperfecta congenita *Medical Journal of Australia* **1** 748–749 (256)

LAWRENCE JS (1970) Paget's disease in population samples *Annals of the Rheumatic Diseases* **29** 562 (241)

LAWRENCE GD LOEFFLER RG MARTIN LG CONNOR TB (1973) Immobilization hypercalcemia *Journal of Bone and Joint Surgery* **55** A 87–94 (75, 127)

LAZOR MZ ROSENBERG LE (1964) Mechanism of adrenal steroid reversal of hypercalcemia in multiple myeloma *New England Journal of Medicine* **270** 749–755 (75)

LeDouarin N Le Lievre C (1972) Demonstration of the neural origin of the ultimobranchial body glandular cells in the avian embryo. In *Endocrinology 1971* ed Taylor S pp 153–163 London: Heinemann (18)

Lee CA Lloyd HM (1971) Bone collagen and calcium metabolism in normocalcemic and hypercalcemic patients with breast cancer *Cancer* 27 1099–1105 (114)

Lee CM McElhinney WT Gall EA (1955) Unusual manifestations of parathyroid adenoma *Archives of Surgery* 71 475–485 (87)

Leedham PW Pollock DJ (1970) Intrafollicular amyloid in primary hyperparathyroidism *Journal of Clinical Pathology* 23 811–817 (82)

Leeson PM Fourman P (1966a) Increased sensitivity to vitamin D after vitamin-D poisoning *Lancet* 1 1182–1185 (117, 118, 119, 159)

Leeson PM Fourman P (1966b) Acute pancreatitis from vitamin-D poisoning in a patient with parathyroid deficiency *Lancet* 1 1185–1186 (Another case is reported in a letter by Dr WML Turner on page 1423) (69)

Lemann J Donatelli AA (1964) Calcium intoxication due to primary hyperparathyroidism *Annals of Internal Medicine* 60 447–461 (108)

Lennon EJ (1969) Metabolic acidosis: A factor in the pathogenesis of azotemic osteodystrophy? *Archives of Internal Medicine* 124 557–562 (196)

Lesh JB Aldred JP Bastian JW Kleszynski RR (1974) Clinical experience with porcine and salmon calcitonins. In *Endocrinology 1973* ed Taylor S London: Heinemann (251)

Lever JV Paterson CR Morgan DB (1967) Calcium infusion test in osteomalacia: an appraisal *British Medical Journal* 3 281–282 (187)

Levison V (1970) The treatment of Paget's disease of bone by radiotherapy *Annals of Physical Medicine* 10 230–235 (250)

Levitt M Gessert C Finberg L (1973) Inorganic phosphate (laxative) poisoning resulting in tetany in an infant *Journal of Pediatrics* 82 479–481 (146)

Lewin PK Reid M Reilly BJ Swyer PR Fraser D (1971) Iatrogenic rickets in low-birth-weight infants *Journal of Pediatrics* 78 207–210 (167)

Lewy JE Cabana EC Repetto HA Canterbury JM Reiss E (1972) Serum parathyroid hormone in hypophosphatemic vitamin D-resistant rickets *Journal oj Pediatrics* 81 294–300 (211)

Liberman UA DeVries A (1971) Idiopathic hypercalciuria: a state of compensated hyperparathyroidism? *Revue Européenne d'Etudes Cliniques et Biologiques* 16 860–865 (134)

Lichtenstein L (1970) *Diseases of bones and joints* St Louis: C V Mosby (270)

Lightwood R (1952) Idiopathic hypercalcaemia in infants with failure to thrive *Archives of Disease in Childhood* 27 302–303. Also *Proceedings of the Royal Society of Medicine* 45 401 (121)

Lim P Jacob E Khoo OT (1969) Handling of induced hypercalcaemia in hyperthyroidism *British Medical Journal* 4 715–717 (279)

Lin S-R Levy W Go EB Lee I Wong WK (1973) Unusual osteosclerotic changes in sarcoidosis simulating osteoblastic metastases *Radiology* 106 311–312 (120)

LINDE J HANSEN JM SIERSBAEK-NIELSEN K FUGLSANG-FREDRIKSEN V (1971) Bone density in patients receiving long-term anticonvulsant therapy *Acta Neurologica Scandinavica* **47** 650–651 (174)

LINDGÄRDE F (1972) Potentiometric determination of serum ionized calcium in a normal human population *Clinica Chimica Acta* **40** 477–484 (37)

LINDGÄRDE F ZETTERVALL O (1973) Hypercalcemia and normal ionized serum calcium in a case of myelomatosis *Annals of Internal Medicine* **78** 396–399 (115)

LIPSON A (1970) Nutritional rickets in Sydney *Medical Journal of Australia* **1** 1221–1223 (168)

LIPSON RL WILLIAMS LE (1968) The 'connective tissue disorder' of hyperparathyroidism *Arthritis and Rheumatism* **11** 198–205 (89)

LITTLEDIKE ET ARNAUD CD (1971) The influence of plasma magnesium concentrations on calcitonin secretion in the pig *Proceedings of the Society for Experimental Biology and Medicine* **136** 1000–1006 (20)

LIVESLEY B (1971) Non-cardiac morphological stigmata of congenital heart disease *Postgraduate Medical Journal* **47** 800–803 (32)

LJUNGBERG O (1972) Argentaffin cells in human thyroid and parathyroid and their relationship to C-cells and medullary carcinoma *Acta Pathologica et Microbiologica Scandinavica* Section A **80** 589–599 (217)

LJUNGBERG O DYMLING J-F (1972) Pathogenesis of C-cell neoplasia in thyroid gland *Acta Pathologica et Microbiologica Scandinavica* Section A **80** 577–588 (218)

LLOYD HM (1968) Primary hyperparathyroidism: An analysis of the role of the parathyroid tumor *Medicine* **47** 53–71 (83)

LLOYD HM AITKEN RE FERRIER TM (1965) Primary hyperparathyroidism resembling rickets of late onset *British Medical Journal* **2** 853–856 (110)

LOMNITZ E SEPULVEDA L STEVENSON C BARZELATTO J (1966) Primary hyperparathyroidism simulating rickets *Journal of Clinical Endocrinology and Metabolism* **26** 309–313 (110)

LOOMIS WF (1970) Rickets *Scientific American* **223** 76–91 (23, 165, 166)

LOOSER E (1920) Über Spätrachitis und Osteomalacia: Klinische, rontgenologische und pathologischanatomische Untersuchungen *Deutsche Zeitschrift für Chirurgie* **152** 210–357 (180)

LORDON RE MCPHAUL JJ MCINTOSH DA (1966) Hypoparathyroidism with hypophosphatemia: a clinical paradox due to acquired renal hyperphosphaturia *Annals of Internal Medicine* **64** 1066–1070 (118, 210)

LOSOWSKY MS WALKER BE KELLEHER J (1974) *Malabsorption in Clinical Practice* Edinburgh: Churchill Livingstone (169)

LOTZ M ZISMAN E BARTTER FC (1968) Evidence for a phosphorus depletion syndrome in man *New England Journal of Medicine* **278** 409–415 (210)

LOWE CU TERREY M MACLACHLAN EA (1952) Organic-aciduria, decreased renal ammonia production, hydrophthalmos and mental retardation *American Journal of Diseases of Children* **83** 164–184 (216)

LOWE KG HENDERSON JL PARK WW MCGREAL DA (1954) The idiopathic hypercalcaemic syndromes of infancy *Lancet* **2** 101–110 (123)

LUCAS RB (1955) The jaws and teeth in Paget's disease of bone *Journal of Clinical Pathology* **8** 195–200 (247)

LUDBROOK J WYNN V (1958) Citrate intoxication *British Medical Journal* **2** 523–528 (147)

LUDWIG GD (1962) Hyperparathyroidism in relation to pregnancy *New England Journal of Medicine* **267** 637–642 (108)

LUKERT BP BOLINGER RE MEEK JC (1972) The effect of fluoride on ^{45}Ca kinetics in Paget's disease *Journal of Clinical Endocrinology and Metabolism* **35** 387–391 (250)

LUM G GAMBINO SR (1972) Serum gamma-glutamyl transpeptidase activity as an indicator of disease of liver, pancreas or bone *Clinical Chemistry* **18** 358–362 (46)

LUMB GA MAWER EB STANBURY SW (1971) The apparent vitamin D resistance of chronic renal failure. A study of the physiology of vitamin D in man *American Journal of Medicine* **50** 421–441 (24)

LYNCH SR SEFTEL HC WAPNICK AA CHARLTON RW BOTHWELL TH (1970) Some aspects of calcium metabolism in normal and osteoporotic Bantu subjects with special reference to the effects of iron overload and ascorbic acid depletion *South African Journal of Medical Sciences* **35** 45–56 (236)

MACCUISH AC MUNRO JF LAMB WL (1970) Reversible renal tubular defects in gluten enteropathy with osteomalacia *British Medical Journal* **2** 343–344 (186)

MACDONALD AM (1958) Hypercalcaemia in infants and young animals *Proceedings of the Nutrition Society* **17** 74–77 (123)

MACGILLIVRAY JB ANDERSON CJB (1971) Medullary carcinoma of the thyroid with parathyroid adenoma and hypercalcaemia *Journal of Clinical Pathology* **24** 851–855 (95, 218)

MACMANUS J HEATON FW LUCAS PW (1971) A decreased response to parathyroid hormone in magnesium deficiency *Journal of Endocrinology* **49** 253–258 (145)

MACPHERSON RI KROEKER M HOUSTON CS (1972) Hypophosphatasia *Journal of the Canadian Association of Radiologists* **23** 16–26 (180, 266, 267, 269)

MADHAVAN T FRAME B BLOCK MA (1970) Influence of surgical correction of primary hyperparathyroidism on associated hypertension *Archives of Surgery* **100** 212–214 (92)

MALLICK NP BERLYNE GM (1968) Arterial calcification after vitamin-D therapy in hyperphosphataemic renal failure *Lancet* **2** 1316–1320 (204)

MALONE DNS HORN DB (1971) Acute hypercalcaemia and renal failure after antacid therapy *British Medical Journal* **1** 709–710 (126)

MANCHANDA SS LAL H (1972) The challenge of rickets in Punjab *Indian Journal of Pediatrics* **39** 52–57 (168)

MANIOS SG ANTENER I (1966) A study of vitamin D metabolism in idiopathic hypercalcemia of infancy *Acta Paediatrica Scandinavica* **55** 600–608 (126)

MARCUS R WILBER JF AURBACH GD (1971) Parathyroid hormone-sensitive adenyl cyclase from the renal cortex of a patient with pseudohypoparathyroidism *Journal of Clinical Endocrinology and Metabolism* **33** 537–541 (161)

MARKOVITZ M (1971) Medullary carcinoma of the thyroid with hypercalcitoninemia and hypocalcemia *Arizona Medicine* **28** 26–27 (219)

MAROTEAUX P et al (1971) Nomenclature for constitutional (intrinsic) diseases of bones *Pediatrics* **47** 431–434 (253)

MARSDEN P ANDERSON J DOYLE D MORRIS BA BURNS DA (1971) Familial hyperparathyroidism *British Medical Journal* **3** 87–90 (80)

MARSHALL RW NORDIN BEC (1971) The state of inorganic phosphorus in plasma and its relation to other ions. In *Phosphate et métabolisme phosphocalcique* ed Hioco DJ 128–138 Paris: Sandoz (29)

MARSHALL RW COCHRAN M ROBERTSON WG HODGKINSON A NORDIN BEC (1972) The relation between the concentration of calcium salts in the urine and renal stone composition in patients with calcium-containing renal stones *Clinical Science* **43** 433–441 (133)

MARTIN TJ GREENBERG PB MICHELANGELI V (1973) Synthesis of human parathyroid hormone by cultured cells: evidence for release of prohormone by some adenomata *Clinical Science* **44** 1–8 (116)

MASSRY SG COBURN JW POPOVTZER MM SHINABERGER JH MAXWELL MH KLEEMAN CR (1969) Secondary hyperparathyroidism in chronic renal failure *Archives of Internal Medicine* **124** 431–441 (201)

MASSRY SG COBURN JW KLEEMAN CR (1970) Evidence for suppression of parathyroid gland activity by hypermagnesemia *Journal of Clinical Investigation* **49** 1619–1629 (15)

MASSRY SG COBURN JW LEE DBN JOWSEY J KLEEMAN CR (1973) Skeletal resistance to parathyroid hormone in renal failure *Annals of Internal Medicine* **78** 357–364 (196)

MATES J (1969) External factors in the genesis of urolithiasis. In *Renal stone research symposium* ed Hodgkinson A Nordin BEC 59–64 London: Churchill (136)

MATRAJT-DENYS H TUN-CHOT S BORDIER P HIOCO D CLARK MB PENNOCK J DOYLE FH FOSTER GV (1971) Effect of calcitonin on vitamin A-induced changes in bone in the rat *Endocrinology* **88** 129–137 (128)

MATTSSON S (1972) The reversibility of disuse osteoporosis—experimental studies in the adult rat *Acta Orthopaedica Scandinavica* Suppl **144** 1–135 (233, 235)

MAUTALEN CA (1970) Total urinary hydroxyproline excretion after administration of vitamin D to patients with hypoparathyroidism *Journal of Clinical Endocrinology and Metabolism* **31** 595–599 (158)

MAWER EB BACKHOUSE J TAYLOR CM LUMB GA STANBURY SW (1973) Failure of formation of 1,25-dihydroxycholecalciferol in chronic renal insufficiency *Lancet* **1** 626–628 (193)

MAYNE V MCCREDIE D (1972) Rickets in Melbourne *Medical Journal of Australia* **2** 873–875 (See also the subsequent letter on p. 1468) (168)

McCance RA Widdowson EM (1960) *The composition of foods* Medical Research Council, Special Report Series No 297 London: HM Stationery Office (61)

McCollum EV (1967) The paths to the discovery of vitamins A and D *Journal of Nutrition* **91** 11–16 (22)

McConnell TH (1971) Fatal hypocalcemia from phosphate absorption from laxative preparation *Journal of the American Medical Association* **216** 147–148 (146)

McDonald KM (1972) Responsiveness of bone to parathyroid extract in siblings with pseudohypoparathyroidism *Metabolism* **21** 521–531 (161)

McEnery PT Silverman FN West CD (1972) Acceleration of growth with combined vitamin D-phosphate therapy of hypophosphataemic resistant rickets *Journal of Pediatrics* **80** 763–774 (214)

McGarity WC Miles AE Hoffman JC (1971) Angiographic diagnosis and localization of endocrine tumors *Annals of Surgery* **173** 583–592 (103)

McGeown MG Bull GM (1957) The pathogenesis of urinary calculus formation *British Medical Bulletin* **13** 53–57 (137)

McKenna RJ Schwinn CP Soong KY Higginbotham NL (1964) Osteogenic sarcoma arising in Paget's disease *Cancer* **17** 42–66 (245)

McKie BD (1969) Hypocalcaemia and prolonged curarization *British Journal of Anaesthesia* **41** 1091–1094 (143)

McKusick VA (1972) *Heritable disorders of connective tissue* 4th edition St Louis: CV Mosby (253, 254, 256, 258, 259, 260, 264, 270)

McMillan DE Freeman RB (1965) The milk alkali syndrome: a study of the acute disorder with comments on the development of the chronic condition *Medicine* **44** 485–501 (126)

McMurrich JP (1930) *Leonardo da Vinci the anatomist* Baltimore: Williams Wilkins (32)

McNutt DR Fudenberg HH (1972) Bone-marrow biopsy and osteoporosis *New England Journal of Medicine* **286** 46 (59)

Mears DC (1972) Effects of parathyroid hormone and thyrocalcitonin on the membrane potential of osteoclasts *Endocrinology* **88** 1021–1028 (21)

Meema HE Meema S (1963) Measurable roentgenologic changes in some peripheral bones in senile osteoporosis *Journal of the American Geriatrics Society* **11** 1170–1182 (227)

Meema HE Meema S (1968) Prevention of postmenopausal osteoporosis by hormone treatment of the menopause *Canadian Medical Association Journal* **99** 248–251 (233)

Meema HE Meema S (1972) Comparison of microradioscopic and morphometric findings in the hand bones with densitometric findings in the proximal radius in thyrotoxicosis and in renal osteodystrophy *Investigative Radiology* **7** 88–96 (198, 279)

Meema HE Bunker ML Meema S (1965) Loss of compact bone due to menopause *Obstetrics and Gynecology* **26** 333–343 (236)

MÉHES K KLUJBER L LASSU G KAJTÁR P (1972) Hypophosphatasia: screening and family investigations in an endogamous Hungarian village *Clinical Genetics* **3** 60–66 (266, 269)

MEHLS O MÜLLER B SCHÄRER K (1971) Pseudomangelrachitis *Montasschrift für Kinderheilkunde* **119** 429–430 (176)

MELICK RA BAIRD CW (1970) The effect of 'Parenabol' on patients with osteoporosis *Medical Journal of Australia* **2** 960–962 (234)

MELICK RA MARTIN TJ (1971) Assay of parathyroid hormone in disturbances of calcium metabolism *Australian and New Zealand Journal of Medicine* **2** 146–153 (47)

MELICK RA MARTIN TJ HICKS JD (1972) Parathyroid hormone production and malignancy *British Medical Journal* **2** 204–205 (116)

MELNICK I LANDES RR HOFFMAN AA BURCH JF (1971) Magnesium therapy for recurring calcium oxalate urinary calculi *Journal of Urology* **105** 119–122 (139)

MELTZER LE PALMON FP PAIK YK CUSTER RP (1962) Acute pancreatitis secondary to hypercalcemia of multiple myeloma *Annals of Internal Medicine* **57** 1008–1012 (69)

MELVIN KE CASTLEMAN B (1971) Persistent hypercalcaemia after removal of a parathyroid tumor *New England Journal of Medicine* **285** 1422–1429 (105, 112)

MELVIN KE MILLER HH TASHJIAN AH (1971) Early diagnosis of medullary carcinoma of the thyroid gland by means of calcitonin assay *New England Journal of Medicine* **285** 1115–1120 (218, 219)

MERSHON JC DIETRICH JG (1966) Hereditary Addison's disease and multiple endocrine adenomatosis in a kindred *Annals of Internal Medicine* **65** 252–258 (94)

MESSNER RP SMITH HT SHAPIRO FL GREGORY DH (1969) The effect of hemodialysis, vitamin D and renal homotransplantation on the calcium malabsorption of chronic renal failure *Journal of Laboratory and Clinical Medicine* **74** 472–481 (196, 197)

MEUNIER P VIGNON G BENARD J EDOUARD C COURPRON P PORTE J (1972) La lecture quantitative de la biopsie osseuse, moyen de diagnostic et d'étude de 106 hyperparathyroïdies primitives, secondaires et paranéoplastiques *Revue du Rhumatisme* **39** 635–644 (87, 116)

MICHIE W STOWERS JM DUNCAN T PEGG CAS HAMER-HODGES DW HEMS G BEWSHER PD HEDLEY AJ (1971) Mechanism of hypocalcaemia after thyroidectomy for thyrotoxicosis *Lancet* **1** 508–514 (151, 280)

MILHAUD G TUBIANA M PARMENTIER C COUTRIS G (1968) Epithélioma de la thyroïde sécrétant de la thyrocalcitonine *Comptes Rendus des Séances de l'Academie des Sciences, Paris, Series D* **266** 608–610 (217)

MILHAUD G CALMETTES C JULIENNE A THARAUD D BLOCH-MICHEL H CARVAILLON JP COLIN R MOUKHTAR MS (1972) A new chapter in human pathology: calcitonin disorders and therapeutic use. In *Calcium parathyroid hormone and the calcitonins* Ed. Talmage RV Munson PL 56–70 Amsterdam: Excerpta Medica (219)

MITCHELL RG (1967) Modern views on rickets and hypercalcaemia in infancy *World Review of Nutrition and Dietetics* **8** 207–243 (121)

MITCHELL ABS GLASS D GILL AM (1971) Osteomalacia following vagotomy and pyloroplasty *Postgraduate Medical Journal* **47** 233–237 (172)

MITTAL MM GUPTA NC SHARMA ML (1971) Osteomalacia in neurofibromatosis *Journal of the Association of Physicians of India* **19** 823–825 (210)

MIZRAHI A LONDON RD GRIBETZ D (1968) Neonatal hypocalcemia—its causes and treatment *New England Journal of Medicine* **278** 1163–1165 (147)

MOE PJ SKJAEVELAND A (1969) Therapeutic studies in osteopetrosis *Acta Paediatrica Scandinavica* **58** 593–600 (265)

MONCRIEFF MW CHANCE GW (1969) Nephrotoxic effect of vitamin D therapy in vitamin D refractory rickets *Archives of Diseases in Childhood* **44** 571–579 (214)

MONIF GRG SAVORY J (1972) Iatrogenic maternal hypocalcemia following magnesium sulfate therapy *Journal of the American Medical Association* **219** 1469–1470 (146)

MONRO P (1970) Effect of treatment on renal function in severe osteomalacia due to Wilson's disease *Journal of Clinical Pathology* **23** 487–491 (209)

MORGAN DB (1973) Ageing and osteoporosis, in particular spinal osteoporosis *Clinics in Endocrinology and Metabolism* **2** 187–201 (232)

MORGAN DB NEWTON-JOHN HF (1969) Bone loss and senescence *Gerontologia* **15** 140–154 (229)

MORGAN DB PATERSON CR WOODS CG PULVERTAFT CN FOURMAN P (1965a) Search for osteomalacia in 1228 patients after gastrectomy and other operations on the stomach *Lancet* **2** 1085–1088 (172)

MORGAN DB PATERSON CR WOODS CG PULVERTAFT CN FOURMAN P (1965b) osteomalacia after gastrectomy: A response to very small doses of vitamin D *Lancet* **2** 1089-1091 (24, 27, 172, 186, 190)

MORGAN DB PULVERTAFT CN FOURMAN P (1966) Effects of age on the loss of bone after gastric surgery *Lancet* **2** 772–773 (237)

MORGAN DB SPIERS FW PULVERTAFT CN FOURMAN P (1967) The amount of bone in the metacarpal and the phalanx according to age and sex *Clinical Radiology* **18** 101–108 (223, 224, 225, 228)

MORGAN HG DRYBURGH FJ WILSON R PROTHERO K WHITE J MANN TS (1968) The hypercalcaemia of adolescents *Calcified Tissue Research* **2** Suppl 89–89B (127)

MORGAN DB HUNT G PATERSON CR (1970) The osteomalacia syndrome after stomach operations *Quarterly Journal of Medicine* NS **39** 395-410 (30, 173, 177, 180, 183, 185)

MORII H TANAE A IBAYASHI H NAKAO K (1971) Effects of calcitonin in metastatic bone carcinoma, osteoporosis, polyostotic fibrous dysplasia and hypercalcemia *Endocrinologia Japonica* **18** 81–90 (272)

MOSES AM SPENCER H (1969) Hypercalcemia in patients with malignant lymphoma *Annals of Internal Medicine* **59** 531–536 (115)

MOULIAS R GOUST JM MULLER-BERAT CN (1971) Hypoparathyroidism and cell-mediated immunity *Lancet* **1** 1239 (152)

MUENTER MD WHISNANT JP (1968) Basal ganglia calcification, hypoparathyroidism, and extrapyramidal motor manifestations *Neurology* **18** 1075–1083 (153)

MUGGIA FM HEINEMANN HO (1970a) Hypercalcemia associated with neoplastic disease *Annals of Internal Medicine* **73** 281–290 (70, 113)

MUGGIA FM HEINEMANN HO (1970b) Hypercalcaemia in cancer *Annals of Internal Medicine* **73** 1048–1049 (77)

MÜHLBAUER RC RUSSELL RGG WILLIAMS DA FLEISCH H (1971) The effects of diphosphonates, polyphosphates and calcitonin on 'immobilisation osteoporosis' in rats *European Journal of Clinical Investigation* **1** 336–344 (233)

MÜHLETHALER JP SCHÄRER K ANTENER I (1967) Akuter Hyperparathyreoidismus bei primärer Nebenschilddrüsenhyperplasie *Helvetica Paediatrica Acta* **22** 529–557 (109)

MUIRHEAD W (1967) Hormonal treatment of hypercalcemia caused by bone metastases *Canadian Medical Association Journal* **97** 569–572 (75, 77)

MULDOWNEY FP CARROLL DV DONOHOE JF FREANEY R (1971) Correction of renal bicarbonate wastage by parathyroidectomy *Quarterly Journal of Medicine* NS **40** 487–498 (67, 91)

MULDOWNEY FP DONOHOE JF CARROLL DV POWELL D FREANEY R (1972) Parathyroid acidosis in uraemia *Quarterly Journal of Medicine* NS **41** 321–342 (196)

MULLER H (1969) Sex, age and hyperparathyroidism *Lancet* **1** 449–450 (79)

MULLIGAN RM (1947) Metastatic calcification *Archives of Pathology* **43** 177–230 (70)

MUNSON PL GRAY TK (1970) Function of thyrocalcitonin in normal physiology *Federation Proceedings* **29** 1206–1208 (20)

MURATA I HIRONO T SAEKI Y NAKAGAWA S (1970) Cadmium enteropathy, renal osteomalacia ('Itai itai' disease in Japan) *Bulletin de la Société Internationale de Chirurgie* **29** 34–42 (176)

MURIE N FERRAND B ETIENNE P (1973) Le cancer des parathyroïdes: revue générale de 109 observations *Nouvelle Presse Médicale* **2** 1293–1296 (111)

MURPHY KJ (1967) Bilateral renal calculi and aminoaciduria after excessive intake of Worcestershire sauce *Lancet* **2** 401–403 (137)

MURPHY HM (1972) Calcitonin-like activity in the circulation of osteopetrotic grey-lethal mice *Journal of Endocrinology* **53** 139–150 (220)

MURRAY RO JACOBSON HG (1971) *The Radiology of Skeletal Disorders* Edinburgh: Churchill Livingstone (243, 264, 275, 278)

MURRAY TM PEACOCK M POWELL D MONCHIK JM POTTS JT (1972) Non-autonomy of hormone secretion in primary hyperparathyroidism *Clinical Endocrinology* **1** 235–246 (98)

NADARAJAH A HARTOG M REDFERN B THALASSINOS N WRIGHT AD JOPLIN GF FRASER TR (1968) Calcium metabolism in acromegaly *British Medical Journal* **4** 797–801 (275)

NAGANT DE DEUXCHAINES C KRANE SM (1964) Paget's disease of bone: clinical and metabolic observations *Medicine* **43** 233–266 (241, 248)

NAGANT DE DEUXCHAISNES C KRANE SM (1967) The treatment of adult phosphate diabetes and Fanconi Syndrome with neutral sodium phosphate *American Journal of Medicine* **43** 508–543 (11, 214)

NAIKEN VS (1971) Did Beethoven have Paget's disease of bone *Annals of Internal Medicine* **74** 995–999 (also *Clinical Orthopaedics* **89** (1972) 103–105) (246)

NASSIM JR SAVILLE PD COOK PB MULLIGAN L (1959) The effects of vitamin D and gluten-free diet in idiopathic steatorrhoea *Quarterly Journal of Medicine* NS **28** 141–162 (170)

NATIONAL FOOD SURVEY COMMITTEE (1964) *Domestic food consumption and expenditure 1962* London: HM Stationery Office (23)

NEELON FA DREZNER M BIRCH BM LEBOVITZ HE (1973) Urinary cyclic adenosine monophosphate as an aid in the diagnosis of hyperparathyroidism *Lancet* **1** 631–634 (68)

NELP WB DENNEY JD MURANO R HINS GM WILLIAMS JL RUDD TG PALMER HE (1972) Absolute measurement of total body calcium (bone mass) *in vivo Journal of Laboratory and Clinical Medicine* **79** 430–438 (57)

NEMOY NJ STAMEY TA (1971) Surgical, bacteriological and biochemical management of 'infection stones' *Journal of the American Medical Association* **215** 1470–1476 (139)

NEUMAN WF (1969) The *milieu interieur* of bone: Claude Bernard revisited *Federation Proceedings* **28** 1846–1850 (2)

NEVILLE PF DE LUCA HF (1966) The synthesis of $(1,2\text{-}^3\text{H})$ vitamin D_3 and the tissue localization of a $0.25\text{-}\mu\text{g}$ (10 IU) dose per rat *Biochemistry* **5** 2201–2207 (26)

NEWTON-JOHN HF MORGAN DB (1968) Osteoporosis: disease or senescence? *Lancet* **1** 232–233 (230)

NEWTON-JOHN HF MORGAN DB (1970) The loss of bone with age osteoporosis and fractures *Clinical Orthopaedics* **71** 229–252 (31, 221, 225, 227, 228, 229)

NIALL HD KEUTMAN HT TREGEAR GW O'RIORDAN JLH AURBACH GD POTTS JT (1973) Personal communication (14)

NICHOLS BL MONTANDON C POTTS E (1970) Nutritional rickets among indigent children in Houston *Texas Medicine* **66** 74–77 (168)

NICOLAYSEN R EEG-LARSEN N MALM OJ (1953) Physiology of calcium metabolism *Physiological Reviews* **33** 424–444 (10)

NIELSEN OV ALEXANDERSEN V (1971) Malignant osteopetrosis in ancient Nubia *Danish Medical Bulletin* **18** 125–128 (261)

NIELSEN SP JØRGENSEN FS (1972) Mechanism of the hypocalcaemic action of parenterally administered magnesium *Acta Endocrinologica* **70** 476–486 (146)

NIKLASSON E (1970) Familial early hypoparathyroidism associated with hypomagnesaemia *Acta Paediatrica Scandinavica* **59** 715–719 (156)

NILSSON BE (1970) Spinal osteoporosis and femoral neck fracture *Clinical Orthopaedics* **68** 93–95 (227)

NISBET DI BUTLER EJ ROBERTSON JM BANNATYNE CC (1970) Osteodystrophic diseases of sheep. IV. Osteomalacia and osteoporosis in lactating ewes on West Scotland hill farms *Journal of Comparative Pathology* **80** 535–542 (32)

NOLPH KD STOLZ M MAHER JF (1971) Calcium-free peritoneal dialysis. Treatment of vitamin D intoxication *Archives of Internal Medicine* **128** 809–814 (78)

NONIDEZ JF (1932) The origin of the 'parafollicular' cell, a second epithelial component of the thyroid gland of the dog *American Journal of Anatomy* **49** 479–505 (18)

NORDIN BEC (1973) *Metabolic bone and stone disease* Edinburgh: Churchill Livingstone (226)

NORDIN BEC BULUSU L (1968) A modified index of phosphate excretion *Postgraduate Medical Journal* **44** 93–97 (66)

NORDIN BEC FRASER R (1956) A calcium-infusion test *Lancet* **1** 823–826 (172, 187)

NORDIN BEC PEACOCK M (1969) Role of kidney in regulation of plasma-calcium *Lancet* **2** 1280–1283 (16)

NORDIN BEC SMITH DA (1964) The relation between calcium balance and hydroxyproline excretion in osteoporosis *Proceedings of the Royal Society of Medicine* **57** 868–870 (191)

NORDIN BEC YOUNG MM OXBY C BULUSU L (1968) Calculation of calcium absorption rate from plasma radioactivity *Clinical Science* **35** 177–182 (56)

NORDIO S DONATH A MACAGNO F GATTI R (1971) Chronic hypomagnesemia with magnesium-dependent hypocalcemia *Acta Paediatrica Scandinavica* **60** 441–448, 449–455 (145)

NORMAN AW (1971) Evidence for a new kidney-produced hormone, 1,25-dihydroxycholecalciferol, the proposed biologically active form of vitamin D *American Journal of Clinical Nutrition* **24** 1346–1351 (24)

NORMAN AW (1972) Problems relating to the definition of an international unit for vitamin D and its metabolites *Journal of Nutrition* **102** 1243–1246 (23)

NORRIS EH (1947) The parathyroid adenoma: A study of 322 cases *International Abstracts of Surgery* **84** 1–41 (79)

O'DUFFY JD (1970) Hypophosphatasia associated with calcium pyrophosphate dihydrate deposits in cartilage *Arthritis and Rheumatism* **13** 381–388 (267)

OESER H KROKOWSKI E (1963) Quantitative analysis of inorganic substances in the body. A method using X-rays of different qualities *British Journal of Radiology* **36** 274–279 (223)

OGG CS (1969) Calcium metabolism in chronic renal failure *British Journal of Urology* **41** 97–102 (195)

OHLSSON L (1970) Renal function in hyperparathyroidism *Acta Endocrinologica* **63** 161–174 (92, 105, 106)

OLAH AJ (1973) Quantitative relations between osteoblasts and osteoid in primary hyperparathyroidism, intestinal malabsorption and renal osteodystrophy *Virchows Archiv: Abteilung A: Pathologische Anatomie* **358** 301–308 (86)

OLAMBIWONNU NO EBBIN AJ FRASIER SD (1972) Primary hypoparathyroidism associated with ring chromosome 18 *Journal of Pediatrics* **80** 833–835 (160)

OLDHAM SB FISCHER JA CAPEN CC SIZEMORE GW ARNAUD CD (1971) Dynamics of parathyroid hormone secretion in vitro *American Journal of Medicine* **50** 650–657 (15)

OLDHAM SB FISCHER JA SIZEMORE GW ARNAUD CD (1972) Calcium-dependent enzymatic conversion of glandular to secreted parathyroid hormone. In *Calcium parathyroid hormone and the calcitonins* ed Talmage RV Munson PL 213–218 Amsterdam: Excerpta Medica (14)

OLEFSKY J KEMPSON R JONES H REAVEN G (1972) 'Tertiary' hyperparathyroidism and apparent 'cure' of vitamin-D-resistant rickets after removal of an ossifying mesenchymal tumor of the pharynx *New England Journal of Medicine* **286** 740–745 (210)

OLSON EB DE LUCA HF POTTS JT (1972) Calcitonin inhibition of vitamin D-induced intestinal calcium absorption *Endocrinology* **90** 151–157 (26)

OMDAHL JL DE LUCA HF (1971) Strontium induced rickets: metabolic basis *Science* **174** 949–951 (175)

OMDAHL JL DE LUCA HF (1973) Regulation of vitamin D metabolism and function *Physiological Reviews* **53** 327–372 (25)

OMDAHL JL THORNTON PA (1972) Intestinal calcium absorption and calcium-binding protein: influence of dietary calcium *Proceedings of the Society for Experimental Biology and Medicine* **139** 975–980 (26)

OMDAHL JL GRAY RW BOYLE IT KNUTSON J DE LUCA HF (1972) Regulation of metabolism of 25-hydroxycholecalciferol by kidney tissue *in vitro* by dietary calcium *Nature New Biology* **237** 63–64 (25)

OMENN GS ROTH SI BAKER WH (1969) Hyperparathyroidism associated with malignant tumors of nonparathyroid origin *Cancer* **24** 1004–1012 (115)

O'NEILL RT MIKUTA JJ (1970) Reversible hypercalcemia in sqaumous cell carcinoma of the vagina *Obstestrics and Gynecology* **36** 458–461 (116)

ORIMO H FUJITA T YOSHIKAWA M (1971) Effect of calcitonin on the development of immobilization osteoporosis in rat *Endocrinologia Japonica* **18** 117–121 (233)

ORIMO H FUJITA T YOSHIKAWA M (1972) Increased sensitivity of bone to parathyroid hormone in ovariectomized rats *Endocrinology* **90** 760–763 (16)

O'RIORDAN JLH PAGE J KERR DNS WALLS J MOORHEAD J CROCKETT RE FRANZ H RITZ E (1970) Hyperparathyroidism in chronic renal failure and dialysis osteodystrophy *Quarterly Journal of Medicine* NS **39** 359–376 (195, 196)

O'RIORDAN JLH WATSON L WOODHEAD JS (1972) Secretion of parathyroid hormone in primary hyperparathyroidism *Clinical Endocrinology* **1** 149–155 (47, 63, 84)

ORME RL (1971) Idiopathic hypoparathyroidism in a neonate *Proceedings of the Royal Society of Medicine* **64** 727–728 (160)

ORME MCL'E CONOLLY ME (1971) Hypoparathyroidism after iodine 131 treatment of thyrotoxicosis *Annals of Internal Medicine* **75** 136–137 (See also the subsequent correspondence on pages 647, 648, and 808) (151)

ORRELL DH (1971) Albumin as an aid to the interpretation of serum calcium *Clinica Chimica Acta* **35** 483–489 (38)

OTTENJANN R (1971) Hypercalcaemia and gastric secretion *German Medicine* **1** 62–64 (93)

OZSOYLU S KAYA G (1971) Pseudo-vitamin D deficiency rickets *Turkish Journal of Pediatrics* **13** 1–8 (176)

PAK CYC (1973) Sodium cellulose phosphate: mechanism of action and effect on mineral metabolism *Journal of Clinical Pharmacology* **13** 15–27 (139)

PAK CYC OHATA M (1973) Quantitative assessment of various forms of therapy for nephrolithiasis. In *Proceedings of the International Symposium on Renal Stone Research, Madrid 1972* ed Delatte LC Basle: Karger (139)

PAK CYC WORTSMAN J BENNETT JE DELEA CS BARTTER FC (1968) Control of hypercalcemia with cellulose phosphate *Journal of Clinical Endocrinology and Metabolism* **28** 1829–1832 (78)

PAK CYC DE LUCA HF CHAVEZ DE LOS RIOS JM SUDA T RUSKIN B DELEA CS (1970) Treatment of vitamin D-resistant hypoparathyroidism with 25-hydroxycholecalciferol *Archives of Internal Medicine* **126** 239–247 (159)

PAK CYC EAST D SANZENBACHER L RUSKIN B COX J (1972a) A simple and reliable test for the diagnosis of hyperparathyroidism *Archives of Internal Medicine* **129** 48–55 (100, 134)

PAK CYC EAST DA SANZENBACHER LJ DELEA CS BARTTER FC (1972b) Gastrointestinal calcium absorption in nephrolithiasis *Journal of Clinical Endocrinology and Metabolism* **35** 261–270 (56)

PAK CYC DE LUCA HF BARTTER FC HENNEMAN DH FRAME B SIMOPOULUS A DELEA CS (1972c) Treatment of vitamin D-resistant rickets with 25-hydroxycholecalciferol *Archives of Internal Medicine* **129** 894–899 (211)

PALOYAN E SCANU A STRAUS FH PICKLEMAN JR PALOYAN D (1970) Familial pheochromocytoma, medullary thyroid carcinoma and parathyroid adenomas *Journal of the American Medical Association* **214** 1443–1447 (95, 218)

PALVA I SALOKANNEL SJ (1972) Hypercalcaemia in acute leukaemia *Blut* **24** 209–214 (115)

PAPADIMITRIOU M GINGELL JC CHISHOLM GD (1968) Hypercalcaemia from calcium ion-exchange resin in patients on regular haemodialysis *Lancet* **2** 948–949 (202)

PARFITT AM (1969a) Study of parathyroid function in man by EDTA infusion *Journal of Clinical Endocrinology and Metabolism* **29** 569–580 (151, 156)

PARFITT AM (1969b) Soft-tissue calcification in uremia *Archives of Internal Medicine* **124** 544–556 (200)

PARFITT AM (1971) The incidence of hypoparathyroid tetany after thyroid operations. Relationship to age, extent of resection and surgical experience *Medical Journal of Australia* **1** 1103–1107 (150)

PARFITT AM (1972a) The spectrum of hypoparathyroidism *Journal of Clinical Endocrinology and Metabolism* **34** 152–158 (151, 155, 156, 163)

PARFITT AM (1972b) Thiazide-induced hypercalcemia in vitamin D-treated hypoparathyroidism *Annals of Internal Medicine* **77** 557–563 (127, 159)

PARFITT AM DENT CE (1970) Hyperthyroidism and hypercalcaemia *Quarterly Journal of Medicine* NS **39** 171–187 (280)

PARFITT AM FRAME B (1972) Treatment of rickets and osteomalacia *Seminars in Drug Treatment* **2** 83–115 (187, 287)

PARFITT AM NASSIM JR COLLINS J HILB A (1962) Metabolic studies in a case of fibrocystic disease of the pancreas *Archives of Disease in Childhood* **37** 25–33 (237)

PARFITT AM HIGGINS BA NASSIM JR COLLINS JA HILB A (1964) Metabolic studies in patients with hypercalciuria *Clinical Science* **27** 463–482 (97, 139)

PARFITT AM MASSRY SG WINFIELD AC DE PALMA JR GORDON A (1971) Disordered calcium and phosphorus metabolism during maintenance hemodialysis *American Journal of Medicine* **51** 319–330 (199, 202)

PARFITT AM MASSRY SG WINFIELD AC (1972) Osteopenia and fractures occurring during maintenance hemodialysis *Clinical Orthopaedics* **87** 287–302 (199)

PARK EA (1939) Observations on the pathology of rickets with particular reference to the changes at the cartilage-shaft junctions of the growing bones *Harvey Lectures* **34** 157–213 (179)

PARK EA (1954) The influence of severe illness on rickets *Archives of Disease in Childhood* **29** 369–380 (179)

PARSONS JA ROBINSON CJ (1971) Calcium shift into bone causing transient hypocalcaemia after injection of parathyroid hormone *Nature* **230** 581–582 (16)

PARSONS V PARSONS V PORTER A LUND C (1970) An acceptable slow-release phosphate preparation 'slow P' *Postgraduate Medical Journal* **46** 417–421 (73)

PATERSON CR LOSOWSKY MS (1967) The bones in chronic liver disease *Scandinavian Journal of Gastroenterology* **2** 293–300 (173)

PATERSON CR WOODS CG MORGAN DB (1968) Osteoid in metabolic bone disease *Journal of Pathology and Bacteriology* **95** 449–456 (61)

PATERSON CR DOWNIE WW HEDLEY AJ (1972) Hypercalcaemia: some problems of diagnosis and management *Practitioner* **209** 811–816 (118)

PATTERSON CN STONE HB (1970) Stapedectomy in van der Hoeve's syndrome *Laryngoscope* **80** 544–558 (258)

PAUNIER L BORGEAUD M WYSS M (1972) Acute effect of aldosterone on tubular calcium and magnesium reabsorption *Helvetica Medica Acta* **36** 265–275 (283)

PAYNE WR (1952) The blood chemistry in idiopathic hypercalcaemia *Archives of Disease in Childhood* **27** 302 (121)

PAYNE RL FITCHETT CW (1965) Hyperparathyroid crisis *Annals of Surgery* **161** 737–747 (108)

PEACOCK M ROBERTSON WG NORDIN BEC (1969) Relation between serum and urinary calcium with particular reference to parathyroid activity *Lancet* **1** 384–386 (50, 96, 156)

PEARSE AGE (1968) The thyroid parenchymatous cell of Baber, and the nature and function of their C-cell successors in thyroid, parathyroid and ultimo-branchial bodies. In *Calcitonin* ed Taylor S 98–109 London: Heinemann (18)

PEARSE AGE POLAK JM (1972) The neural crest origin of the endocrine polypeptide cells of the APUD series. In *Endocrinology 1971* ed Taylor S 145–152 London: Heinemann (18)

PEARSON KD WELLS SA KEISER HR (1973) Familial medullary carcinoma of thyroid, adrenal phaeochromocytoma and parathyroid hyperplasia. A syndrome of multiple endocrine neoplasia *Radiology* **107** 249–256 (218)

PEDERSEN KO (1972) Binding of calcium to serum albumin *Scandinavian Journal of Clinical and Laboratory Investigation* **7** 75–83 (37)

PELLEGRINO ED BILTZ RM (1965) The composition of human bone in uremia *Medicine* **44** 397–418 (6)

PENNOCK JM KALU DN CLARK MB FOSTER GV DOYLE FH (1972) Hypoplasia of bone induced by immobilization *British Journal of Radiology* **45** 641–646 (235)

PERLIA CP GUBISCH NJ WOLTER J EDELBERG D DEDERICK MM TAYLOR SG (1970) Mithramycin treatment of hypercalcemia *Cancer* **25** 389–394 (76)

PETERSON PA (1971) Isolation and partial characterization of a human vitamin D-binding plasma protein *Journal of Biological Chemistry* **246** 7748–7754 (24)

PHANG JM KALES AN HAHN TJ (1968) Effect of divided calcium intake on urinary calcium excretion *Lancet* **2** 84–85 (48)

PHILLIPS RM BUSH OB HALL HD (1972) Massive osteolysis (phantom bone, disappearing bone) *Oral Surgery Oral Medicine Oral Pathology* **34** 886–896 (239)

PIERSON JD CRAWFORD JD (1972) Dietary dependent neonatal hypocalcaemia *American Journal of Diseases of Children* **123** 472–474 (148)

PINALS RS JABBS JM (1972) Type-IV hyperlipoproteinaemia and transient osteoporosis *Lancet* **2** 929 (239)

PINGGERA WF POPOVTZER MM (1972) Uremic osteodystrophy: The therapeutic consequences of effective control of serum phosphorus *Journal of the American Medical Association* **222** 1640–1642 (205)

PIRANI BBK MACGILLIVRAY I DUNCAN RO (1972) Serum heat stable alkaline phosphatase in normal pregnancy and its relationship to urinary oestriol and pregnanediol excretion, placental weight and baby weight *Journal of Obstetrics and Gynaecology* **79** 127–132 (44)

PLETKA P BERNSTEIN DS HAMPERS CL MERRILL JP SHERWOOD LM (1971) Effects of magnesium on parathyroid hormone secretion during chronic haemodialysis *Lancet* **2** 462–463 (See also the subsequent correspondence on page 879) (196)

PLIMPTON CH GELLHORN A (1956) Hypercalcemia in malignant disease without evidence of bone destruction *American Journal of Medicine* **21** 750–759 (115)

POLGA JP BALIKIAN JP (1971) Partially calcified functioning parathyroid adenoma *Radiology* **99** 55–56 (103)

POLLOCK RA WATSON RL (1971) Malignant hyperthermia associated with hypocalcemia *Anesthesiology* **34** 188–194 (41, 147)

POPE FM (1971) Blue sclerotics in iron deficiency *Lancet* **2** 1160 (258)

POPOVTZER MM PINGGERA WF HUTT MP ROBINETTE J HALGRIMSON CG STARZL TE (1972) Serum parathyroid hormone levels and renal handling of phosphorus in patients with chronic renal disease *Journal of Clinical Endocrinology and Metabolism* **35** 213–218 (52)

PORTER RW WELLS CH (1964) Urinary concentrating ability changes and associated renal tissue sodium concentration changes induced by calcium excess *Texas Reports on Biology and Medicine* **22** 165–169 (69)

POSEN S (1970) Turnover of circulating enzymes *Clinical Chemistry* **16** 71–84 (46)

POSEN S JEROME E (1971) Some problems concerning urinary calculi *Practitioner* **207** 600–608 (137, 138)

POTCHEN EJ WATTS HG AWWAD HK (1967) Parathyroid scintiscanning *Radiologic Clinics of North America* **5** 267–275 (103)

POTTS JT (1974) Recent advances in the chemistry and physiology of parathyroid hormones. In *Endocrinology 1973* ed Taylor S London: Heinemann (14)

POTTS JT DEFTOS LJ (1969) Parathyroid hormone, thyrocalcitonin, vitamin D, bone and bone mineral metabolism In *Duncan's Diseases of Metabolism*, 6th edition ed Bondy PK Vol 2 Ch 19 pp 904–1082 Philadelphia: Saunders (13)

POTTS JT KEUTMANN HT NIALL HD TREGEAR GW (1971a) The chemistry of parathyroid hormone and the calcitonins *Vitamins and Hormones* **29** 41–93 (18, 19)

POTTS JT MURRAY TM PEACOCK M NIALL HD TREGEAR GW KEUTMANN HT POWELL D DEFTOS LJ (1971b) Parathyroid hormone: sequence, synthesis, immunoassay studies *American Journal of Medicine* **50** 639–649 (14, 47)

POWELL GD PEARSALL PR WIGLEY JEM (1948) Calciferol in the treatment of cutaneous tuberculosis *British Medical Journal* **1** 386–389 (118)

POWELL D SINGER FR MURRAY TM MINKIN C POTTS JT (1973) A new syndrome of hypercalcaemia with cancer. In *Clinical Aspects of metabolic bone disease* ed Frame B Parfitt AM Duncan H 670–673 Amsterdam: Excerpta Medica (116)

PRAKASH O AHUJA MMS (1971) Calcium-45 absorption and excretion in nutritional osteomalacia *Indian Journal of Medical Research* **58** 730–738 (186)

PRATI RC ALFREY AC HULL AR (1972) Spironolactone-induced hypercalciuria *Journal of Laboratory and Clinical Medicine* **80** 224–230 (133)

PREECE MA FORD JA McINTOSH WB DUNNIGAN MG TOMLINSON S O'RIORDAN JLH (1973) Vitamin-D deficiency among Asian immigrants to Britian *Lancet* **1** 907–910 (168, 185)

PRESCOTT RJ HEDLEY AJ PATERSON C (1973) Serum alkaline phosphatase in rickets *British Medical Journal* **2** 47 (43)

PRESTON ET (1972) Avulsion of both quadriceps tendons in hyperparathyroidism *Journal of the American Medical Association* **221** 406–407 (90)

PRESTON FS ADICOFF A (1962) Hyperparathyroidism with avulsion of three major tendons *New England Journal of Medicine* **266** 968–973 (90)

PRETORIUS PJ POTGIETER M DE J (1971) Hypothyroidism and hypercalcaemia: report of a cretin showing manifestations of idiopathic infantile hypercalcaemia *South African Medical Journal* **45** 753–757 (278)

PRIEN EL (1971) The riddle of urinary stone disease *Journal of the American Medical Association* **216** 503–507 (129)

PRIEN EL PRIEN EL (1973) Optical crystallographic analysis of urinary stones. In *Proceedings of the International Symposium on Renal Stone Research, Madrid 1972* ed Delatte LC Basle: Karger (131)

PRINGLE A SMITH EKM (1964) Renal vein thrombosis in acute hyperparathyroidism *British Medical Journal* **2** 675–676 (107, 108)

PRITCHARD JJ (1972a) General histology of bone. In *The Biochemistry and Physiology of Bone* ed Bourne GH (2nd edition) Vol 1 1–20 New York: Academic Press (3)

PRITCHARD JJ (1972b) The osteoblast. In *The Biochemistry and Physiology of Bone* ed Bourne GH (2nd edition) Vol 1 21–43 New York: Academic Press (2)

PURNELL DC (1971) Laboratory aids in the diagnosis of hypoparathyroidism. In *Laboratory diagnosis of endocrine disease* ed Sunderman FW Sunderman FW 310–318 St Louis: WH Green; London: Hilger (156)

PURNELL DC SMITH LH SCHOLZ DA ELVEBACK LR ARNAUD CD (1971) Primary hyperparathyroidism: a prospective clinical study *American Journal of Medicine* **50** 670–678 (47, 102, 105, 106)

PUSCHETT JB MORANZ J KURNICK WS (1972) Evidence for a direct action of cholecalciferol and 25-hydroxycholecalciferol on the renal transport of phosphate, sodium and calcium *Journal of Clinical Investigation* **51** 373–385 (27)

PUTMAN JM (1972) A routine method for determining plasma ionised calcium and its application to the study of congenital heart disease in children *Clinica Chimica Acta* **32** 33–41 (39)

PYBUS J FELDMAN FJ BOWERS GN (1970) Measurement of total calcium in serum by atomic absorption spectrophotometry, with use of a strontium internal reference *Clinical Chemistry* **16** 998–1007 (36)

PYGOTT F (1957) Paget's disease of bone: the radiological incidence *Lancet* **1** 1170–1171 (240, 241)

PYRAH L HODGKINSON A ANDERSON CK (1966) Primary hyperparathyroidism *British Journal of Surgery* **53** 245–316 (80, 85, 86, 90, 92, 93, 97, 106, 111)

RADDE IC HÖFFKEN B PARKINSON DK SHEEPERS J LUCKHAM A (1971) Practical aspects of a measurement technique for calcium ion activity in plasma *Clinical Chemistry* **17** 1002–1006 (39)

RAINA V (1972) Normal osteoid tissue *Journal of Clinical Pathology* **25** 229–232 (60)

RAISZ LG TRUMMEL CL HOLICK MF DE LUCA HF (1972a) 1,25-dihydroxychole-calciferol: a potent stimulator of bone resorption in tissue culture *Science* **175** 768–769 (27)

RAISZ LG AU WYW SIMMONS H MANDELSTAM P (1972b) Calcitonin in human serum *Archives of Internal Medicine* **129** 889–893 (47)

RAISZ LG TRUMMEL CL WENER JA SIMMONS H (1972c) Effect of glucocorticoids on bone resorption in tissue culture *Endocrinology* **90** 961–967 (282)

RAJASURIYA K PEIRIS OA RATNAIKE VT DE FONSEKA CP (1964) Parathyroid adenomas in childhood *American Journal of Diseases of Children* **107** 442–449 (110)

RAMALINGASWAMI V AURORA AL (1961) Nutritional aspects of calculus disease of the urinary tract *Federation Proceedings* **20** Suppl 7 317–322 (137)

RAMAN A (1970a) Determination of ionized calcium in serum with a calcium electrode *Biochemical Medicine* **3** 369–375 (39)

RAMAN A (1970b) Effect of adrenalectomy on ionic and total plasma calcium in rats *Hormone and Metabolic Research* **2** 181–183 (281)

RAMAN A (1971) The calcium fractions of normal serum *Clinical Biochemistry* **4** 141–146 (39)

RAO KM (1970) Concurrent hyperthyroidism and hyperparathyroidism *British Journal of Surgery* **57** 868–869 (280)

RAPOPORT A CRASSWELLER PO HUSDAN H FROM GLA ZWEIG M JOHNSON MD (1967) The renal excretion of hydrogen ion in uric acid stone formers *Metabolism* **16** 176–188 (135)

RASHKIND WJ GOLINKO R ARCASOY M (1961) Cardiac findings in idiopathic hypercalcemia of infancy *Journal of Pediatrics* **58** 464–469 (123)

RASMUSSEN H (ed) (1970) *International encyclopedia of Pharmacology and Therapeutics. Section 51 Vol 1: Parathyroid Hormone Thyrocalcitonin and Related Drugs* Oxford: Pergamon (1)

RASMUSSEN H and others (1970) Unpublished. Cited by Yendt (1970) (Also personal communication from H Rasmussen 1973) (126)

RAVAULT PP LEJEUNE E BOUVIER M MAITREPIERRE J BOCHU M QUENEAU P (1970) L'Ostéoporose circonscrite des os longs au cours de la maladie de Paget *Journal de Radiologie et d'Electrologie* **51** 499–502 (243)

RAVENNI G RUBEGNI M DEL GIOVANE L (1962) L' idrossiprolinuria nel soggetto normale *Bolletina della Societa Italiana di Biologia Sperimentale* **38** 263–266 (55)

REEDER DD JACKSON BM BAN J CLENDINNEN BG DAVIDSON WD THOMPSON JC (1970) Influence of hypercalcemia on gastric secretion and serum gastrin concentrations in man *Annals of Surgery* **172** 540–546 (93)

REES JKH COLES GA (1969) Calciphylaxis in man *British Medical Journal* **2** 670–672 (201)

REEVE J VEALL N (1972) Radioisotope studies of calcium metabolism and their interpretation *Clinics in Endocrinology and Metabolism* **1** 185–196 (57)

REINBERG A SIDI E (1959) Tétanie chronique et eczéma constitutionnel *Annales d'Endocrinologie* **20** 186–191 (143)

REINHOLD JG NASR K LAHIMGARZADEH A HEDAYATI H (1973) Effects of purified phytate and phytate-rich bread upon metabolism of zinc calcium phosphorus, and nitrogen in man *Lancet* **1** 283–288 (168)

REISS E CANTERBURY JM (1971) Genesis of hyperparathyroidism *American Journal of Medicine* **50** 679–685 (47, 63)

REISS E CANTERBURY JM KANTER A (1969) Circulating parathyroid hormone concentration in chronic renal insufficiency *Archives of Internal Medicine* **124** 417–422 (195)

REISS E CANTERBURY JM BERCOVITZ MA KAPLAN EL (1970) The role of phosphate in the secretion of parathyroid hormone in man *Journal of Clinical Investigation* **49** 2146–2149 (15)

REITE M DAVIS K SOLOMONS C OTT J (1972) Osteogenesis imperfecta: psychological function *American Journal of Psychiatry* **128** 1540–1546 (259)

REYNOLDS EH HALLPIKE JF PHILLIPS BM MATTHEWS DM (1965) Reversible absorptive defects in anticonvulsant megaloblastic anaemia *Journal of Clinical Pathology* **18** 593–598 (174)

RHANEY K MITCHELL RG (1956) Idiopathic hypercalcaemia of infants *Lancet* **1** 1028–1032 (123)

RHODES BA GREYSON ND HAMILTON CR WHITE RI GIARGIANA FA WAGNER HN (1972) Absence of anatomic arteriovenous shunts in Paget's disease of bone *New England Journal of Medicine* **287** 686–689 (247)

RICHARDS AJ (1970) Hypercalcaemia in thyrotoxicosis with and without hyperparathyroidism *Postgraduate Medical Journal* **46** 440–446 (280)

RICHARDS P WRONG OM (1972) Dominant inheritance in a family with familial renal tubular acidosis *Lancet* **2** 998–999 (215)

RICHARDS P CHAMBERLAIN MJ WRONG OM (1972) Treatment of osteomalacia of renal tubular acidosis by sodium bicarbonate alone *Lancet* **2** 994–997 (216)

RICHENS A ROWE DJF (1970) Disturbance of calcium metabolism by anticonvulsant drugs *British Medical Journal* **4** 73–76 (See also the subsequent correspondence on pages 559, 803 and 804) (174)

RIGGS BL JOWSEY J (1972) Treatment of Paget's disease with fluoride *Seminars in Drug Treatment* **2** 65–68 (250)

RIGGS BL KELLY PJ KINNEY VR SCHOLZ DA BIANCO AJ (1967) Calcium deficiency and osteoporosis *Journal of Bone and Joint Surgery* **49A** 915–924 (231)

RIGGS BL ARNAUD CD GOLDSMITH RS TAYLOR WF McGALL JT SESSLER AD (1971a) Plasma kinetics and acute effects of pharmacologic doses of porcine calcitonin in man *Journal of Clinical Endocrinology* **33** 115–127 (20)

RIGGS BL ARNAUD CD REYNOLDS JC SMITH LH (1971b) Immunologic differentiation of primary hyperparathyroidism from hyperparathyroidism due to nonparathyroid cancer *Journal of Clinical Investigation* **50** 2079–2083 (47, 116)

RIGGS BL JOWSEY J KELLY PJ HOFFMAN DL (1972a) Treatment for postmenopausal and senile osteoporosis *Medical Clinics of North America* **56** 989–997 (233, 234)

RIGGS BL RANDALL RV WAHNER HW JOWSEY J KELLY PJ SINGH M (1972b) The nature of the metabolic bone disorder in acromegaly *Journal of Clinical Endocrinology and Metabolism* **34** 911–918 (275)

RIGGS BL ARNAUD CD JOWSEY J GOLDSMITH RS KELLY PJ (1973a) Parathyroid function in primary osteoporosis *Journal of Clinical Investigation* **52** 181–184 (231)

RIGGS BL JOWSEY J KELLY PJ HOFFMAN DL ARNAUD CD (1973b) Studies on pathogenesis and treatment in postmenopausal and senile osteoporosis *Clinics in Endocrinology and Metabolism* **2** 317–332 (234)

RILEY CJ (1970) Chronic milk-alkali syndrome associated with prolonged excessive intake of 'Moorland' tablets *Practitioner* **205** 657–660 (126)

RITZ E KREMPIEN R MEHLS O MALLUCHE H STROEBEL Z ZIMMERMAN H (1973) Skeletal complications of renal insufficiency and maintenance haemodialysis *Nephron* **10** 195–207 (197, 200)

RIVETT JD ROBINSON JM (1972) Hypercalcaemia associated with an ovarian carcinoma of mesonephromatous type *Journal of Obstetrics and Gynaecology of the British Commonwealth* **79** 1047–1052 (116)

ROBERTSON I (1969) Survey of clinical rickets in the infant population in Cape Town 1967–1968 *South African Medical Journal* **43** 1072–1076 (168)

ROBERTSON I (1970) Follow-up study of clinical rickets in Cape Town infants *South African Medical Journal* **44** 368 (167, 168)

ROBERTSON WG MORGAN DB (1972) The distribution of urinary calcium excretions in normal persons and stone-formers *Clinica Chimica Acta* **37** 503–508 (48, 134)

ROBERTSON WG PEACOCK M (1972) Calcium oxalate crystalluria and inhibitors of crystallization in recurrent renal stone-formers *Clinical Science* **43** 499–506 (133)

ROBINSON RA (1964) Observations regarding compartments for tracer calcium in the body. In *Bone Biodynamics* ed Frost HM 423–439 Boston: Little Brown London: Churchill (11)

ROBINSON CJ RAFFERTY B PARSONS JA (1972) Calcium shift into bone: a calcitonin-resistant primary action of parathyroid hormone studied in rats *Clinical Science* **42** 235–241 (20)

RODRIGUEZ RP WICKSTROM JK (1971) Osteogenesis imperfecta: A preliminary report on resurfacing of long bones with intramedullary fixation by an extensible intramedullary device *Southern Medical Journal* **64** 169–176 (261)

ROGÉ J DREYFUS P DORFMANN H MARCHE C PIRONNEAU A BORDIER P SILVÉRÉANO-DE-ROISSARD F ZECHOVSKY N JUSTIN-BESANÇON L (1973) Ostéomalacie malabsorption intestinale polyadénopathies et polyarthrite inflammatoire par phénomène d'anse stagnante *Semaine des Hôpitaux de Paris* **49** 163–174 (170)

ROGERS LA FETTER BF PEETE WPJ (1969) Parathyroid cyst and cystic degeneration of parathyroid adenoma *Archives of Pathology* **88** 476–479 (83)

ROMANUS R HEIMANN P NILSSON O HANSSON G (1973) Surgical treatment of hyperparathyroidism *Progress in Surgery* **12** 22–76 (104)

ROSE GA (1967) Some thoughts on osteoporosis and osteomalacia *Scientific Basis of Medicine Annual Reviews* 252–275 (170, 233)

ROSE GA (1972) A simple and rapid method for the measurement of plasma ultrafiltrable and ionized calcium *Clinica Chimica Acta* 37 343–349 (39)

ROSE GA HARRISON AR (1973) The incidence investigation and treatment of idiopathic hypercalciuria. In *Proceedings of the International Symposium on Renal Stone Research Madrid 1972* ed Delatte LC Basle: Karger (134)

ROSE GA REED GW SMITH AH (1965) Isotopic method for measurement of calcium absorption from the gastro-intestinal tract *British Medical Journal* 1 690–692 (56)

ROSEN JF HAYMOVITS A (1972) Liver lysosomes in congenital osteopetrosis *Journal of Pediatrics* 81 518–527 (263)

ROSENBERG LE SCRIVER CR (1969) Disorders of amino acid metabolism. In *Duncan's Diseases of Metabolism* 6th edition Ed Bondy PK 366–515 Philadelphia: Saunders (209)

ROSENSTREICH SJ RICH C VOLWILER W (1971) Deposition in and release of vitamin D_3 from body fat: evidence for a storage site in the rat *Journal of Clinical Investigation* 50 679–687 (24)

ROSENTHAL FD ROY S (1972) Hypertension and hyperparathyroidism *British Medical Journal* 4 396–397 (92)

ROSIN AJ (1970) Clinical features and detection of osteomalacia in the elderly *Postgraduate Medical Journal* 46 131–136 (169, 190)

ROSLER A RABINOWITZ D (1973) Magnesium-induced reversal of vitamin-D resistance in hypoparathyroidism *Lancet* 1 803–805 (See also the subsequent letter by Dr.ME Scott on page 1005). (159)

ROSSI P CARILLO FJ JOHNSTON B (1971) Angiography in the diagnosis of parathyroid carcinoma *New England Journal of Medicine* 284 198–201 (103)

ROTH SI (1971) Recent advances in parathyroid gland pathology *American Journal of Medicine* 50 612–622 (81)

ROTH SI MARSHALL RB (1969) Pathology and ultrastructure of the human parathyroid glands in chronic renal failure *Archives of Internal Medicine* 124 397–407 (200)

ROUND JM (1972) Rickets in Glasgow Pakistanis *British Medical Journal* 3 114 (42, 43)

RUBENS RD HOFFMANN DC HARCOURT-WEBSTER JN BROOKE BN (1969) Dissimilar adenomas in four parathyroids presenting as primary hyperparathyroidism *Lancet* 1 596–598 (104)

RUSSELL RGG (1965) Excretion of inorganic pyrophosphate in hypophosphatasia *Lancet* 2 461–464 (53, 269)

RUSSELL JGB (1973a) *Radiology in obstetrics and antenatal paediatrics* London: Butterworths (260)

RUSSELL RGG (1973b) Pyrophosphate in renal stone disease. In *Proceedings of the International Symposium on Renal Stone Research, Madrid 1972*, ed. Delatte LC Basle: Karger (132)

RUSSELL JGB (1973c) Personal communication (167)

RUSSELL RGG FLEISCH H (1970) Inorganic pyrophosphate and pyrophosphatases in calcification and calcium homeostasis *Clinical Orthopaedics* **69** 101–117 (7, 42)

RUSSELL RGG HODGKINSON A (1969) The urinary excretion of inorganic pyrophosphate in hyperparathyroidism, hyperthyroidism, Paget's disease and other disorders of bone metabolism *Clinical Science* **36** 435–443 (53, 280)

RUSSELL RGG WADSTROM LB LINDSTEDT S CARE AD BISAZ S FLEISCH H (1969) The origin of inorganic pyrophosphate in urine *Clinical Science* **37** 419–129 (53)

RUSSELL RGG BISAZ S DONATH A MORGAN DB FLEISCH H (1971) Inorganic pyrophosphate in plasma in normal persons and in patients with hypophosphatasia, osteogenesis imperfecta and other disorders of bone *Journal of Clinical Investigation* **50** 961–969 (54, 259, 269)

RYAN WG (1973) Mithramycin in Paget's disease of bone *Lancet* **1** 1319 (251)

RYCKEWAERT A SOLNICA J LANHAM C DE SÈZES (1966) Manifestations articulaires de l'hyperparathroïde *Presse Médicale* **74** 2599–2603 (89)

RYCKEWAERT A KUNTZ D TEYSSEDOU J-P TUN CHOT S BORDIER P HIOCO D (1972) Étude histologique de l'os chez des sujets ostéoporotiques en traitement prolongé par le flourure de sodium *Revue du Rhumatisme* **39** 627–634 (234)

SACHS CE BOURDEAU AM (1971) Bovine serum albumin (BSA)-calcium binding studies with a calcium selective liquid membrane electrode *Clinical Orthopaedics* **78** 24–29 (37)

SAFRIT HF STITT H ROSNER W (1970) Angiographic localization of an adenoma in an aberrant parathyroid gland *New England Journal of Medicine* **282** 209–210 (103)

SAGAR S ESTRADA RL KAYE M (1972) Dihydrotachysterol and vitamin D resistance in renal failure *Archives of Internal Medicine* **130** 768–769 (204)

SALGADO R BARCIA JM PATARO VF (1971) Hiperparatiroidismo por adenoma paratiroideo mediastínico radiólogicamente evidente *Prensa Médica Argentina* **58** 896–902 (103)

SAMUELS BI DOWDY AH LECKY JW (1972) Parathyroid thermography *Radiology* **104** 575–578 (103)

SANDERSON PH MARSHALL F WILSON RE (1960) Calcium and phosphorus homeostasis in the parathyroidectomized dog; evaluation by means of ethylenediamine tetraacetate and calcium tolerance tests *Journal of Clinical Investigation* **39** 662–670 (12, 17)

SARASIN C (1941) Osteomalacie und hypochrome Anaemie nach Magenresektion *Gastroenterologia* (Basel) **66** 182–197 (171)

SAVAGE RH (1969) The calcitonin story *Guy's Hospital Reports* **118** 433–457 (17)

SAVILLE PD (1965) Changes in bone mass with age and alcoholism *Journal of Bone and Joint Surgery* **47A** 492–499 (237)

SCADDING JG (1967) *Sarcoidosis* London: Eyre and Spottiswoode (121)

SCADDING JG and others (1969) A case of sarcoidosis with cryptococcal meningitis *British Medical Journal* **4** 729–732 (120)

SCANDELLARI C CONTE N FEDERSPIL G FREZZATO S TRISOTTO A (1972) A propos du mécanisme de l'effet hypocalcémiant du glucagon chez l'homme. Études à l'aide de calcium radio-actif *Annales d'Endocrinologie* **33** 464–470 (144)

SCHAAF M PAYNE CA (1966) Effect of diphenylhydantoin and phenobarbital on overt and latent tetany *New England Journal of Medicine* **274** 1228–1233 (34, 153)

SCHAEFER K KRAFT D VON HERRATH D OPITZ A (1972) Intestinal absorption of vitamin D_3 in epileptic patients and phenobarbital-treated rats *Epilepsia* **13** 509–519 (174)

SCHANTZ A CASTLEMAN B (1973) Parathyroid carcinoma: a study of 70 cases *Cancer* **31** 600–605 (111)

SCHMID F (1967) Osteopathien bei antiepileptischer Dauerbehandlung *Fortschritte der Medizin* **85** 381–382 (174)

SCHMIDT J (1962) Osteopetrosis myxoedematosa mit Nephrolithiasis *Zeitschrift für Kinderheilkunde* **86** 602–618 (278)

SCHMORL G (1932) Uber Osteitis deformans Paget *Virchows Archiv für Pathologische Anatomie* **283** 694–751 (240)

SCHNEIDER SH (1971) Hyperparathyroidism masked by Cushing's syndrome *Arizona Medicine* **28** 259–261 (284)

SCHNEIDER H-J HEIDE K (1971) Mikrothermische Untersuchungen zur phasenalalytischen Identifizierung von Harnsteinen *Zeitschrift für Urologie* **64** 323–329 (131)

SCHRÖDER G (1964) Eine klinisch-erbbiologische Untersuchungen des Krankengutes in Westfalen *Zeitschrift für Menschliche Verebungsund Konstitutionslehre* **37** 632–676 (253)

SCHULMAN JD WONG VG BRADLEY KH SEEGMILLER JE (1970a) A simple technique for the biochemical diagnosis of cystinosis *Journal of Pediatrics* **76** 289–292 (209)

SCHULMAN JD SCHNEIDER JA BRADLEY KH SEEGMILLER JE (1970b) Heterozygote studies in cystinosis *Clinical Chimica Acta* **29** 73–76 (209)

SCOTT JT DIXON AStJ BYWATERS EGL (1964) Association of hyperuricaemia and gout with hyperparathyroidism *British Medical Journal* **1** 1070–1073 (89, 98)

SCRIVER CR CAMERON D (1969) Pseudohypophosphatasia *New England Journal of Medicine* **281** 604–606 (269)

SEEDAT YK VINIK AI STEWART-WYNNE EG (1970) Propranolol and serum calcium in thyrotoxicosis *British Medical Journal* **3** 525–526 (280)

SEEGMILLER JE (1968) Xanthine stone formation *American Journal of Medicine* **45** 780–783 (135)

SEEGMILLER JE (1973) Metabolic bases of renal lithiasis from overproduction of uric acid. In *Proceedings of the International Symposium on Renal Stone Research, Madrid 1972* ed Delatte LC Basle: Karger (135)

SEELIG MS (1969) Vitamin D and cardiovascular renal and brain damage in infancy and childhood *Annals of the New York Academy of Sciences* **147** 537–582 (117, 126)

SEELIG MS (1970) Are American children still getting an excess of vitamin D? *Clinical Pediatrics* **9** 380–383 (23, 117)

SELLE JG ALTEMEIER WA FULLEN WD GOLDSMITH RE (1972) Cholelithiasis in hyperparathyroidism *Archives of Surgery* **105** 369–374 (96)

SELZMAN HM FECHNER RE (1967) Oxyphil adenoma and primary hyperparathy roidism *Journal of the American Medical Association* **199** 359–361 (81)

SERRE H SIMON L SANY C SANY J LAMBOLEY C LAVEIL G (1972) Le devenir chez l'adulte du rachitisme vitamino-résistant *Revue du Rhumatisme* **39** 681–690 (213)

SEVITT LH WRONG OM (1968) Hypercalcaemia from calcium resin in patients with chronic renal failure *Lancet* **2** 950–951 (202)

SHAFER RB GREGORY DH (1972) Calcium malabsorption in hyperthyroidism *Gastroenterology* **63** 235–239 (279)

SHAH BG DRAPER HH (1966) Depression of calcium absorption in parathyroidectomized rats *American Journal of Physiology* **211** 963–966 (16)

SHAI F BAKER RK WALLACH S (1971) The clinical and metabolic effects of porcine calcitonin on Paget's disease of bone *Journal of Clinical Investigation* **50** 1927–1940 (250)

SHAI F BAKER RK ADDRIZZO JR WALLACH S (1972) Hypercalcemia in mycobacterial infection *Journal of Clinical Endocrinology* **34** 251–256 (127)

SHARMA OP LAMON J WINSOR D (1972) Hypercalcemia and tuberculosis *Journal of the American Medical Association* **222** 582 (127)

SHARRARD WJW (1971) *Paediatric orthopaedics and fractures* Oxford: Blackwell (32)

SHAW WH (1971) A study of the renal excretion of calcium by the production of a constant level of hypercalcemia in normal and abnormal human subjects *Canadian Journal of Physiology & Pharmacology* **49** 469–478 (49)

SHAW MT DAVIES M (1968) Primary hyperparathyroidism presenting as spinal cord compression *British Medical Journal* **4** 230–231 (86)

SHAW JCL JONES A GUNTHER M (1973) Mineral content of brands of milk for infant feeding *British Medical Journal* **2** 12–15 (148)

SHELLING DH HOPPER KB (1936) Calcium and phosphorus studies. XII: Six years clinical experience in the prevention and treatment of rickets, tetany and allied diseases *Bulletin of the Johns Hopkins Hospital* **58** 137 (191)

SHENOLIKAR IS (1970) Absorption of dietary calcium in pregnancy *American Journal of Clinical Nutrition* **23** 63–67 (8)

SHERLOCK S (1968) Chronic cholangitides: aetiology, diagnosis and treatment *British Medical Journal* **3** 515–521 (170, 173)

SHERLOCK S (1970) Nutritional complications of biliary cirrhosis *American Journal of Clinical Nutrition* **23** 640–644 (173)

SHERMAN LA PFEFFERBAUM A BROWN EB (1970) Hypoparathyroidism in a patient with longstanding iron storage disease *Annals of Internal Medicine* **73** 259–261 (152)

SHERWOOD LM HERRMAN I BASSETT CA (1970) Parathyroid hormone secretion *in vitro*: regulation by calcium and magnesium ions *Nature* **225** 1056–1058 (15)

SHIEBER W (1970) Why hypocalcemia in pancreatitis? *American Journal of Surgery* **120** 685–686 (144)

SHEIBER W BIRGE SJ AVIOLI LV TEITELBAUM SL (1971a) Normocalcemic hyperparathyroidism with 'normal' parathyroid glands *Archives of Surgery* **103** 299–302 (134)

SHIEBER W KINGSBURY R BAUE AE (1971b) The role of the thyroid gland in the hypocalcemia of acute pancreatitis *Surgical Forum* **22** 333–334 (144)

SIDDIQUI J KERR DNS (1971) Complications of renal failure and their response to dialysis *British Medical Bulletin* **27** 153–159 (199)

SIDDIQUI AA WILSON DR (1972) Primary hyperparathyroidism and proximal tubular acidosis: Report of two cases *Canadian Medical Association Journal* **106** 654–659 (67, 91)

SIEGLER DIM (1970) Idiopathic Addison's disesae presenting with hypercalcaemia *British Medical Journal* **2** 522 (282)

SIGURDSSON G WOODHOUSE NJY TAYLOR S JOPLIN GF (1973) Stilboestrol diphosphate in hypercalcaemia due to parathyroid carcinoma *British Medical Journal* **1** 27–28 (77, 112)

SILBERBERG M SILBERBERG R (1971) Steroid hormones and bone. *The Biochenistry and Physiology of Bone*, 2nd edition ed Bourne GH Vol 3 pp 401–484 New York: Academic Press (274)

SILVA OL BECKER KL (1973) Treatment of hypercalcemia with synthetic salmon calcitonin *Archives of Internal Medicine* **132** 337–339 (77)

SIMPSON GR DALE E (1972) Serum levels of phosphorus, magnesium and calcium in women utilising combination oral or long-acting injectable progestational contraceptives *Fertility and Sterility* **23** 326–330 (28)

SIMPSON W KERR DNS HILL AVL SIDDIQUI JY (1973) Skeletal changes in patients on regular haemodialysis *Radiology* **107** 313–320 (199)

SINGER FR NEER RM MURRAY TM KEUTMANN HT DEFTOS LJ POTTS JT (1970) Mithramycin treatment of intractable hypercalcemia due to parathyroid carcinoma *New England Journal of Medicine* **283** 634–636 (76, 112)

SINGER FR ALDRED JP NEER RM KRANE SM POTTS JT BLOCH KJ (1972) An evaluation of antibodies and clinical resistance to salmon calcitonin *Journal of Clinical Investigation* **51** 2331–2338 (77, 251)

SINGER FR POWELL D MINKIN C BETHUNE JE BRICKMAN A COBURN JW (1973) Hypercalcemia in reticulum cell sarcoma without hyperparathyroidism or skeletal metastases *Annals of Internal Medicine* **78** 365–369 (116)

SINGER FR NEER R GOLZMAN D KRANE SM POTTS JT (1974) Treatment of Paget's disease of bone with salmon calcitonin. In *Endocrinology 1973* ed Taylor S London: Heinemann (251)

SINGH M JOWSEY J (1970) Failure of calcitonin to prevent disuse osteopenia: an experimental study in rabbits *Endocrinology* **87** 183–186 (233)

SINGH M RIGGS BL BEABOUT JW JOWSEY J (1972) Femoral trabecular-pattern index for evaluation of spinal osteoporosis *Annals of Internal Medicine* **77** 63–67 (222)

SINGLETON AO ALLUMS J (1970) Identification of parathyroid glands by toluidine blue staining *Archives of Surgery* **100** 372–375 (103)

SIRCUS W BRUNT PW WALKER RJ SMALL WP FALCONER CWA THOMSON CG (1970) Two cases of 'pancreatic cholera' with features of peptide-secreting adenomatosis of the pancreas *Gut* **11** 197–205 (95)

SISSON GA VANDER AARDE SB (1971) Control of hypoparathyroidism after extensive neck surgery *Archives of Otolaryngology* **93** 249–255 (151, 157)

SIZEMORE GW GO VLW KAPLAN EL SANZENBACHER LJ HOLTERMULLER KH ARNAUD CD (1973) Relations of calcitonin and gastrin in the Zollinger-Ellison syndrome and medullary carcinoma of the thyroid *New England Journal of Medicine* **288** 641–644 (47)

SJÖBERG HE NILSSON LH (1970) Retention of oral ^{47}Ca in patients with intestinal malabsorption: regional enteritis and pancreatic insufficiency *Scandinavian Journal of Gastroenterology* **5** 265–272 (56, 170)

SKJOLDBERG H NIELSEN HM (1971) Peroperative staining of parathyroid adenomas by intravenous infusion of toluidine blue *Acta Chirurgica Scandinavica* **137** 213–219 (103)

SLATOPOLSKY E CAGLER S GRADOWSKA L CANTERBURY J REISS E BRICKER NS (1972) On the prevention of secondary hyperparathyroidism in experimental chronic renal disease using 'proportional reduction' of dietary phosphorus intake *Kidney International* **2** 147–151 (195, 205)

SLAYTON RE SHNIDER BI ELIAS E HORTON J PERLIA CP (1971) New approach to the treatment of hypercalcemia. The effect of short-term treatment with mithramycin *Clinical Pharmacology and Therapeutics* **12** 833–837 (76)

SMEENK D VAN DEN BRAND IBAM (1965) De invloed van de lichaamshouding op hematocriet en het gehalte aan eiwit, calcium, cholesterol en PBI van het bloed *Nederlands Tijdschrift voor Geneeskunde* **109** 1798–1800 (38)

SMILEY WK MAY E BYWATERS EGL (1957) Ocular presentations of Still's disease and their treatment *Annals of the Rheumatic Diseases* **16** 371–383 (33)

SMITH R (1967) Total urinary hydroxyproline in primary hyperparathyroidism An assessment of its clinical significance *Clinica Chimica Acta* **18** 47–50 (100)

SMITH LH (1968) ed *Symposium on stones. American Journal of Medicine* **45** 649–783 (129)

SMITH LH (1972) The diagnosis and treatment of metabolic stone disease *Medical Clinics of North America* **56** 977–988 (129)

SMITH R DENT CE (1969) Vitamin D requirements in adults: Clinical and metabolic studies on seven patients with nutritional osteomalacia *Bibliotheca Nutrito et Dieta* **13** 44–45 (24)

SMITH LH HOFFMAN AF (1973) Acquired hyperoxaluria, nephrolithiasis and intestinal disease In *Proceedings of the International Symposium on Renal Stone Research Madrid 1972* ed Delatte LC Basle: Karger (134)

SMITH LH McCALL JT (1973) The chemical nature of crystal inhibitors isolated from human urine. In *Proceedings of the International Symposium on Renal Stone Research Madrid 1972* ed Delatte LC Basle: Karger (132)

SMITH RB PETRUSCAK J (1972) Succinylcholine, digitalis and hypercalcemia *Anesthesia and Analgesia* **51** 202–205 (103)

SMITH PH ROBERTSON WG (1969) Stone formation in the immobilised patient. In *Renal stone research symposium* ed Hodgkinson A Nordin BEC 85–92 London: Churchill (136)

SMITH R STERN G (1967) Myopathy, osteomalacia and hyperparathyroidism *Brain* **90** 593–602 (31, 90)

SMITH FE REINSTEIN H BRAVERMAN LE (1965) Cork stoppers and hypercalcemia *New England Journal of Medicine* **272** 787–788 (37)

SMITH FG ALEXANDER DP BUCKLE RM BRITTON HG NIXON DA (1972a) Parathyroid hormone in foetal and adult sheep: the effect of hypocalcaemia *Journal of Endocrinology* **53** 339–348 (28)

SMITH DM JOHNSTON CC YU P-L (1972b) In *vivo* measurement of bone mass *Journal of the American Medical Association* **219** 325–329 (223)

SMITH R RUSSELL RGG BISHOP MC WOODS CG BISHOP M (1973a) Paget's disease of bone: experience with a diphosphonate (disodium etidronate) in treatment *Quarterly Journal of Medicine* NS **42** 235–256 (248, 251)

SMITH DA FRASER SA WILSON GM (1973b) Hyperthyroidism and calcium metabolism *Clinics in Endocrinology and Metabolism* **2** 333–354 (279, 281)

SMITH LH THOMAS WC ARNAUD CD (1973c) Orthophosphate therapy in calcium renal lithiasis. In *Proceedings of the International Symposium on Renal Stone Research Madrid 1972* ed Delatte LC Basle: Karger (139)

SNAPPER I KAHN A (1960) Tubular reabsorption of phosphorus in avitaminosis D *Clinical Orthopaedics* **17** 297–302 (186)

SOFIELD HA MILLAR EA (1959) Fragmentation, realignment and intramedullary rod fixation of deformities of the long bones in children: a ten-year appraisal *Journal of Bone and Joint Surgery* **41A** 1371–1391 (260)

SOLHEIM K (1969) Osteogenesis imperfecta *Journal of Oslo City Hospitals* **19** 193–199 (255)

SOLOMONS CC STYNER J (1969) Osteogenesis imperfecta: effect of magnesium administration on pyrophosphate metabolism *Calcified Tissue Research* **3** 318–326 (54)

SØRENSEN OH FRIIS T HINDBERG I NEILSEN SP (1970) The effect of calcitonin injected into hypercalcaemic and normocalcaemic patients *Acta Medica Scandinavica* **187** 283–290 (76, 77)

SØRENSEN OH HINDBERG I MADSEN SN (1972) Secondary hyperparathyroidism in young rats given prolonged treatment with calcitonin *Acta Endocrinologica* **71** 313–320 (219)

SOTANIEMI EA HAKKARAINEN HK PURANEN JA LAHTI RO (1972) Radiologic bone changes and hypocalcemia with anticonvulsant therapy in epilepsy *Annals of Internal Medicine* **77** 389–394 (174)

SOUILLET G GERMAIN D FREDERICH A DAVID M MEUNIER P FAVROT B SANN L VALANCOGNE A BRUNAT M (1973) Hypercalcémie et hypocalcémie dans les leucoses aiguës de l'enfant *Lyon Médical* **229** 301–315 (147)

SPAULDING SW WALSER M (1970) Treatment of experimental hypercalcemia with oral phosphate *Journal of Clinical Endocrinology* **31** 531–538 (73)

SPAULDING WB YENDT ER (1964) Prolonged vitamin D intoxication in a patient with hypoparathyroidism *Canadian Medical Association Journal* **90** 1049–1054 (119)

SPENCER H LEWIN I FOWLER J SAMACHSON J (1969) Influence of dietary calcium intake on Ca^{47} absorption in man *American Journal of Medicine* **46** 197–205 (56)

SRIVASTAVA TP GUPTA OP (1969) Otosclerosis and osteogenesis imperfecta *Journal of Laryngology and Otology* **2** 1195–1204 (258)

STAMP TCB (1971) The hypocalcaemic effect of intravenous phosphate administration *Clinical Science* **40** 55–65 (73)

STAMP TCB (1973) Vitamin D metabolism: recent advances *Archives of Disease in Childhood* **48** 1–7 (25)

STAMP TCB STACEY TE (1970) Evaluation of theoretical renal phosphorus threshold as an index of renal phosphorus handling *Clinical Science* **39** 505–516 (51)

STAMP TCB ROUND JM ROWE DJF HADDAD JG (1972) Plasma levels and therapeutic effect of 25-hydroxycholecalciferol in epileptic patients taking anticonvulsant drugs *British Medical Journal* **4** 9–12 (174)

STANBURY SW (1972) Azotaemic renal osteodystrophy: A review with special reference to the problems encountered in dialysed patients and after transplantation *Clinical Endocrinology* **1** 267 (192)

STANBURY SW LUMB GA (1966) Parathyroid function in chronic renal failure *Quarterly Journal of Medicine* NS **35** 1–23 (201)

STANBURY SW LUMB GA NICHOLSON WF (1960) Elective subtotal parathyroidectomy for renal hyperparathyroidism *Lancet* **1** 793–799 (205)

STEENDIJK R (1971) Metabolic bone disease in children *Clinical Orthopaedics* **77** 247–275 (212)

STEIN RC (1971) Hypercalcemia in leukemia *Journal of Pediatrics* **78** 861–863 (115)

STEINBERG D OSOFSKY M RUBIN AD (1971) Acute phase of chronic granulocytic leukemia *New York State Journal of Medicine* **71** 583–586 (115)

STEPHEN JML STEPHENSON P (1971) Alkaline phosphatase in normal infants *Archives of Disease in Childhood* **46** 185–188 (42, 43)

STEPHENS AD WATTS RWE (1971) The treatment of cystinuria with N-acetyl-D-penicillamine, a comparison with the results of D-penicillamine treatment *Quarterly Journal of Medicine* NS **40** 355–370 (135)

STEVENSON CJ BOTTOMS E SHUSTER S (1970) Skin collagen in osteogenesis imperfecta *Lancet* **1** 860–861 (255)

STEWART WK MITCHELL RG MORGAN HG LOWE KG THOMSON J (1964) The changing incidence of rickets and infantile hypercalcaemia as seen in Dundee *Lancet* **1** 679–682 (167)

STICKLER GB BEABOUT JW RIGGS BL (1970) Vitamin D-resistant rickets: clinical experience with 41 typical familial hypophosphatemic patients and 2 atypical nonfamilial cases *Mayo Clinic Proceedings* **45** 197–218 (207, 212, 213, 214)

STICKLER GB JOWSEY J BIANCO AJ (1971) Possible detrimental effect of large doses of vitamin D in familial hypophosphatemic vitamin D-resistant rickets *Journal of Pediatrics* **79** 68–71 (214)

STOKER DJ WYNN V (1966) Effect of posture on the plasma cholesterol level *British Medical Journal* **1** 336–338 (38)

STORCK G BJÖRNTORP P (1971) Chemical composition of fat necrosis in experimental pancreatitis in the rat *Scandinavian Journal of Gastroenterology* **6** 225–230 (144)

STOTE RM SMITH LH WILSON DM DUBE WJ GOLDSMITH RS ARNAUD CD (1972) Hydrochlorothiazide effects on serum calcium and immunoreactive parathyroid hormone concentrations *Annals of Internal Medicine* **77** 587–591 (127)

STOWERS JM MICHIE W FRAZER SC (1967) A critical evaluation of the trisodium-edetate test for hypoparathyroidism after thyroidectomy *Lancet* **1** 124–127 (This paper should be read with the subsequent correspondence on pages. 442, 513 and 620 together with the paper by Professor P Fourman and others *Lancet* (1967) **2** 914–915) (151)

STREETO JM (1969) Acute hypercalcemia simulating basilar-artery insufficiency *New England Journal of Medicine* **280** 427–429 (69)

SUCHETT-KAYE AI (1970) Paget's disease of bone *Gerontologia Clinica* **12** 241–255 (244)

SUH SM FRASER D KOOH SW (1970) Pseudohypoparathyroidism: responsiveness to parathyroid extract induced by vitamin D_2 therapy *Journal of Clinical Endocrinology and Metabolism* **30** 609–614 (161)

SUH SM CSIMA A FRASER D (1971) Pathogenesis of hypocalcemia in magnesium depletion: normal end-organ responsiveness to parathyroid hormone *Journal of Clinical Investigation* **50** 2668–2678 (146)

SUH SM TASHJIAN AH MATSUO N PARKINSON DK FRASER D (1973) Pathogenesis of hypocalcemia in primary hypomagnesemia: normal end-organ responsiveness to parathyroid hormone, impaired parathyroid gland function *Journal of Clinical Investigation* **52** 153–160 (146)

SUKI WN YIUM JJ VON MINDEN M SALLER-HEBERT C EKNOYAN G MARTINEZ-MALDONADO M (1970) Acute treatment of hypercalcemia with furosemide *New England Journal of Medicine* **283** 836–840 (73, 74)

SUSSMAN HH (1970) Source of increased serum alkaline phosphatase activity in Paget's disease *Clinica Chimica Acta* **27** 121–124 (248)

SUTOR DJ O'FLYNN JD (1973) Matrix formation on crystalline material *in vivo* In *Proceedings of the International Symposium on Renal Stone Research Madrid 1972* ed Delatte LC Basle: Karger (131)

Sutor DJ Wooley SE MacKenzie KR Wilson R Scott R Morgan HG (1971) Urinary tract calculi—a comparison of chemical and crystallographic analyses *British Journal of Urology* **43** 149–153 (131)

Sutton RAL (1970) Plasma magnesium concentration in primary hyperparathyroidism *British Medical Journal* **1** 529–533 (98)

Sutton RAL Watson L (1969) Urinary excretion of calcium and magnesium in primary hyperparathyroidism *Lancet* **1** 1000–1003 (132)

Svane S (1964) Hypercalcemia in malignant disease without evidence of bone destruction *Acta Medica Scandinavica* **175** 353–357 (116)

Swan CHJ Cooke WT (1973) Fibrogenesis imperfecta ossium. In *Clinical aspects of metabolic bone disease* ed Frame B Parfitt AM Duncan H 465–468 Amsterdam: Excerpta Medica (272)

Swash M Rowan AJ (1972) Electroencephalographic criteria of hypocalcemia and hypercalcemia *Archives of Neurology* **29** 218–228 (70, 143)

Swinton NW Clerkin EP Flint LD (1972) Hypercalcemia and familial pheochromocytoma *Annals of Internal Medicine* **76** 455–457 (95, 116)

Szabó E (1973) Polarizing microscopic studies on the fine structure of renal stones. In *Proceedings of the International Symposium on Renal Stone Research Madrid 1972* ed Delatte LC Basle: Karger (131)

Szymendera J (1970) *Bone mineral metabolism in cancer* Berlin: Springer-Verlag; London: Heinemann (113, 115)

Tabaee-Zadeh MJ Frame B Kapphahn K (1972) Kinesiogenic choreoathetosis and idiopathic hypoparathyroidism *New England Journal of Medicine* **286** 762–763. (Another case is mentioned in a letter **287** 569–570) (153)

Tabaqchali S (1970) The pathophysiological role of small intestinal bacterial flora *Scandinavian Journal of Gastroenterology* **5** Suppl. 6 139–163 (170)

Taguchi Y (1970) Management of urinary calculi: updated *Canadian Medical Association Journal* **102** 154–156 (138)

Takeuchi J (1973) Etiology of Itai-itai disease. Personal communication (176)

Tamm HS Nolph KD Maher JF (1971) Factors affecting plasma calcium concentration during hemodialysis *Archives of Internal Medicine* **128** 769–773 (202)

Tan CM Ramana A (1972) Maternal-fetal calcium relationships in man *Quarterly Journal of Experimental Physiology* **57** 56–59 (28)

Tan KL Tock EPC (1971) Osteogenesis imperfecta congenita *Australian Paediatric Journal* **7** 49–53 (256)

Tan CM Ramana A Sinnathyray TA (1972) Serum ionic calcium levels during pregnancy *Journal of Obstetrics and Gynaecology of the British Commonwealth* **79** 694–697 (28)

Tanaka Y De Luca HF Omdahl J Holick MF (1971) Mechanism of action of 1,25-dihydroxycholecalciferol on intestinal calcium transport *Proceedings of the National Academy of Sciences* **68** 1286–1288 (26)

TASHJIAN AH VOELKEL EF LEVINE L GOLDHABER P (1972) Evidence that the bone resorption-stimulating factor produced by mouse fibrosarcoma cells is prostaglandin E_2: a new model for the hypercalcemia of cancer *Journal of Experimental Medicine* **136** 1329–1343 (116)

TAYLOR WH (1972) Renal calculi and self-medication with multivitamin preparations containing vitamin D *Clinical Science* **42** 515–522 (133)

TAYLOR RL LYNCH HJ WYSOR WG (1963) Seasonal influence of sunlight on the hypercalcemia of sarcoidosis *American Journal of Medicine* **34** 221–227 (120)

TAYLOR AL DAVIS BB PAWLSON LG JOSIMOVICH JB MINTZ DH (1970) Factors influencing the urinary excretion of 3′,5′-adenosine monophosphate in humans *Journal of Clinical Edocrinology* **30** 316–324 (15)

TEOTIA SPS TEOTIA M (1973) Secondary hyperparathyroidism in patients with endemic skeletal fluorosis *British Medical Journal* **1** 637–640 (110)

TEOTIA M TEOTIA SPS KUNWAR KB (1971) Endemic skeletal fluorosis *Archives of Disease in Childhood* **46** 686–691 (264)

TEPPER LB HARDY HL CHAMBERLIN RI (1961) *Toxicity of beryllium compounds* Amsterdam: Elsevier (128)

TEREE TM KLEIN L (1968) Hypophosphatasia: clinical and metabolic studies *Journal of Pediatrics* **72** 41–50 (269, 270)

TEREE TM FRIEDMAN AB KEST LM FETTERMAN GH (1970) Cystinosis and proximal tubular nephropathy in siblings *American Journal of Diseases of Children* **119** 481–487 (208)

THACKER WC WELLS VH HALL ER (1971) Parathyroid cyst of the mediastinum *Annals of Surgery* **174** 969–975 (83)

THALASSINOS N JOPLIN GF (1968) Phosphate treatment of hypercalcaemia due to carcinoma *British Medical Journal* **4** 14–19 (72, 75)

THALASSINOS NC JOPLIN GF (1970) Failure of corticosteroid therapy to correct the hypercalcaemia of malignant disease *Lancet* **2** 537–538 (64, 75)

THIELE J REALE E GEORGII A (1973) Electronenmikroskopische Befunde an Epithelkörperadenomen unterschiedlicher endokriner Aktivität *Virchows Archiv: Abteilung B: Zellpathologie* **12** 168–188 (81)

THOMAS WC (1971) Effectiveness and mode of action of orthophosphates in patients with calcareous renal calculi *Transactions of the American Clinical and Climatological Association* **83** 113–124 (139)

THOMAS WC FRY RM (1970) Parathyroid adenomas in chronic rickets *American Journal of Medicine* **49** 404–407 (213)

THOMAS WC WISWELL JG CONNOR TB HOWARD JE (1958a) Hypercalcemic crisis due to hyperparathyroidism *American Journal of Medicine* **24** 229–239 (107)

THOMAS WC CONNOR TB MORGAN HG (1958b) Some observations on patients with hypercalcemia exemplifying problems in differential diagnosis especially in hyperparathyroidism *Journal of Laboratory and Clinical Medicine* **52** 11–19 (64)

THOMAS WC CONNOR TB MORGAN HG (1959) Diagnostic considerations in hypercalcemia *New England Journal of Medicine* **260** 591–596 (66)

THOMPSON NW HARNESS JK (1970) Complications of total thyroidectomy for carcinoma *Surgery Gynecology and Obstetrics* **131** 861–868 (151)

THOMPSON GR LEWIS B BOOTH CC (1966) Vitamin-D absorption after partial gastrectomy *Lancet* **1** 457–458 (173)

THOMPSON JS PALMIERI GMA ELIEL LP CRAWFORD RL (1972) The effect of porcine calcitonin on osteoporosis induced by adrenal cortical steroids *Journal of Bone and Joint Surgery* **54A** 1490–1500 (282)

THURSTON H GILMORE GR SWALES JD (1972) Aluminium retention and toxicity in chronic renal failure *Lancet* **1** 881–883 (205)

TOBIN JS (1970) Physical medicine for the osteoporotic patient. In *Osteoporosis* ed Barzel US 133–139 New York: Grune Stratton (234)

TOFT H ROIN J (1971) Effect of frusemide administration on calcium excretion *British Medical Journal* **1** 437–438 (74, 147)

TOMKIN GH WEIR DG (1972) Indicanuria after gastric surgery *Quarterly Journal of Medicine* NS **41** 191–203 (173)

TRANSBØL I HORNUM I HAHNEMANN S HASNER E ØHLENSCHLAEGER H DIEMER H LOCKWOOD K (1970a) Tubular reabsorption of calcium in the differential diagnosis of hypercalcaemia *Acta Medica Scandinavica* **188** 505–522 (39, 49 66, 68, 96, 97, 98, 99, 116, 118)

TRANSBØL I HAHNEMANN S HORNUM I (1970b) Ionized ultrafiltrable and total calcium in serum in hyperparathyroidism *Acta Endocrinologica* **65** 385–400 (97)

TROUGHTON O SINGH SP (1972) Heart failure and neonatal hypocalcaemia *British Medical Journal* **4** 76–79 (143)

TSAI HC WONG RG NORMAN AW (1972) Studies on calciferol metabolism: IV subcellular localization of 1,25-dihydroxy-vitamin D_3 in intestinal mucosa and correlation with increased calcium transport *Journal of Biological Chemistry* **247** 5511–5519 (26)

TSANG RC KLEINMAN LI SUTHERLAND JM LIGHT IJ (1972) Hypocalcemia in infants of diabetic mothers *Journal of Pediatrics* **80** 384–395. (See also the subsequent correspondence *ibid* (1972) **81** 633–634) (148)

TSUCHIYA K (1969) Causation of ouch-ouch disease (Itai-itai byō) *Keio Journal of Medicine* **18** 181–194 195–211 (176)

TURBEY WJ PASSARO E (1972) Hyperparathyroidism in the Zollinger-Ellison syndrome *Archives of Surgery* **105** 62–66 (95)

TUVEMO T GUSTAVSON K-H (1972) Idiopathic hypoparathyroidism in a girl with Turner's Syndrome *Acta Paediatrica Scandinavica* **61** 724–728 (162)

TWYCROSS RG MARKS V (1970) Symptomatic hypercalcaemia in thyrotoxicosis *British Medical Journal* **2** 701–703 (280)

ULSTROM RA BROWN DM (1972) Hypercalcemia as a complication of parenteral alimentation *Journal of Pediatrics* **81** 419–421 (128)

URIST MR (1972) Growth hormone and skeletal tissue metabolism. In *The Biochemistry and Physiology of Bone* 2nd edition ed Bourne GH Vol. 2 pp 155–195 New York: Academic Press (274)

UTHMAN AA AL-SHAWAFF M (1969) Paget's disease of the mandible *Oral Surgery Oral Medicine and Oral Pathology* **28** 866–870 (244)

UTIAN WH (1971) Oestrogens and osteoporosis *South African Medical Journal* **45** 879–882 (236)

UTLEY PM (1970) Osteopetrosis *Journal of the Tennessee Medical Association* **63** 659–661 (265)

VACHON A VIGON G CHATIN B PANSU D CHAPUY N-C (1970) Insuffisance parathyroïdienne des hemochromatoses *Revue Lyonnaise de Médicine* **19** 543–552 (152)

VAINSEL M (1973) Effects of parathyroid hormone and calcium on renal reabsorption of bicarbonate in children *Biomedicine* **18** 112–117 (16)

VAINSEL M VANDEVELDE G SMULDERS J VOSTERS M HUBAIN P LOEB H (1970) Tetany due to hypomagnesaemia with secondary hypocalcaemia *Archives of Disease in Childhood* **45** 254–258 (145)

VALDÉS-DAPENA MA WEINSTEIN DS (1971) The parathyroids in sudden unexpected death in infants *Acta Pathologica et Microbiologica Scandinavica: Section A* **79** 228–232 (160)

VANASIN B COLMER M DAVIS PJ (1972) Hypocalcemia hypomagnesemia and hypokalemia during chemotherapy of pulmonary tuberculosis *Chest* **61** 496–499 (147)

VANDERHOOFT GA COLEMAN SS (1972) Reversal of skeletal changes in renal osteodystrophy following partial parathyroidectomy and renal allotransplantation *Clinical Orthopaedics* **88** 113–118 (206)

VANDERLINDE RE KOWALSKI P (1971) The clinical biochemistry of phosphorus *Clinical Biochemistry* **4** 76–88 (40)

VAN GERVEN DP ARMELAGOS GJ (1970) Cortical involution in prehistoric Mississippian femora *Journal of Gerontology* **25** 20–22 (228)

VASCONEZ LO MASS MF JURKIEWICZ MJ THOMAS WC (1970) Review of 35 cases of hyperparathyroidism at the University of Florida *Journal of the Florida Medical Association* **57** 36–38 (84)

VAUGHAN JM (1970) *The physiology of bone* Oxford: Oxford University Press (1, 2, 274, 276)

VELLAR ID SHAW J BROSNAN G (1973) Glandula in glandula: the intrathyroid parathyroid *Australian and New Zealand Journal of Surgery* **42** 257–259 (104)

VENDER I LOVELY FW YORK SE (1971) Lamina dura and other metabolic changes in hyperparathyroidism *Journal of the Canadian Dental Association* **37** 261–264 (88)

VERDY M BEAULIEU R DEMERS L STURTRIDGE WC THOMAS P KUMAR MA (1971) Plasma calcitonin activity in a patient with thyroid medullary carcinoma and her children with osteopetrosis *Journal of Clinical Endocrinology and Metabolism* **32** 216–221 (220)

VIANNA NJ (1971) Severe hypophosphataemia due to hypokalemia *Journal of the American Medical Association* **215** 1497–1498 (40, 210)

VINCENT RG MOORE GE WATNE AL (1962) Abnormal behavior following parathyroidectomy *Journal of the American Medical Association* **180** 372–375 (105)

WACKER WEC PARISI AF (1968) Magnesium metabolism *New England Journal of Medicine* **278** 658–663 712–717 772–776 (145)

WAHL AR RÖHER H-D (1973) Pseudohyperparathyreiodismus als paraneoplastisches Syndrom bei einem Fall von Magenkarzinom *Deutsche Medizinische Wochenschrift* **98** 565–568 (116)

WAITE LC VOLKERT WA KENNY AD (1970) Inhibition of bone resorption by acetazolamide in the rat *Endocrinology* **87** 1129–1139 (16)

WALDBOTT GL (1963) Acute fluoride intoxication *Acta Medica Scandinavica* Suppl 400 (147)

WALKER D (1971) Hyperthyroidism and urinary tract calculus *Journal of Urology* **105** 868–869 (133, 280)

WALKER ARP (1972a) The human requirement of calcium: should low intakes be supplemented? *American Journal of Clinical Nutrition* **25** 518–530 (8, 27 61, 144, 238)

WALKER DG (1972b) Congenital osteopetrosis in mice cured by parabiotic union with normal siblings *Endocrinology* **91** 916–920 (220)

WALKER PG (1973) Biochemistry of bone mineralization *Biochemical Society Transactions* **1** 62–67 (6)

WALLACH S (ed) (1972) Drug treatment of bone *Seminars in Drug Treatment* **2** 1–146 (234)

WALLS J LAUDER I ELLIS HA (1972) Chronic renal failure in a patient with parathyroid carcinoma and hyperplasia *Beiträge zur Pathologie* **147** 45–50 (112)

WALSER M (1961) Ion association: VI Interactions between calcium, magnesium inorganic phosphate, citrate and protein in normal human plasma *Journal of Clinical Investigation* **40** 723–730 (10)

WALSER M (1970) Treatment of hypercalcemias *Modern Treatment* **7** 662–674 (74)

WALSER M ROBINSON BHB DUCKETT JW (1963) The hypercalcemia of adrenal insufficiency *Journal of Clinical Investigation* **42** 456–465 (281, 282)

WALTNER JG (1965) Stapedectomy in Paget's disease *Archives of Otolaryngology* **82** 355–358 (246)

WALTON IG STRONG JA (1973) Calcitonin and osteogenic sarcoma *Lancet* **1** 887–888 (246)

WANG C-A REITZ RE POLLARD JJ FLEISCHLI DJ MURRAY TM DEFTOS LJ POTTS JT COPE O (1970) Localization of hyperfunctioning parathyroids *American Journal of Surgery* **119** 462–464 (103)

WAPNICK AA LYNCH SR SEFTEL HC CHARLTON RW BOTHWELL TH JOWSEY J (1971) The effect of siderosis and ascorbic acid depletion on bone metabolism with special reference to osteoporosis in the Bantu *British Journal of Nutrition* **25** 367–376 (236)

WAREMBOURG H DELOMEZ M CARRE A GOSSELIN B DUPUIS C BERTRAND M BOURET G (1972) Association de lésions congénitales et de séquelles d'hypercalcémie idiopathique sous forme de sténoses étagées de la voie aortique et d'une sténose mitrale *Archives des Maladies du Coeur et des Vaisseaux* **65** 1349–1356 (124)

WARSHAW JB LITTLEFIELD JW FISHMAN WH INGLIS NR STOLBACH LL (1971) Serum alkaline phosphatase in hypophosphatasia *Journal of Clinical Investigation* **50** 2137–2142 (269)

WARWICK OH YENDT ER OLIN JS (1961) The clinical features of hypercalcemia associated with malignant disease *Canadian Medical Association Journal* **85** 719–723 (114)

WATNEY PJM CHANCE GW SCOTT P THOMPSON JM (1971) Maternal factors in neonatal hypocalcaemia: a study in three ethnic groups *British Medical Journal* **2** 432–436 (148)

WATSON L (1972) Diagnosis and treatment of hypercalcaemia *British Medical Journal* **2** 150–152 (85)

WATTS RWE (1973) Oxaluria *Journal of the Royal College of Physicians of London* **7** 161–174 (134)

WEBER JC PONS V KODICEK E (1971) The localization of 1,25-dihydroxycholecalciferol in bone cell nuclei of rachitic chicks *Biochemical Journal* **125** 147–153 (27)

WEEKE E FRIIS T (1971) Serum fractions of calcium and phosphorus in uraemia *Acta Medica Scandinavica* **189** 79–85 (201)

WEIDMANN P MASSRY SG COBURN JW MAXWELL MH ATLESON J KLEEMAN CR (1972) Blood pressure effects of acute hypercalcaemia: Studies in patients with chronic renal failure *Annals of Internal Medicine* **76** 741–745 (92)

WEINBERG AG STONE RT (1971) Autosomal dominant inheritance in Albright's hereditary osteodystrophy *Journal of Pediatrics* **79** 996–999 (162, 164)

WEISS A (1971) The scapular sign in rickets *Radiology* **98** 633–636 (179)

WELLS SA KETCHAM AS MARX SJ POWELL D BILEZIKIAN JP SHIMKIN PM PEARSON KD DOPPMAN JL (1973) Preoperative localisation of hyperfunctioning parathyroid tissue: radioimmunoassay of parathyroid hormone in plasma from selectively catheterized thyroid veins *Annals of Surgery* **177** 93–98 (103)

WERMER P (1963) Endocrine adenomatosis and peptic ulcer in a large kindred *American Journal of Medicine* **35** 205–212 (94)

WERNER M TOLLS RE HULTIN JV MELLECKER J (1970) Influence of sex and age on the normal range of eleven serum constituents *Zeitschrift für Klinische Chemie und Klinische Biochemie* **8** 105–115 (36)

WEST TET JOFFE M SINCLAIR L O'RIORDAN JLH (1971) Treatment of hypercalcaemia with calcitonin *Lancet* **1** 675–678 (76)

WESTBURY EJ OMENOGOR P (1970) A quantitative approach to the analysis of renal calculi *Journal of Medical Laboratory Technology* **27** 462–474 (131)

WHELTON MJ KEHAYOGLOU AK AGNEW JE TURNBERG LA SHERLOCK S (1971) [47]Calcium absorption in parenchymatous and biliary liver disease *Gut* **12** 978–983 (236)

364 REFERENCES

WHITEHEAD RG (1965) Hydroxyproline creatinine ratio as an index of nutritional status and rate of growth *Lancet* **2** 567–570 (54)

WHITELAW AGL COHEN SL (1973) Ectopic production of calcitonin *Lancet* **2** 443 (219)

WIELAND RG HENDRICKS FH AMAT Y LEON F GUTIERREZ L JONES JC (1971) Hypervitaminosis A with hypercalcaemia *Lancet* **1** 698 (128)

WILLIAMS ED (1966) Histogenesis of medullary carcinoma of the thyroid *Journal of Clinical Pathology* **19** 114–118 (217)

WILLIAMS JA NICHOLSON GI (1963) A modified bone biopsy drill for outpatient use *Lancet* **1** 1408. (The trephine is obtainable from Edwards Surgical Supplies 289 City Road London EC1) (57, 58)

WILLIAMS ED BROWN CL DONIACH I (1966) Pathological and clinical findings in a series of 67 cases of medullary carcinoma of the thyroid *Journal of Clinical Pathology* **19** 103–113 (218)

WILLIAMS H EARNEST D ADMIRAND W (1973) Mechanisms of hyperoxaluria in bowel disease. In *Proceedings of the International Symposium on Renal Stone Research Madrid 1972* ed Delatte LC Basle: Karger (134)

WILLS MR (1970a) Fundamental physiological role of parathyriod hormone in acid-base homoeostasis *Lancet* **2** 802–804 (15)

WILS MR (1970b) The effect of diurnal variation on total plasma calcium concentration in normal subjects *Journal of Clinical Pathology* **23** 772–777 (37, 40)

WILLS MR (1971a) Normocalcaemic primary hyperparathyroidism *Lancet* **1** 849–852 (82, 101)

WILLS MR (1971b) Value of plasma chloride concentration and acid-base status in the differential diagnosis of hyperparathyroidism from other causes of hypercalcaemia *Journal of Clinical Pathology* **24** 219–227 (66, 67, 116, 118)

WILLS MR (1971c) *Biochemical consequences of chronic renal failure* Aylesbury: Harvey Miller & Medcalf (192, 196)

WILLS MR (1973a) Calcium homeostasis in health and disease. In *Recent Advances in Medicine* ed Baron DN Compston N Dawson AM 16th edition 57–102 Edinburgh: Churchill Livingstone (64, 65)

WILLS MR (1973b) Intestinal absorption of calcium *Lancet* **1** 820–823 (8)

WILLS MR LEWIN MR (1971) Plasma calcium fractions and the protein-binding of calcium in normal subjects and in patients with hypercalcaemia and hypocalcaemia *Journal of Clinical Pathology* **24** 856–866 (37)

WILLS MR McGOWAN GK (1964) Plasma-chloride levels in hyperparathyroidism and other hypercalcaemic states *British Medical Journal* **1** 1153–1156 (66, 97)

WILLS MR ZISMAN E WORTSMAN J EVENS RG PAK CYC BARTTER FC (1970) The measurement of intestinal calcium absorption by external radioisotope counting: application to study of nephrolithiasis *Clinical Science* **39** 95–106 (56)

WILNER D SHERMAN RS (1966) Roentgen diagnosis of Paget's disease (osteitis deformans) *Medical Radiography and Photography* **42** 35–78 (243)

WINKELMAN J NADLER S DEMETRIOU J PILEGGI VJ (1972) The clinical usefulness of alkaline phosphatase isoenzyme determinations *American Journal of Clinical Pathology* **57** 625–633 (46)

WINKELMANN RK KEATING FR (1970) Cutaneous vascular calcification, gangrene and hyperparathyroidism *British Journal of Dermatology* **83** 263–267 (85)

WINTERFELDT EA EYRING EJ VIVIAN VM (1970) Ascorbic-acid treatment for osteogenesis imperfecta *Lancet* **1** 1347–1348 (260)

WOLF L-M COURTOIS H SCHRUB J-C (1973) Hypercalcémie et thiazides *Semaine des Hôpitaux de Paris* **49** 1239–1242 (127)

WONG RG MYRTLE JF TSAI HC NORMAN AW (1972) Studies on calciferol metabolism: V The occurrence and biological activity of 1,25-dihydroxyvitamin D_3 in bone *Journal of Biological Chemistry* **247** 5728–5735 (27)

WOOD SJ THOMAS J BRAIMBRIDGE MV (1973) Mitral valve disease and open heart surgery in osteogenesis imperfecta tarda *British Heart Journal* **35** 103–106 (259)

WOODARD HQ MARCOVE RC (1969) A comparison of the chemistry of blood from bone and peripheral veins *Clinical Orthopaedics* **66** 254–264 (46, 248)

WOODHOUSE NJY (1972) Paget's disease of bone *Clinics in Endocrinology and Metabolism* **1** 125–141 (46, 240, 248, 249)

WOODHOUSE NJY REINER M BORDIER P KALU DN FISHER M FOSTER GV JOPLIN GF MACINTYRE I (1971a) Human calcitonin in the treatment of Paget's bone disease *Lancet* **1** 1139–1143 (250)

WOODHOUSE NJY DOYLE FH JOPLIN GF (1971b) Vitamin-D deficiency and primary hyperparathyroidism *Lancet* **2** 283–287 (101)

WOODHOUSE NJY FISHER MT SIGURDSSON G JOPLIN GF MACINTYRE I (1972) Paget's disease in a 5-year-old: acute response to human calcitonin *British Medical Journal* **4** 267–269 (240, 270)

WOODS CG (1972) *Diagnostic orthopaedic pathology* Oxford: Blackwell (60, 155)

WOODS CG MORGAN DB PATERSON CR GOSSMANN HH (1968) Measurement of osteoid in bone biopsy *Journal of Pathology and Bacteriology* **95** 441–447 (60, 178)

WOODS CG BISHOP MC NICHOLSON GD (1972) Bone histological changes occurring after haemodialysis treatment for chronic renal failure *Journal of Pathology* **107** 137–143 (200)

WORMSLEY KG (1972) Pancreatic exocrine function in patients with gastric ulceration before and after gastrectomy *Lancet* **2** 682–684 (173)

WRIGHT AD JOPLIN GF DIXON HG (1969) Post-partum hypercalcaemia in treated hypoparathyroidism *British Medical Journal* **1** 23–25 (159, 160)

WU BC PILLAY VKG HAWKER CD ARMBRUSTER KFW SHAPIRO HS ING TS (1972) Hypercalcaemia in acute renal failure of acute alcoholic rhabdomyolysis *South African Medical Journal* **46** 1631–1633 (128)

WYNNE-DAVIES R (1973) *Heritable disorders in orthopaedic practice* Oxford: Blackwell (253, 264, 266)

YARBRO JW KENNEDY BJ BARNUM CP (1966) Mithramycin inhibition of ribonucleic acid synthesis *Cancer Research* **26** 36–39 (75, 251)

YENDT ER (1970a) Vitamin D: part II In *International encyclopedia of pharmacology and therapeutics Section 51 Vol 1 Parathyroid hormone, thyrocalcitonin and related drugs* ed Ramussen H 139–195 Oxford: Pergamon (24, 116, 118, 119, 125)

YENDT ER (1970b) Renal calculi *Canadian Medical Association Journal* **102** 479–489 (129, 131)

YENDT ER GAGNÉ RJA (1968) Detection of primary hyperparathyroidism with special reference to its occurrence in hypercalciuric females with 'normal' or borderline serum calcium *Canadian Medical Association Journal* **98** 331–336 (36, 97, 134)

YENDT ER GUAY GF GARCIA DA (1970) The use of thiazides in the prevention of renal calculi *Canadian Medical Association Journal* **102** 614–620 (139)

YOUNG DA LAMAN ML (1972) Radiodense skeletal lesions in Boeck's sarcoid *American Journal of Roentgenology, Radium Therapy and Nuclear Medicine* **114** 553–558 (120)

YOUNG CM CHALMERS FW CHURCH HN CLAYTON MM TUCKER RE WERTS AW FOSTER WD (1952) A comparison of dietary study methods *Journal of the American Dietetic Association* **28** 124–128 (61)

YOUNG CM CHALMERS FW CHURCH HN CLAYTON MM MURPHY GC TUCKER RE (1953) Subjects' estimation of food intake and calculated nutritive value of the diet *Journal of the American Dietetic Association* **29** 1216–1220 (61)

YU PNG (1952) The electrocardiographic changes associated with hypercalcemia and hypocalcemia *American Journal of the Medical Sciences* **224** 413–423 (70)

YU JS WALKER-SMITH JA BURNARD ED (1971a) Rickets: a common complication of neonatal hepatitis *Medical Journal of Australia* **1** 790–792 (173)

YU JS OATES RK WALSH KH STUCKEY SJ (1971b) Osteopetrosis *Archives of Disease in Childhood* **46** 257–263 (265)

ZAREMBSKI PM (1972) Personal communication (37)

ZAREMBSKI PM HODGKINSON A (1969) Some factors influencing the urinary excretion of oxalic acid in man *Clinica Chimica Acta* **25** 1–10 (134)

ZIMMERMAN HB (1962) Osteosclerosis in chronic renal disease *American Journal of Roentgenology* **88** 1152–1169 (199)

ZIMMERMAN RE GRIFFITHS HJ D'ORSI C (1973) Bone mineral measurement by means of photon absorption *Radiology* **106** 561–564 (223)

ZIMMET P (1968) Role of magnesium in tetany *New England Journal of Medicine* **279** 109–110 (35, 145)

ZORAB PA (1969) Normal creatinine and hydroxyproline excretion in young persons *Lancet* **2** 1164–1165 (55)

ZULL JE REPKE DW (1972) Tissue localization of tritiated parathyroid hormone thyroparathyroidectomized rats *Journal of Biological Chemistry* **247** 2195–2199 (15)

Index